John A. Stew
14. II. 00.

BEYOND THE UNCONSCIOUS

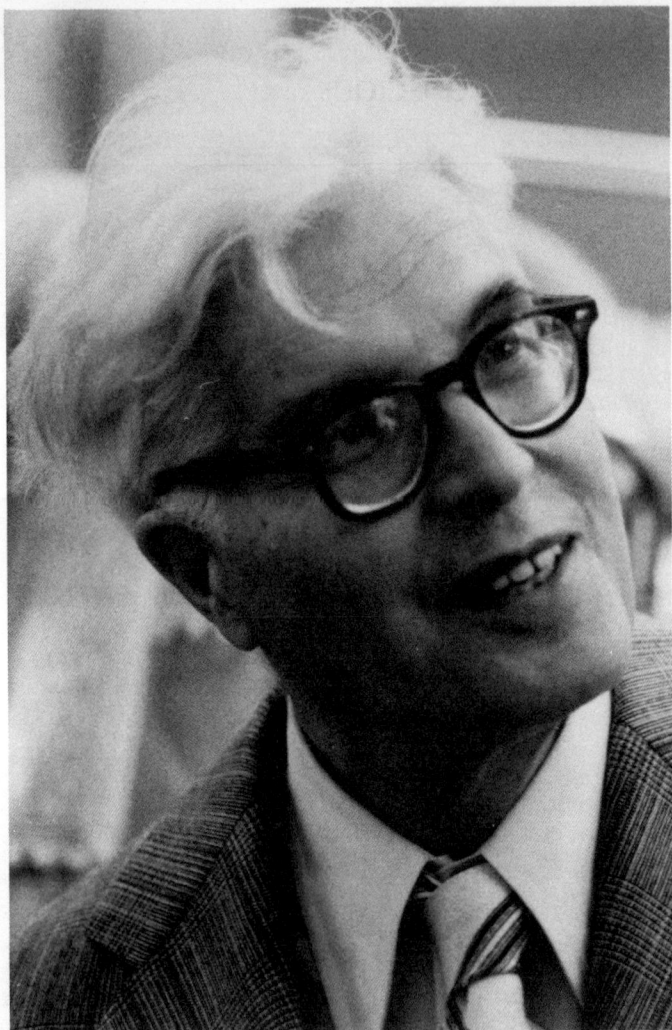

BEYOND THE UNCONSCIOUS

ESSAYS OF
HENRI F. ELLENBERGER IN THE
HISTORY OF PSYCHIATRY

Introduced and Edited by
Mark S. Micale

Translations from the French by
Françoise Dubor and Mark S. Micale

PRINCETON UNIVERSITY PRESS   PRINCETON, NEW JERSEY

Library of Congress Cataloging-in-Publication Data

Ellenberger, Henri F. (Henri Frédéric), 1905–
    Beyond the unconscious : essays of Henri F. Ellenberger in the history
of psychiatry / introduced and edited by Mark S. Micale ; translations
from the French by Françoise Dubor and Mark S. Micale.
        p.   cm.
    Selected essays translated from the French.
    Includes bibliographical references and index.
    ISBN 0-691-08550-1 (cl)
    1. Psychiatry—History.   2. Ellenberger, Henri F. (Henri Frédéric),
1905–   .   I. Micale, Mark S., 1957–   .   II. Title.
    [DNLM: 1. Ellenberger, Henri F. (Henri Frédéric), 1905–   .
2. Psychoanalysis—history—essays.   3. Psychoanalytic Theory—
essays.   WM 11.1 E45b]
    RC438.E635   1993
    616.89'009—dc20
    DNLM/DLC
    for Library of Congress   92-48967

This book has been composed in Sabon

Princeton University Press books are printed
on acid-free paper, and meet the guidelines
for permanence and durability of the Committee
on Production Guidelines for Book Longevity
of the Council on Library Resources

Printed in the United States of America

10 9 8 7 6 5 4 3 2 1

Frontispiece: Henri F. Ellenberger, 1978, age 73. (Courtesy of
Henri and Emilie Ellenberger)

Contents

Preface and Acknowledgments _____

THE SWISS medical historian Henri F. Ellenberger is best remembered today as the author of *The Discovery of the Unconscious*, published in 1970.[1] A brilliant, encyclopedic study of psychiatric theory and therapy from primitive times to the middle of the twentieth century, Ellenberger's book was widely regarded upon publication as a major, masterly work. Twenty years later, it remains simply indispensable to research in many areas of the history of psychology, psychiatry, and psychoanalysis.

In addition to *The Discovery of the Unconscious*, Ellenberger, across a span of some thirty years, has produced many shorter writings in psychiatric history. Before publication of his classic, Ellenberger had written a monograph as well as approximately twenty articles on historical subjects. Furthermore, since 1970 Ellenberger has continued to work quietly and has written another fifteen essays of a historical nature. Oddly, however, whereas readers in the history of the mental sciences are closely familiar with Ellenberger's large study, few individuals, including specialists, are aware of his essays. A majority of these historical articles were originally published in specialized medical periodicals, quite a few of them outside of the United States, while several others appeared in volumes that are currently out of print. Ellenberger's monograph—a short but factually dense and highly interesting history of psychiatry in Switzerland published in 1954—is all but impossible to locate today. Moreover, and for reasons that are themselves significant, Ellenberger personally and professionally has been largely invisible since the appearance of *The Discovery of the Unconscious*. Indeed, many people, North Americans and Europeans alike, have the impression that he is no longer alive.

This situation is as curious as it is undeserved. Many of Ellenberger's scattered historical writings deal with subjects of considerable interest and importance. Not infrequently, they are based on pioneering research in the original sources, and they often reveal the same series of outstanding qualities that marks *The Discovery of the Unconscious*. Nor is this all. Over the last decade and a half, the fields of the history of psychiatry, psychology, and psychoanalysis have begun to develop extremely rapidly. More young practitioners, from an impressive range of disciplinary backgrounds, generating an ever greater quantity of scholarly material on a broad range of subject matters, are entering these fields all the time. Furthermore, the

---

[1] Ellenberger, *The Discovery of the Unconscious: The History and Evolution of Dynamic Psychiatry* (New York, Basic Books, 1970).

debates waged within these scholarly circles have often been followed by readers in many other areas of the sciences and humanities. What was once an antiquarian pastime of historically minded physicians and social scientists is in the process of becoming an independent field of historical inquiry with considerable cultural resonance. An important part of such a development must be the discovery and critical interpretation of the intellectual origins of these fields of study, and in this process of disciplinary self-definition, the work of Ellenberger figures prominently. Indeed, as I will propose, Ellenberger in a striking number of ways anticipates directly many of the most significant developments in present-day psychiatric historiographies. In other respects, his writings point forward to fresh areas of inquiry still awaiting historical exploration.

Fortunately, as these disciplines develop, Ellenberger is beginning to receive the kind of professional appreciation he deserves. A scholarly conference recently held in Toronto, Canada, devoted to the history of psychoanalysis, was dedicated to Ellenberger.[2] And in October 1990, at the first meeting of the European Association of the History of Psychiatry in 's Hertogenbosch, the Netherlands, where nearly two hundred psychiatric historians from a dozen countries gathered for the first time, Ellenberger was enthusiastically elected honorary chairman of the organization. Most significant have been developments in France. From a lifetime of research in European libraries and archives, Ellenberger amassed a formidable collection of historical materials, including roughly two thousand books and over thirty crates of printed and archival documents. In 1986, Ellenberger, with the guidance of his son, Michel, offered the bulk of his personal library and archives to the Société Internationale d'Histoire de la Psychologie et de la Psychanalyse in Paris. The French, who had received *The Discovery of the Unconscious* less ambiguously than the American medical community (where the current of Freudian revisionism running through the work caused many reviewers to qualify their accolades), received the offer with notable enthusiasm. In March 1992, a special Centre de Recherche et de Documentation, designated officially as the Institut Henri Ellenberger, opened in the main library building of Sainte Anne Hospital in the French capital. This center will house the contents of Ellenberger's rich collection in combination with other historical materials in what is certain to become a major resource for historians in the future.[3]

---

[2] The proceedings of the conference have been published as Toby Gelfand and John Kerr, eds. *Freud and the History of Psychoanalysis* (Hillsdale, N.J., Analytic Press, 1992).

[3] Also, the French edition of Ellenberger's major work, *A la découverte de l'inconscient: Histoire de la psychiatrie dynamique* (Villeurbanne, Simep-Éditions, 1974), is in the process of being reissued.

These recent occurrences, while admirable, are essentially honorific in nature. They suggest that a detailed and informed reappraisal of the substance of Ellenberger's historical work itself is now in order. Such a reassessment should extend beyond *The Discovery of the Unconscious* (which in its English paperback form has remained readily available since 1981) to include Ellenberger's lesser-known historical writings. In 1978, a French-Canadian miscellany of Ellenberger's essays was published.[4] But the selection of essays in this work was incomplete and eccentric, and the book is now out of print. Moreover, the collection lacked the factual and interpretive scholarly apparatus necessary to place and fully to appreciate Ellenberger's work. It seems clear that a more substantial presentation is desirable, and *Beyond the Unconscious* is the result of this need.

The present volume is designed to offer the most pertinent and important of Ellenberger's historical essays to English-language audiences, both medical and nonmedical. Fourteen of Ellenberger's approximately thirty-five essays have been chosen for republication. These essays divide roughly into four thematic categories: Freud and the early intellectual history of psychoanalysis; figures and philosophies in the history of the mental sciences (including pieces on Jean-Martin Charcot, Pierre Janet, and Hermann Rorschach); the role of the "great patients" in the history of psychology and psychoanalysis; and topics in the cultural history of medicine. With the exception of the entry on Charcot, these essays contain historical material not to be found in the large book. The articles in the collection span Ellenberger's career, the earliest dating from 1954, the most recent from 1991. Five of the essays were originally written and published in French and appear here in translation for the first time. As with all of Ellenberger's writings, the chronological emphasis in these works is on the nineteenth and twentieth centuries, while the focus culturally and geographically remains on the central and western European experiences with instructive comparative glances toward North America and Asia.

The articles in the book are preceded by a substantial biohistoriographical introduction. In these pages, I sketch Ellenberger's life and career, review the contents and critical reception of *The Discovery of the Unconscious*, and discuss the major themes running through his historical essays. I also attempt here to establish Ellenberger's importance for the contemporary study of psychiatric history and to suggest, rather more interpretively, the cultural significance of his work. The volume contains as well three appendices, the last of which records Ellenberger's complete histori-

---

[4] Ellenberger, *Les mouvements de libération mythique et autres essais sur l'histoire de la psychiatrie* (Montreal, Éditions Quinze, 1978), which later appeared in an Italian translation as *I movimenti di liberazione mitica* (Naples, Liguori, 1986).

cal writings. Finally, the appendices are followed by a wide-ranging bibliographical essay, which is intended both to indicate the current state of
scholarship on the subjects about which Ellenberger wrote and to trace out
his influence on a later generation of researchers and writers.

With an ample analytical introduction and a detailed bibliography, it
has proved unnecessary to remark extensively in a direct textual way on
Ellenberger's essays. I have commented annotatively only occasionally—
all in all, no more than twenty times—in places either where the text
required clarification or where a biographical circumstance of the author
seemed interesting or relevant. Stylistically, these writings, like their author, are clear, straightforward, and utterly without affectation. Edi-
torially, therefore, my interventions are also rather sparse. In the early
essays from the 1950s, written when Ellenberger had recently come to the
United States to work at the Menninger Clinic and was still learning English, the diction is at times awkward. This I have altered accordingly. Also,
in certain articles Ellenberger tends to write in short, clipped paragraphs,
which might have seemed strange to North American and British audiences, so I have taken the liberty of combining these paragraphs. In numerous places, I have as well made brief excisions, indicated by ellipses,
where the information presented was repetitive or extraneous. Moreover,
in preparation for this volume, Ellenberger himself has made scattered
factual corrections in his articles and has stylistically revised a number of
them. Otherwise, the essays appear here as they did upon initial
publication.

In assembling the materials for this project, I received the encouragement
and assistance of many people. As with *The Discovery of the Unconscious*
in the 1960s, this shorter work received crucially important financial assistance from the Historical Section of the National Institutes of Health in
Bethesda, Maryland (Grant no. 1 R01 LM04938-01). I would like on this
score to acknowledge in particular the support of Gerald Grob and Barbara Rosenkrantz and, later, the thoughtful, decisive intervention of
Jeanne Brand. At an early stage, Richard Wolfe, Frank Sulloway, and Eugene Taylor encouraged the project. As so often before, Peter Gay provided sage advice. In Paris, Dr. Olivier Husson regularly kept me apprised
of the progress of the Institut Henri Ellenberger while Michel Ellenberger,
from his special vantage point, gave a close and informed reading to the
biographical sections of the Introduction of the book. Kelly E. Burket
cooperatively provided extensive materials from the Menninger Archives
about Ellenberger's career, and Rose-May Nahabet, of the Department of
Criminology at the University of Montreal, graciously offered the same
service. Larry Friedman answered questions about the professional atmosphere at the Menninger Clinic during the 1950s, and Philip Holzman and

Dr. Irving Kartus reminisced freely about Ellenberger and the Menninger Clinic during this same period. Dr. Stanley Jackson helped me to place Ellenberger in the Canadian psychiatric community of the 1960s. Diana Wylie, my colleague in the History Department at Yale University, graciously attempted to educate me about South African history and culture at the turn of the century.

Further, in assessing the status of Ellenberger's work for scholars today and in gathering references for the bibliographical essay, I have spoken informally over the past two years with many individuals. In a long and stimulating conversation, Paul Stepansky shared his thoughts with me about Ellenberger's writings on Alfred Adler as well as Ellenberger's accomplishments generally. Adam Crabtree kindly allowed me to consult portions of his forthcoming work on the history of Mesmerism and animal magnetism. Dr. Gerhard Fichtner, at the Institute of Medical History in Tübingen, placed at my disposal his splendid computerized bibliographical programs, and Onno van der Hart, of the University of Amsterdam, alerted me to the new medical literature on Pierre Janet. My friends George Mora, Michael Neve, and John Kerr kindly read the introductory essay and made perceptive observations. In addition, I have had valuable conversations or correspondence with Mireille Cifali, Geoffrey Cocks, Angela Graf-Nold, Dr. James Phillips, Sonu Shamdasani, Eugene Taylor, and Fernando Vidal. In preparing the manuscript, Sarah Trapnell provided excellent typographical service under short notice while Paul Dambowic perused many of these pages with an expert editorial eye. It has also been a professional pleasure working with Françoise Dubor in translating the French-language essays in the collection. Moreover, at Princeton University Press I want enthusiastically to thank Emily Wilkinson, who tolerated a number of delays with this manuscript, who graciously accommodated a generous selection of essays, and who then shepherded the book through the process of publication.

Far and away, however, my greatest acknowledgment of thanks goes to Dr. Ellenberger himself and his wife Emilie. Under severely constraining medical circumstances, during long and unforeseen delays, through the mail, and in personal conversations, Dr. Ellenberger has provided for this project an abundance of information about his life and work. To be able to present to him this volume in completion gives me the greatest satisfaction.

"Moritz Benedikt (1835–1920)," reprinted with permission from *Confrontations psychiatriques*, 11 (1973), 183–200.

"La conférence de Freud sur l'hystérie masculine (15 octobre 1886). Étude critique," reprinted with permission from *L'information psychiatrique*, 44, no. 10 (1968), 921–29.

"Charcot and the Salpêtrière School," reprinted with permission from *American Journal of Psychotherapy*, 19, no. 2 (April 1965), 253–67.

"Pierre Janet, philosophe," reprinted with permission from *Dialogue: Canadian Philosophical Review/Revue philosophique canadienne*, 12, no. 2 (June 1973), 254–87.

"The Scope of Swiss Psychology," from *Perspectives in Personality Theory*, edited by Henry P. David and Helmut von Bracken. Copyright 1957 by Basic Books, Inc. Reprinted by permission of Basic Books, a division of HarperCollins Publishers.

"The Life and Work of Hermann Rorschach (1884–1922)," reprinted with permission from the *Bulletin of the Menninger Clinic*, 18, no. 5 (September 1954), 173–219. Copyright 1954 by The Menninger Foundation, Topeka, Kansas, U.S.A.

"La psychiatrie et son histoire inconnue," reprinted with permission from *L'union médicale du Canada*, 90, no. 3 (March 1961), 281–89.

"The Story of 'Anna O.': A Critical Review with New Data," *Journal of the History of the Behavioral Sciences*, 8, no. 3 (July 1972), 267–79; and "The Pathogenic Secret and Its Therapeutics," *Journal of the History of the Behavioral Sciences*, 2, no. 1 (January 1966), 29–42. Copyright 1966 and 1972 by the Clinical Psychology Publishing Co., Inc., Brandon, Vermont 05733.

"C. G. Jung and the Story of Helene Preiswerk: A Critical Study with New Documents," reprinted with permission from *History of Psychiatry*, 2, no. 5 (March 1991), 41–52.

"Les illusions de la classification psychiatrique," reprinted with permission from *L'évolution psychiatrique*, 28, no. 2 (April–June 1963), 221–42; and "L'histoire d'"Emmy von N.,'" reprinted with permission from *L'évolution psychiatrique*, 42, no. 3 (July–September 1977), 519–40.

"The Concept of Creative Illness," reprinted with permission from *The Psychoanalytic Review*, 55, no. 3 (1968), 442–56.

BEYOND THE UNCONSCIOUS

Introduction

Henri F. Ellenberger and the Origins of European Psychiatric Historiography

The Biographical View

Henri Frédéric Ellenberger was born on November 6, 1905, in southern Africa. Ellenberger issued from a large French-speaking Swiss family from the town of Yverdon in the Vaud canton near Lake Neuchâtel. Since the middle of the nineteenth century the family had worked as European Protestant missionaries at various locations in the south of Africa. Ellenberger's grandfather, who arrived on the African continent in 1861, initiated the family tradition.[1] In addition to his missionary pursuits, D. Frédéric Ellenberger gathered volumes of information from native sources about the life and customs of the local indigenous peoples and prepared a full account of the early tribal history of the Basuto.[2]

Ellenberger's father, Victor Ellenberger, passed nearly his entire adult life in South Africa, where he worked at a number of sites as a member of the Société des Missions Évangéliques de Paris. Ellenberger *père* seems to have been a remarkable man—a self-taught linguist, naturalist, and social anthropologist. Among other activities, he traveled widely on the African continent, often recording his botanical, zoological, and anthropological observations; he translated into French an African literary masterwork, the epic poem *Chaka* by the Sotho poet Thomas Mofolo, which aroused considerable European interest in native African literatures; and he collected remnants of the ancient Bushmen societies, including rock paintings, which were exhibited at the Musée de l'Homme in Paris in 1930.[3] He also wrote two historical books about the French-speaking Protestant church in Africa.[4]

[1] The story of the family's missionary work is related by Ellenberger's father in Victor Ellenberger, *A Century of Mission Work in Basutoland (1833–1933)*, translated from the French by Edmond M. Ellenberger (Morija, Sesuto Book Depot, 1938).

[2] *History of the Basuto: Ancient and Modern*, compiled by D. Frédéric Ellenberger and written in English by J. C. MacGregor (London, Caston, 1912).

[3] V. Ellenberger, *Sur les hauts—plateaux de Lessouto: Notes et souvenirs de voyages* (Paris, Société des Missions Évangéliques, 1930); Thomas Mofolo, *Chaka, une épopée bantoue*, translated from the Sotho into French by V. Ellenberger (Paris, Gallimard, 1940).

[4] V. Ellenberger, *A Century of Mission Work in Basutoland*; idem, *Landmarks in the Story of the French Protestant Church in Basutoland* (London, Pickering and Inglis, 1933).

Unfortunately, we have less information about Ellenberger's mother. However, we do know that Évangéline Ellenberger (née Christol) also came from a large Protestant missionary family and that her father, Frédéric Christol, wrote one of the first books on African art as well as numerous personal reminiscences about his experiences on the African continent.[5] Ellenberger's mother raised a family of six children in a foreign, difficult, and often dangerous environment where she seems to have shared the interest of other family members in the popular culture of her surroundings.[6] For several generations, the Ellenberger family kept one foot in Europe (they always retained their Swiss citizenship and returned intermittently to France and Switzerland) and the other in Africa, where they worked among the Bantu-speaking Sotho in the colony of Basutoland, a British protectorate within the Union of South Africa.

Henri Frédéric Ellenberger, the historian and author of the essays in this book, was born in a small village along the Zambezi River, in what was then Northern Rhodesia and is now western Zambia, at the missionary outpost there. Ellenberger spent the first nine years of his life, from 1905 to 1914, at several sites in Zambia and South Africa. In retrospect, these early years are significant. With his distinctive family background, Ellenberger developed at an early age a keen and enduring interest in the comparison of foreign cultures. He also had ample opportunity to cultivate his considerable linguistic aptitudes. At home, he learned French and German,[7] while at primary school he was introduced to English and Dutch Afrikaans. In addition, through his father's work, he learned to speak Sotho, a language of the Bantu-speaking people, who were the subjects of his mission.

In 1914, Ellenberger's parents sent their son, then 9 years old, on an extended trip to Europe for his secondary education. Soon after his arrival, however, the First World War broke out, and young Ellenberger was unable to return to his family for over five years. Ellenberger received most of his pre-university schooling at a number of locations in France, where he seems to have performed well academically and to have read widely and independently. For his undergraduate education, Ellenberger studied in the humanities at the University of Strasbourg from 1921 to 1924. Alsace had recently been reclaimed by the French as a result of the war, and Strasbourg combined freely, if uneasily, French and German cultures and languages. In 1924, at the age of 19, Ellenberger received his baccalaureate degree in *lettres-philosophie*.

[5] Frédéric Christol, *L'art dans l'Afrique australe* (Paris, Berger-Levrault, 1911); idem, *Vingt-six ans au sud de l'Afrique* (Paris, Société des Missions Évangéliques, 1930).

[6] Mme. Victor Ellenberger, *Silhouettes zambéziennes* (Paris, Société des Missions Évangéliques, 1920).

[7] While Ellenberger's immediate family came from French-speaking Switzerland, the original place of family birth (*lieu d'origine* or *Heimatort*), an important concept in Swiss citizenship, was Rüderswyl in the German-speaking canton of Bern.

Upon graduation, Ellenberger moved to Paris, where he spent the next ten years. He recalls these years in the French capital as among the happiest and most intellectually stimulating of his life. Soon after his arrival, he enrolled in medical school at the University of Paris, deciding almost immediately upon a specialty in psychiatry. After his general medical course of study, he worked during the late 1920s and early 1930s as an *externe* in a number of Parisian hospitals, and then from 1932 to 1934 as *interne des asiles de la Seine*, including one-year stints at two celebrated French psychiatric establishments, the Salpêtrière and the Sainte Anne asylum. Ellenberger wrote his medical dissertation on the affective states of catatonic psychoses and received his medical degree in 1934.[8] In November 1930 he had married Emilie Esther von Bachst, a young woman of Russian extraction who was then studying painting and the crafts in Paris.

Fond of France but disadvantaged by the hierarchical Parisian medical system, Ellenberger upon graduation from medical school moved to Poitiers in the department of Vienne in west-central France, where he spent the remainder of the 1930s. Here he worked in a small private psychiatric practice as a *spécialiste des maladies nerveuses*. At the same time, he served as consulting neuropsychiatrist at a local private hospital as well as a regional consultant in forensic psychiatry. Ellenberger's years in Poitiers, while predating his historical scholarship, were also significant for his intellectual formation. His medical practice at this time included a large number of refugees from the Spanish Civil War, which gave him an opportunity to develop reading and speaking skills in yet another language. Further, Ellenberger was struck in the region of Poitou by the many popular superstitions and practices that endured among the local people, reminiscent in ways of the habits and mentalities he had encountered earlier among native Africans. Also, during this period Ellenberger maintained a friendship with Arnold Van Gennep, one of the founding figures of French ethnography, who throughout the 1930s published a series of pioneering monographs on the folklore of the French provinces. As a result, Ellenberger now developed a powerful interest in regional anthropological lore. He learned the local *patois*, which enabled him to collect information about the rural populations of Poitou. In his spare time, he read deeply in the literature of European anthropology, and he wrote a book-length manuscript about the folklore of the area.[9]

---

[8] Ellenberger, *Essai sur le syndrome psychologique de la catatonie* (Poitiers, Société Française d'Imprimerie de la Librairie, 1933).

[9] Ellenberger, "Le folklore du Poitou: Département de la Vienne" (unpublished typescript), portions of which later appeared as "Le monde fantastique," *Nouvelle revue des traditions populaires*, 1 (1949), 407–35; 2 (1950), 3–26; "Relevé des pèlerinages du département de la Vienne," *Nouvelle revue des traditions populaires*, 9 (1950), 331–57, 387–415; and "Documents de littérature orale du Poitou," *Arts et traditions populaires*, 8 (1960), 115–42.

Most importantly, Ellenberger at this time conceived the idea of combining his interests in cultural anthropology and medical psychology. As a field of scholarly study, cross-cultural psychiatry scarcely existed in the 1930s. Nonetheless, Ellenberger began systematically to gather data on what he has always preferred to call "ethnopsychiatry," or the comparative study of the past and present experiences of mental illness in different cultures. From the mid-1940s onward, he published articles on suicide, hysteria, schizophrenia, alcoholism, and obsessive-compulsive disorders from a transcultural perspective, and has in fact continued to do so until recently.[10] Long before the field began to develop rapidly in the 1970s, Ellenberger was charting the territory of transcultural psychiatry, a fact that has gone almost entirely unnoticed outside of specialized medical circles.[11]

In the spring of 1941, owing to the political and military situation in France, Ellenberger, along with his wife and their three young children, left Poitiers and returned to Switzerland.[12] Despite his Swiss citizenship, Ellenberger had in fact spent little time actually living in Switzerland and had no professional experience with Swiss medicine. Over the course of the following twelve years, however, this changed. For two years during the early 1940s, he worked as a senior psychiatrist at the Waldau Mental Hospital near Bern. Then, from 1943 to 1952, he served as associate director, or *Oberarzt*, of the Breitenau Mental Hospital in Schaffhausen. A historic town placed picturesquely on the Rhine River near the German border in the north-central part of the country, Schaffhausen was a classic Swiss

[10] The major writings include Ellenberger, "Die Putzwut," *Der Psychologe*, 2 (1950), 91–94, 138–47; "Der Tod aus psychischen Ursachen bei Naturvölkern," *Psyche*, 5 (1951–1952), 333–34; "Der Selbstmord im Lichte der Ethno-Psychiatrie," *Monatsschrift für Psychiatrie und Neurologie*, 125 (1953), 347–61; "Cultural Aspects of Mental Illness," *American Journal of Psychotherapy*, 14 (1960), 158–73; (with E. D. Wittkower, H.B.M. Murphy, and J. Fried), "Crosscultural Inquiry into the Symptomatology of Schizophrenia," *Annals of the New York Academy of Sciences*, 84 (1960), 854–63; "Ethno-psychiatrie," in *Encyclopédie médico-chirurgicale* (Paris, 1965), vol. 1, *Psychiatrie*, 37725 A 10, pp. 1–14, and 37725 B 10, pp. 1–22; "Intérêt et domaine d'application de l'ethno-psychiatrie," *Proceedings of the Fourth World Congress of Psychiatry*, Madrid, Spain (September 5–11, 1966); "Aspects ethno-psychiatriques de l'hystérie," *Confrontations psychiatriques*, 1 (1968), 131–45; "Impressions psychiatriques d'un séjour à Dakar," *Psychopathologie africaine*, 4 (1968), 469–80; "L'alcoolisme à la lumière de la psychiatrie comparée," *L'union médicale du Canada*, 103 (1974), 1914–20; and "Psychiatrie transculturelle," in R. Duguay, H. F. Ellenberger, et al., eds., *Précis pratique de psychiatrie* (Montreal, Chenelière & Stanké, 1981), 625–42.

[11] For an exception to this rule, see Erwin H. Ackerknecht, "Transcultural Psychiatry," in Edwin R. Wallace IV and Lucius C. Pressley, eds., *Essays in the History of Psychiatry* (Columbia, S.C., William S. Hall Psychiatric Institute, 1980), 172.

[12] Ellenberger's children, named Michel, Hélène, and André, had been born, respectively, in 1931, 1933, and 1935. His fourth child, Irène, was born in 1941 after the family's return to Switzerland.

setting. It was also a town associated with the history of psychiatry and psychology, for it was in Schaffhausen that Hermann Rorschach had been born and raised and had initiated a strong national tradition of psycho-diagnostic testing. Equipped with approximately three hundred beds and divided into two large sections for male and female patients, the Breitenau Hospital served as the public psychiatric facility for the town and canton of Schaffhausen. Here, Ellenberger was in charge of the Division for Women, where he worked regularly with a range of patients, including the acutely and chronically psychotic. He also perfected his spoken German, read systematically in the large hospital library, provided service at local military medical facilities, and became active in Swiss societies of psychiatry, psychology, criminology, and culture.

As a state hospital, the Schaffhausen asylum was linked to other cantonal psychiatric institutions in Switzerland. As a result of this arrangement, during the 1940s and early 1950s Ellenberger became acquainted with many of psychiatry's old-timers who had been members of the first generation of Swiss psychiatry and of the famous Swiss psychiatric circle influenced by Sigmund Freud. He met former students of Auguste Forel and Eugen Bleuler. He became acquainted with Manfred Bleuler and Carl Gustav Jung (who by that time had retreated to the nearby town of Küsnacht on the shores of Lake Zurich). He frequently visited Ludwig Binswanger, the well-known existential psychiatrist. And he developed close friendships with Alphonse Maeder, an early member of the Zurich psychoanalytic group and later Jung disciple, with Leopold Szondi, the psychiatrist–geneticist and inventor of the Szondi Test, and with Oskar Pfister, the lay pastor and psychoanalyst who had been on intimate terms for many years with the Freud family. With Pfister—"the grand old man of psychoanalysis," as Ellenberger's generation knew him[13]—Ellenberger underwent an informal training analysis during the early 1950s. He also frequently attended lectures and seminars at the Zurich Psychoanalytic Society and the Psychological Institute in Zurich. At these meetings, Pfister, Maeder, Jung, Szondi, and the others spoke often of their earlier experiences during what sounded to many younger physicians at the time like a past golden age of European psychiatry. Ellenberger in particular listened attentively to these stories and later drew upon this rich store of observation and knowledge. Perhaps most importantly, Ellenberger established during the Schaffhausen years a network of personal and professional contacts in the world of central European psychiatry that, as we will see shortly, proved immensely valuable for his later historical research.

[13] "The Life and Work of Hermann Rorschach (1884–1922)," *Bulletin of the Menninger Clinic*, 18, no. 5 (September 1954), 214.

Ultimately, however, the career of a provincial asylum doctor and administrator frustrated Ellenberger. He recalls the modest salary of his post at Schaffhausen, the endless ward rounds and staff meetings, and the excessive paperwork required under the Swiss hospital system. Moreover, after the preceding decade in France, Ellenberger experienced in Switzerland a certain claustrophobia—a *Kantönligeist* or "little canton spirit," he calls it. Perhaps most significantly, after a number of years at Schaffhausen Ellenberger was chagrined to realize that, without a diploma from a Swiss medical faculty, he was unable to advance to a position at one of the prestigious university psychiatric clinics of Zurich, Basel, Bern, Lausanne, or Geneva. For these reasons, by the early 1950s Ellenberger was open to alternative career opportunities.

Foremost among these opportunities in Ellenberger's mind was America. Following the war, which had impeded the flow of medical and scientific information in both directions across the Atlantic, a strong interest formed in Switzerland in learning about recent developments in psychotherapeutics abroad. In this spirit, Ellenberger was able to procure from the American-Swiss Foundation a grant for a three-month sojourn in the United States in order to lecture on contemporary European psychiatric theories and practices and to return with information about the latest American developments. From September to December 1952, Ellenberger toured widely throughout the United States, speaking at prominent psychiatric establishments in New York, New Haven, Philadelphia, Washington, and Chicago.[14] Included in his travels was a three-week stay in Topeka, Kansas, at the Menninger Clinic. Ellenberger departed from America late in 1952 with a wealth of ideas and observations about life in the New World—and with an offer to join the Menninger staff as a professor of clinical psychiatry on the teaching faculty and as a special assistant to Karl Menninger.

The family partnership between father and sons in Topeka that matured into the Menninger Clinic had begun in 1919 and had grown steadily during the following two decades. During the post–World War II years, the institution was undergoing a rapid expansion of all of its medical services. As Lawrence Friedman recounts in his recent history of the establishment, by the 1950s the clinic was evolving into "the major facility for mental health professional education in the nation."[15] Moreover, during the 1930s and early 1940s, many European physicians had emigrated to the

---

[14] Ellenberger's lecture during this trip, which seems to have charmed his audiences, was later printed as "Current Trends in European Psychotherapy," *American Journal of Psychotherapy*, 7 (1953), 733–53.

[15] Lawrence J. Friedman, *Menninger: The Family and the Clinic* (New York, Knopf, 1990), xi.

United States, and, under the guidance of David Rapaport, no institution had been more active in recruiting central European psychotherapists, particularly psychoanalysts, than the Menninger.[16] With close associations with the Topeka Psychoanalytic Institute, and with a growing number of European psychoanalysts on its staff, the overwhelming theoretical and therapeutic orientation of the institution during this period was Freudian.

Early in 1953, Ellenberger assumed his new post in the United States. At the Menninger, he for the first time moved from the hospital ward and the administrator's office into the classroom. Working now in English, he taught students, mainly young American doctors, at the Menninger School of Psychiatry in various psychiatric subjects. The curriculum log at the Menninger Archives today indicates that he offered lecture courses on "General Psychopathology," "Classic Psychiatric Syndromes," and "Principles of Psychiatric Treatment" as well as seminars devoted to more specialized topics, such as "Alcoholism and Addiction," "The Neuroses," and "Sexual Deviations."

At the same time, Ellenberger found almost immediately that he was valued in Topeka for other reasons, too. With his multilingualism and his extensive knowledge of recent developments in European psychiatry, he was able to serve as a channel for information about contemporary European psychiatry to American practitioners. Throughout the 1950s, the *Bulletin of the Menninger Clinic* is chock-full of lengthy reviews by Ellenberger of the latest French, German, Swiss, Dutch, Spanish, and Russian medical texts. Ellenberger soon discovered that he was also appreciated by his American hosts for his close personal familiarity with many European psychiatric figures. For instance, a strong interest existed in American psychiatric circles at the time in the Rorschach Test, and at the Menninger, Gardner Murphy was conducting extensive experiments in his psychological laboratory with projective diagnostic techniques. Staff members and students were therefore intrigued to learn that Ellenberger personally knew members of the Rorschach family, had lived and practiced in Schaffhausen, and could describe vividly the institutions where Rorschach had worked. In response to this interest, during his first year in Topeka Ellenberger wrote a lengthy article—really a short monograph—about Rorschach based on a reading of Rorschach's complete writings and on personal interviews with Rorschach's family, teachers, and former colleagues.[17] It

---

[16] On the immigration of European psychoanalysts to the United States, refer to Laura Fermi, *Illustrious Immigrants: The Intellectual Migration from Europe, 1930–1941* (Chicago, University of Chicago Press, 1968), chap. 6. For émigré psychiatrists at the Menninger specifically, see Friedman, *Menninger: The Family and the Clinic*, chap. 5.

[17] Ellenberger, "Life and Work of Hermann Rorschach."

was Ellenberger's first piece of historical writing. In much the same way, Ellenberger often lectured during the 1950s to professional audiences in America about Bleuler, Jung, Adler, Pfister, Binswanger, Maeder, Szondi, Minkowski, and others.

Ellenberger had come to the Menninger with a primary research interest in ethnopsychiatry. However, based on this new and unexpected interest in his knowledge of twentieth-century European psychiatric history, he gradually set his research aside. Curriculum records at the Menninger indicate that in the academic year 1955–1956 Ellenberger for the first time organized a lecture course entitled "The History of Dynamic Psychiatry." The course, which consisted of forty one-hour lectures, reviewed the prescientific origins of modern-day psychiatry from primitive medicine to the Enlightenment, then proceeded to the main theoretical models of dynamic psychiatry in the late nineteenth and twentieth centuries, and concluded with reflections on the contemporary state of psychological theory and therapeutics. The new class was a success, and for the next four years Ellenberger offered the course regularly, polishing his lectures on the subject. These lectures, which are preserved today in handwritten notebooks in his personal archives, represent Ellenberger's first attempt to formulate a comprehensive account of the history of psychiatry; they would later contribute directly to *The Discovery of the Unconscious*.[18]

Without a doubt, Ellenberger's years at the Menninger were a highly significant period in his career. But in the long run Ellenberger chose not to remain in the United States. During the 1950s, Ellenberger's family had remained in Switzerland, where his children were educated, which meant that his time with them was largely limited to the summers. Moreover, with a diverse and cosmopolitan Continental background, it is likely that Ellenberger over time tired of life in a provincial midwestern American setting. Also, while Ellenberger practiced on the staff of the Menninger, he never studied for medical certification in any American state, so that his opportunities for professional practice at other locations in the country were very limited. In combination with these factors, we can speculate that Ellenberger ultimately found the theoretical atmosphere at the Menninger less than congenial. Ellenberger's writings and teachings establish at once his deep familiarity with psychoanalytic theory. But in his personal clinical practice, he has always insisted on a theoretical and therapeutic eclecticism. In addition to psychoanalysis, he has also remained keenly interested in phenomenological psychiatry and existential analysis as well as Jungian

---

[18] Two of Ellenberger's course lectures were published at the time: "The Ancestry of Dynamic Therapy," *Bulletin of the Menninger Clinic*, 20, no. 6 (November 1956), 288–99; and "The Unconscious before Freud," *Bulletin of the Menninger Clinic*, 21, no. 1 (January 1957), 3–15, which later appeared with revisions as, respectively, the first and second chapters of *The Discovery of the Unconscious*.

Analytical Psychology, all of which were then at the peak of development in France, Germany, and Switzerland. It is not certain that these enthusiasms were uniformly welcome at the Menninger in the 1950s. Also, here as elsewhere in his career, it is well to recall Ellenberger's Swiss background. The psychoanalytic school in Switzerland included a rich tradition of lay analysis, accommodated religious interests and beliefs (as exemplified by the psychoanalyst–theologian Pfister), and extended creatively toward the humanities, especially philosophy, literature, and pedagogy. To be sure, Ellenberger found the American psychiatric world of the 1950s more open professionally than the European; but it is likely that he also experienced it as somewhat dogmatic, monodoctrinal, and overly medicalized. If he left Switzerland for professional reasons, he departed Topeka for reasons that were personal, cultural, and ideological.

At the same time, there were many things that Ellenberger admired about life in America. He therefore now searched for a setting that would combine features of the Old and New Worlds and where his French-speaking family could join him. In Montreal, Canada, he found the ideal location. In 1959, Ellenberger left the Menninger and traveled to Montreal, where for the next three years he worked at the Allan Memorial Institute, a facility for general family psychiatry associated with McGill University in the English-speaking sector of the city. Then, in the early 1960s, the University of Montreal sought to establish a Department of Criminology within its Faculty of Social Sciences, the first academic program of its kind in Canada. Academic criminology had not previously been a major area of interest for Ellenberger; but in Poitiers and Schaffhausen he had often provided local medicolegal testimony and filed forensic reports. Therefore, in 1962 Ellenberger accepted a position on the faculty of this new department, a return after over two decades to a French-speaking work environment.

At the University of Montreal, Ellenberger for the next fifteen years taught the psychology and biology of criminal behavior to students in both medicine and the social sciences. He offered lecture courses on "Psychiatry for Criminologists," "Biocriminology," "Judicial Psychology," and "The History of Criminology"; and he developed seminars on "Classical Theories of Criminology," "Victimology" (a subdiscipline he helped to pioneer), and "The Normal and the Pathological." From 1962 to 1965, he ranked on the Montreal faculty as *professeur agrégé* and from 1965 to 1976 as *professeur titulaire*. During the period 1964 to 1972 he also worked as a consultant at the Institut Pinel, a maximum-security prison for the violent insane, and beginning in 1972, he served as a staff psychiatrist at the Hôtel-Dieu de Montréal. Ellenberger retired in the spring of 1977, at the age of 72. At that time he was appointed professor emeritus. He has retained his residence in Montreal, and it is there that he lives today.

Precisely when during the course of his career Ellenberger arrived at the idea of writing a major historical study of psychiatry is difficult to ascertain. The decision seems to have been made gradually, most likely during the second half of the 1950s when he was lecturing at the Menninger. To be sure, when Ellenberger set about systematically to research *The Discovery of the Unconscious*, there existed already a small historical literature on psychiatry, and this extant scholarship provides the immediate historiographical context for a critical understanding of Ellenberger's book. The earliest historical writing about psychiatry, which dates from the nineteenth century, was German in provenance and often took the form either of chapters on psychiatry in general medical histories or of introductory historical chapters to psychiatric textbooks. From the 1920s to the 1950s, a number of ambitious biographical compendia appeared that presented the lives and writings of major psychiatric figures in France and Germany.[19] Also, several volumes had been published that traced in linear fashion the history of psychiatric ideas or practices in individual countries.[20] These works provided highly valuable collections of factual material; but, as Ellenberger observed quietly, they tended to be narrative in style and hagiographical in conception as well as at times nationalistic in tone and intent.

Furthermore, book-length historical accounts of psychiatry up to this time were usually cast in one of two historiographical modes—what might be called the humanitarian/rationalist mode and the Freudian/teleological mode. These approaches were combined in what was easily the most influential study of psychiatric history before Ellenberger's volume, Gregory Zilboorg's *A History of Medical Psychology* (1941).[21] Born and brought up in Russia, trained psychoanalytically in Berlin, and then practicing prominently in private practice in New York City, Zilboorg provided the "standard" version of the history of psychiatry for a generation of medical practitioners. Zilboorg's *History of Medical Psychology* had a number of merits: it was international in scope; chronologically, it offered a full history from primitive times to the present; and the book was attractively

---

[19] Theodor Kirchhoff, ed., *Deutsche Irrenärzte: Einzelbilder ihres Lebens und Wirkens*, 2 vols. (Berlin, Verlag Von Julius Springer, 1921, 1924); René Semelaigne, *Les pionniers de la psychiatrie française avant et après Pinel*, 2 vols. (Paris, Baillière, 1930, 1932); Kurt Kolle, ed., *Grosse Nervenärzte*, 3 vols. (Stuttgart, Georg Thieme Verlag, 1956, 1959, 1963).

[20] Albert Deutsch, *The Mentally Ill in America: A History of Their Care and Treatment from Colonial Times* (Garden City, N.Y., Doubleday, Doran and Company, 1937); Denis Leigh, *The Historical Development of British Psychiatry* (Oxford, Pergamon, 1961); Richard Hunter and Ida Macalpine, eds., *Three Hundred Years of Psychiatry, 1535–1860: A History Presented in Selected English Texts* (New York, Oxford University Press, 1963); Henri Baruk, *La psychiatrie française de Pinel à nos jours* (Paris, Presses Universitaires de France, 1967).

[21] Gregory Zilboorg, in collaboration with George W. Henry, *History of Medical Psychology* (New York, Norton, 1941).

written, with many lively, lengthy quotations.[22] Interpretively, Zilboorg offered readers a rendition of psychiatry's history as a monumental clash between the forces of good and evil. He presented three historical foci of achievement: the struggle of the medical humanists of the Renaissance against witchcraft and the demonological view of mental illness; the legendary work of Philippe Pinel during the French Revolution and the Napoleonic period to liberate the insane from an inhumane incarceration; and the career of Freud, dedicated to formulating a comprehensive, scientific theory of the mind and thereby to inaugurating the genuinely modern phase in the history of psychiatry. In Zilboorg's historical picture, as well as other works from the period, psychiatric history represented centrally a movement from ignorance and irrationality to scientific reason, and from cruelty and persecution to organized kindness and enlightenment.[23] Despite occasional delays, the story was a clear, unilinear, and unproblematical progression to the achievement of Freud.[24]

Several historical works of note also appeared in the two decades following Zilboorg's *History of Medical Psychology*. Between 1957 and 1968 (the year in which Ellenberger completed *The Discovery of the Unconscious*), no fewer than six monographs on the general history of psychiatry were published.[25] Ellenberger admired aspects of these books.[26] But two of these volumes represented compilations of essays, and the others were all under two hundred pages in length. In 1961, a second major study appeared in the form of Werner Leibbrand and Annemarie Wettley's *Der Wahnsinn: Geschichte der abendländischen Psychopathologie*.[27] Unfortunately, this volume has never been translated into English and is not well known among readers in Britain and North America; but Ellenberger was very familiar with it and considered it the best historical survey of psychia-

[22] For more on Zilboorg and his historical work, refer to George Mora, "Three American Historians of Psychiatry: Albert Deutsch, Gregory Zilboorg, George Rosen," in Wallace and Pressley, *Essays in the History of Psychiatry*, 6–13.

[23] See also Walter Bromberg, *Man Above Humanity: A History of Psychotherapy* (Philadelphia, Lippincott, 1954); idem, *The Mind of Man: The History of Psychotherapy and Psychoanalysis* (New York, Harper and Brothers, 1959); and J. Schultz, *Psychotherapie: Leben und Werke grosser Ärzte* (Stuttgart, Hippokrates Verlag, 1952).

[24] For the *locus classicus* of this Whig historiography, see the epilogue of Zilboorg's book.

[25] Erwin H. Ackerknecht, *Kurze Geschichte der Psychiatrie* (Stuttgart, Ferdinand & Enke, 1957; English translation, 1959); Mark Altschule, *Roots of Modern Psychiatry* (New York, Grune and Stratton, 1957); Jerome M. Schneck, *A History of Psychiatry* (Springfield, Ill., Charles C. Thomas, 1960); Nigel Walker, *A Short History of Psychotherapy in Theory and Practice* (London, Routledge and Kegan Paul, 1957); Ernest Harms, *Origins of Modern Psychiatry* (Springfield, Ill., Charles C. Thomas, 1967); Baruk, *Psychiatrie française*.

[26] In particular, see his reviews of Ackerknecht in *Bulletin of the History of Medicine*, 32 (1958), 380–81, and Harms in *Bulletin of the History of Medicine*, 43 (1969), 94–95.

[27] Werner Leibbrand and Annemarie Wettley, *Der Wahnsinn: Geschichte der abendländischen Psychopathologie* (Freiburg, Karl Alber, 1961).

try available at the time.[28] Running to nearly seven hundred pages, Leib-brand and Wettley's book was substantial. It did a good job of placing the main events of psychiatric history in the context of general medical history, and, along with Erwin Ackerknecht's study, it was one of the few books of its kind to be written by professional medical historians rather than physicians. Still, Ellenberger felt that the work had serious limitations. Leib-brand and Wettley were excessively concerned with the philosophical aspects of psychiatric theory, and they seemed to place an inordinate emphasis on German medical developments. Despite the length of the book, the historical sources on which it rested were limited to the most basic printed medical texts, and a good third of the book was given over to lengthy quotations from primary texts. Above all, Leibbrand and Wettley displayed a marked lack of concern, if not outright hostility, to the idea and the history of depth psychology.

Finally, in 1962, when Ellenberger was deeply engaged in the research for his own volume, Lancelot Whyte's *The Unconscious before Freud* appeared.[29] Here was a work that dealt squarely with the history of dynamic psychiatry and that privileged the theme of the unconscious. (Whyte, in fact, had drawn his title from Ellenberger's 1957 essay "The Unconscious before Freud.")[30] But, again, the book was very slender, offered essentially a catalogue of quotations, and was structured throughout by a pronounced psychoanalytic historical teleology. In other words, in the late 1950s and early 1960s, when Ellenberger set about the task of reading and writing for a large-scale historical study, there was ample room for a better book on the subject.[31]

Once Ellenberger embarked upon his historical project, he seems almost immediately to have become passionately involved in it. What had hitherto been an occasional and somewhat antiquarian avocation for him quickly became a consuming intellectual pursuit. In fact, one has the impression that from this time onward in his career, Ellenberger's medical practice, which filled his workaday hours, became largely a practical necessity and

[28] See his very favorable assessment of the book in "Histoire de la psychopathologie en Occident," *Critique*, 18 (1962), 641–55.

[29] Lancelot Law Whyte, *The Unconscious before Freud* (Garden City, N.Y., Doubleday, 1962).

[30] Also available at the time on this theme were Edward L. Margetts, "The Concept of the Unconscious in the History of Medical Psychology," *Psychiatric Quarterly*, 27 (1953), 115–38; and Mark D. Altschule, "The Growth of the Concept of Unconscious Cerebration before 1890," in his *Roots of Modern Psychiatry: Essays in the History of Psychiatry*, 2d ed., rev. and enl. (New York, Grune and Stratton, 1965), chap. 4.

[31] For a comprehensive bibliography of the psychiatric historical literature when Ellenberger began writing *The Discovery of the Unconscious*, refer to George Mora, "The History of Psychiatry: A Cultural and Bibliographical Survey," *Psychoanalytic Review*, 52 (1965), 298–328.

that his absorbing interest now lay in historical scholarship. However, Ellenberger at this point soon came to realize the amount of time and application entailed in a large scholarly enterprise. From the beginning, he was determined to base his study on extensive reading in fresh primary source materials, but this of course required research in European libraries and archives. However, to his great and continual frustration, he found over the next decade that, despite repeated requests, he was unable to obtain sabbatical leave from his medical labors in Canada in order to pursue historical research abroad.

As a result, over the years Ellenberger developed a distinctive and ingenious strategy for research. During the academic year, he lived in Montreal, tending full-time to his duties as a teaching and institutional psychiatrist. He then spent the long summer months of every year in Europe. For these trips, he prepared meticulously with an extensive correspondence with overseas librarians and archivists. During these carefully planned expeditions each year, Ellenberger moved relatively rapidly from one research location to the next. He also regularly combined his reading in libraries with visits to sites significant in the history of psychiatry and with extensive personal interviews with friends, colleagues, and family members of the figures he was studying. His daily travelogues, which he maintained for later reading by his family, record his scholarly activities during these trips: a conversation with Alfred Adler's daughter in New York City, a visit to Ernest Jones in his country home outside of London, a tour with Manfred Bleuler through the Burghölzli Hospital in Zurich, an expedition to Küsnacht to examine Jung's private library, a trip to the newly opened Freud House Museum in Vienna, an excursion to a private sanatorium along Lake Constance where a famous patient of Josef Breuer's had been treated, and so on.

Nor were Ellenberger's scholarly peregrinations limited to the major western and central European countries. His travel diary for the summer of 1961, for instance, reads "Psychiatric Impressions from Latin American Countries." It records his experiences of meeting physicians, lecturing (in Spanish) in several countries, and exploring public and private mental-health facilities in South America. In 1968, he took a similar trip to northern Africa, and during the summer of 1970 he visited a dozen and a half psychiatric facilities in the Netherlands, Denmark, and Sweden.[32] Furthermore, in many places that he visited Ellenberger was careful to establish

---

[32] Other documents pertaining to Ellenberger's research activities are included in his personal archives, which are now housed at the Institut Henri Ellenberger. These materials include a vast correspondence with friends, colleagues, historians, librarians, and archivists across Europe conducted in search of texts and manuscripts. Ellenberger's daily travel diaries remain in the possession of the Ellenberger family. However, for an excerpt see Appendix B.

good working relations with local physicians, medical historians, and library staff, which allowed him to continue his research subsequently through the mail.

Ellenberger's diaries indicate that he traveled in this manner from the mid-1950s until 1981. Through this combination of activities, he was able over the years to amass an enormous quantity of data about his subject. In 1965, in the evenings after his day's work in the classroom and hospital ward, he began to write up his material. This same year, he was awarded a modest three-year grant from the National Institute of Mental Health in the United States, which allowed him to procure the services of a typist to assist in the preparation of his book. Three years later, in December 1968, he completed a full manuscript, and early in 1970 his book appeared in print.

The Discovery of the Unconscious: Anatomy of a Historical Masterwork

With its 10 chapters, 932 pages, and 2,611 footnotes, *The Discovery of the Unconscious* is indeed a book to grapple with. The subtitle of the book states clearly the subject matter of the work: the history and evolution of dynamic psychiatry. Ellenberger never formally defines dynamic psychiatry in the book but rather describes it, massively, over the course of a thousand pages. Elsewhere in his writings, he characterizes this branch of medicine by contrasting it with its principal rival psychological traditions. It is dynamic, or depth, psychiatry and psychology that interests him—as opposed to the rational, commonsense psychologies of the eighteenth and nineteenth centuries, organic psychiatries that trace mental illnesses to pathophysiological disturbances of the brain, descriptive Kraepelinian psychiatry, or Pavlovian and Skinnerian behavioral psychologies.[33] Furthermore, at the center of the history of dynamic psychiatry, in Ellenberger's interpretation, lies the study of a dual model of the mind, divided fundamentally between conscious and unconscious mentation. The goal of his study, which Ellenberger also declares clearly at the outset, is threefold: to establish a factually accurate historical account of psychiatric history; to present the origins and idea content of "the great dynamic psychiatric systems" of the past; and to analyze the scientific and cultural meanings of these systems.[34]

---

[33] Ellenberger, "Ancestry of Dynamic Therapy," 288; "The Evolution of Depth Psychology," in Iago Galdston, ed., *Historic Derivations of Modern Psychiatry* (New York, McGraw-Hill, 1967), 159–60.

[34] Ellenberger, *Discovery of the Unconscious*, v–vi.

Ellenberger sets out the guiding methodological principles of his work in the preface as well as in a separate article published at the same time.[35] He had been struck by the fact that nearly everything written to date about psychiatry and its history was the product of students, partisans, or rivals of particular theories or schools. As a result, he observes, the historical literature on this topic, far more than that about other branches of medicine or science, is replete with tendentious and polemical formulations, to say nothing of simple factual errors. Ellenberger used Philippe Pinel, whom he admires greatly, as an example. No figure was more important in the history of the field; and yet no dependable biography of Pinel existed, only a string of contemporary personal anecdotes, repeated as factual stories, and elevated over time into historical legend.[36] In a similar vein, Ellenberger contends that almost none of the translations into other languages of past psychiatric writings are reliable. As a consequence, he develops a series of simple but important countermeasures that he follows throughout his historical work: at all times verify factual materials, including the most basic facts of biography; gather information from primary source materials rather than secondary literature; read comprehensively and chronologically in the *oeuvre* of a past author; and use first editions of texts in the language in which they were written.

In his prefatory comments to *The Discovery of the Unconscious*, Ellenberger also establishes the range of his study. Previous works had offered essentially linear intellectual histories of psychiatry, accounts of medical doctrine as found in the best-known printed medical texts of the past. Ellenberger, too, places an intellectual-historical explication of his subject at center stage; but he will present this story, he explains, in the round, in its many defining historical contexts. He will combine a traditional study of the theoretical content of past theories of dynamic psychiatry with a consideration of the personality of the theorist, the professional setting, the ambient cultural and intellectual environment, the social and political context, and the clinical factors impinging upon the theoretician. Ellenberger's is to be a multidimensional historical portrait of psychiatry.

Organizationally, Ellenberger divides his work into three large sections. The first five chapters of the book deal with the intricate intellectual and cultural prehistory of modern-day psychiatry. The following four chapters, forming the bulk of the book, present detailed studies of the four major twentieth-century dynamic theoreticians. A closing chapter reviews all of the preceding information synthetically. A criticism frequently lodged

---

[35] Ellenberger, "Methodology in Writing the History of Dynamic Psychiatry," in George Mora and Jeanne L. Brand, eds., *Psychiatry and Its History: Methodological Problems in Research* (Springfield, Ill., Charles C. Thomas, 1970), 26–40.

[36] Ibid., 27–28.

against *The Discovery of the Unconscious* is that the book is swollen and shapeless. On first glance, the chapter headings seem repetitive, and one result has been a tendency for readers to use the work only as a kind of sourcebook of factual information. As I will discuss in greater detail, such an approach is particularly unfortunate because it obscures the important interpretive lines running through the work. Moreover, the impression of repetition and disorganization is largely the result of a presentational deficiency in the American edition of the work, which lists in the table of contents only the major chapter headings, excluding the many subsections of each chapter that differentiate the chapters from one another. An examination of these chapter subheadings, which are included in the French edition of the book, reveals that *The Discovery of the Unconscious* is in fact expertly organized (see Appendix A).

Considering the high inherent interest of *The Discovery of the Unconscious*, the central place of the text in Ellenberger's intellectual career, and its numerous interconnections with his historical essays, it is valuable to survey the contents of the book. The opening chapter of *The Discovery of the Unconscious*, entitled "The Ancestry of Dynamic Psychiatry," presents a discussion of primitive medicine in prehistoric Western societies and in present-day preliterate populations. Zilboorg had presented primitive medicine as a background of superstition and irrationality against which to define the coming of the medical Enlightenment. However, for Ellenberger the shamans and medicine men of primitive peoples had been the first true practitioners of psychotherapy.[37] Drawing widely on historical and anthropological evidence from African, Australian, Siberian, Japanese, and Native American societies, he isolates ten varieties of primitive mental healing. Much of primitive psychotherapy, he demonstrates, was based on the concept of invasion by a foreign disease entity and the magical or ritualistic extraction of the pathogenic object. He proposes that primitive medicine men operated in essence as intuitive psychosomaticians and as such were often highly successful. Their curative techniques were wholly rational within the belief systems of their time, and they usually involved structured ritualized activities engaged in by a specially designated charismatic healer who performed his cure in a public, communal setting. Many

[37] The publication in 1951 of the first volume of Henry Sigerist's *History of Medicine* initiated a widespread interest in primitive medical practices. Sigerist's authoritative volume was followed by an influential article by Erwin Ackerknecht arguing specifically for the significance of psychological healing among primitive populations. See Henry E. Sigerist, *History of Medicine*, 2 vols. (New York, Oxford University Press, 1951), vol. 1, *Primitive and Archaic Medicine*, especially chap. 2; and Erwin H. Ackerknecht, "Psychopathology, Primitive Medicine, and Primitive Culture," *Bulletin of the History of Medicine*, 14 (1943), 30–67.

of these early curative procedures, Ellenberger speculates, involved the induction of hypnotic or quasi-hypnotic states.[38]

Following his analysis of primitive medicine, Ellenberger considers a series of other related past therapeutic practices from diverse cultural settings. These include ceremonial temple healing and "philosophical psychotherapy" in the ancient world; the Catholic experiences of confession, demonic possession, and exorcism; and the Protestant practice of the "Cure of Souls."[39] The explanatory worldviews of these practices, he observes, were very different one from the other; but the psychological factors and forces at play in these methods were often notably similar to those of latter-day scientific psychotherapies. Far from representing an undifferentiated background of ignorance and superstition, many of these teachings offered "a surprisingly high degree of insight into what are usually considered the most recent discoveries in the realm of the human mind."[40] Where previous Whig historians, then, had envisioned a radical value-laden dichotomy between primitivist, religious, and philosophical beliefs and modern science, Ellenberger perceived profound continuities across twenty-five centuries of theory and practice.[41]

An interesting feature of all historical accounts of psychiatry concerns the chronological point at which they begin. What do psychiatric historians interpret as the most important themes in the development of the discipline? Whom do they offer as the founding figures of the field? And where do they locate the key, transformational episodes in psychiatry's past? For Ellenberger, the royal road to the discovery of the unconscious lay through the study of hypnosis, and this hypnotic exploration of the human mind was initiated in the 1770s by the Viennese physician Franz Anton Mesmer. Ellenberger believes that in the exploration of unconscious mental life, Mesmer was a figure of premier importance. Mesmer's work of the late eighteenth century, he shows, was elaborated upon in Europe and North America during the following hundred years by a diversity of medical and nonmedical writers, including animal magnetists, hypnotists, and lay healers. During the 1890s, this heritage of Mesmeric work was picked up, systematized, and scientized by the first major dynamic psychiatric theorists. Chapters 2, 3, and 4 of *The Discovery of the Unconscious* represent chronologically parallel but thematically distinct studies of this important line of evolution from Mesmer to the late nineteenth century.

The second chapter of the book, "The Emergence of Dynamic Psychia-

---

[38] Ellenberger, *Discovery of the Unconscious*, 4–12.

[39] Ibid., 13–22, 40–43, 43–46.

[40] Ibid., 3.

[41] In Ellenberger, *Discovery of the Unconscious*, see Table 1–3, p. 47, which explicitly compares these past and present therapeutic modes.

try," provides a straightforward descriptive narrative of the figures and texts involved in this century-long sequence of research. Ellenberger dates the beginnings of dynamic psychiatry specifically from 1775, when Mesmer clashed with Father Johann Joseph Gassner, a country priest from Württemberg. During the 1770s, Gassner had became widely known for his dramatic public cures of local townspeople, which he conducted as traditional Catholic exorcisms. Mesmer adopted Gassner's procedures; but he effectively naturalized Gassner's work by explaining the alleged recoveries they produced according to fashionable Newtonian theories of the day. Ellenberger then relates colorfully the well-known stories of Mesmer's theories of animal magnetism, of the fashionable Mesmeric cults in which well-to-do Parisian ladies gathered around magnetized *baquets* of water, and of the censorship of Mesmer's activities by a royal commission in 1784.[42]

According to Ellenberger, the next link in this historical chain was furnished by the Marquis de Puységur, a provincial nobleman and high-ranking military officer from Lorraine, France. Puységur had begun as a disciple of Mesmer; however, he soon broke with the orthodox Mesmerists when he made the crucial realization that the cures brought about by Mesmer were not the product of a pseudophysical magnetic fluid but an unknown psychological force operating between the magnetist and the magnetized. By psychologizing the concept of the magnetic *rapport*, Ellenberger argues, Puységur in effect discovered the first channel for psychotherapeutic action between doctor and patient, and for this he deserves a position equal to Mesmer's as the originator of modern dynamic psychiatry. Puységur subsequently practiced his technique on local peasants in the village square of Buzancy near his family estate in the Ardennes where local people joined hands around a large magnetized elm tree.[43] Later in his career, he advocated the use of magnetism in hospitals to treat the insane.

To be sure, the work of Mesmer and Puységur had been discussed by previous medical historians; but Ellenberger characteristically probes further. He discovers that, while Mesmerism had been officially suppressed in 1784, popular interest in animal magnetism flourished until the middle of the following century. In France, the Abbé Faria, François Joseph Noizet, J.P.F. Deleuze, Alexandre Bertrand, and Antoine and Prosper Despine continued Mesmer's research. Between 1815 and 1850, Ellenberger finds, no fewer than nine journals of "magnetic medicine" appeared, and across eastern France, where the influence of Puységur remained strong, societies of animal magnetism cropped up ubiquitously. Using articles from local newspapers and rare compendia of published cases by local physicians

42 Ibid., 53–69.
43 Ibid., 70–74. See also Appendix B.

housed at the University Library of Strasbourg, Ellenberger studies the medical and popular-cultural history of the Mesmerist movement during this period. Furthermore, he brings to light the great interest in Mesmerism in the German lands between 1790 and 1820. In Prussia and Bavaria, for instance, animal magnetism was interpreted according to the dominant Romantic philosophies of the day, as a kind of quasi-pantheistic force, and was studied closely in the universities and with governmental support.

With the coming of scientific positivism at mid-century and the movement toward organicism in the mental sciences, the study of hypnotic psychological phenomena, Ellenberger explains, suffered an eclipse on the European continent. However, in England and Scotland during the 1840s, John Elliotson, James Braid (who coined the term *hypnotism*), and James Esdaile explored the possibility of "Mesmeric anesthesia," or the use of hypnosis for inducing sleep during surgical operations. During these same years, a wave of spiritism began to sweep across large parts of the United States, spreading eventually to Europe and bringing in its wake the practices of séances and mediumship. Another approach to the study of the mind and its unconscious activities was pursued.[44]

The revival of the medical study of hypnosis, and the immediate lead into twentieth-century psychological dynamism, Ellenberger shows next, took place back in France with the appearance of two competing schools of research during the final quarter of the century. In Paris, Jean-Martin Charcot, at the height of international fame for his neurological research, became interested in hypnosis and employed hypnotic techniques in widely publicized experiments on patients with fixed hysterical symptoms. Drawing on a wide range of contemporary medical and popular writings, Ellenberger paints a memorable descriptive portrait of Charcot's scientific work and cultural milieu during the French *fin de siècle*.[45] Simultaneous with Charcot's work in the French capital were developments in Nancy. In the 1860s, A. A. Liébeault, a country doctor familiar with the ideas of Noizet and Bertrand, treated with somnambulic trances poor people from the Lorraine countryside suffering from all manner of mental and physical ailments. Liébeault met with considerable success. The following decade, many of his practices were picked up and developed by Hippolyte Bernheim, a distinguished internist on the medical faculty at the nearby University of Nancy, who in turn formed an informal school of followers around him.[46] With Charcot and Bernheim, the study of hypnotic phenomena, censored officially in France since the late Enlightenment, was integrated into mainstream academic medicine. For Ellenberger, therefore, the back-

---

[44] Ibid., 81–85.

[45] Ibid., 89–101. See also Chapter 4, "Charcot and the Salpêtrière School."

[46] Ellenberger, *Discovery of the Unconscious*, 85–89.

ground to modern psychiatry began with the secularization of the Catholic practices of exorcism in the latter half of the eighteenth century, advanced though the work of Mesmer and Puységur on animal magnetism, extended through an array of lay and professional practitioners of hypnotism across the nineteenth century, and culminated in the writings of Charcot, Bernheim, and their students.[47]

At first glance, it might seem that the work of Mesmer, Puységur, and their followers represented little more than a chapter in the history of charlatanry; but Ellenberger avers otherwise. In the third chapter of *The Discovery of the Unconscious*, "The Background of Dynamic Psychiatry," he proposes innovatively that the cumulative knowledge produced by several generations of Mesmerists, magnetizers, and hypnotists represented a full-fledged system of psychology and psychiatry. Ellenberger goes so far as to refer to these teachings as "the first dynamic psychiatry."[48] Drawing on the abundant nineteenth-century literature of animal magnetism and hypnotism (including monographs by medical Mesmerists, polemical pamphlet literature, Mesmeric textbooks, and the autobiographies of popular magnetists), he reconstructs the salient features of this early psychological dynamism. In the main, the first dynamic psychiatry was the result of experiments made on hypnotized patients. This knowledge was not systematic and theoretical but descriptive and observational. Furthermore, clinical description during the nineteenth century tended to cluster around three or four basic conditions and syndromes—early in the century, around the so-called magnetic diseases, such as artificially induced somnambulism, lethargy, and catalepsy; then around multiple personality, or *dédoublement de la personnalité*; and finally, during the closing quarter of the century, around the diagnosis of hysteria, which synthesized these earlier clinical categories and led directly into the "scientific" psychodynamic theories as they are known presently.

Cumulatively, Ellenberger continues, the writings of Mesmer, Puységur, and their followers document a dual model of the mind, the existence of conscious and unconscious ego activities, and a belief in the psychogenesis of many emotional and physical conditions. Their works also reveal the utilization of the unconscious for specific psychotherapeutic purposes.

[47] Similar historical trajectories had been described by other historians of psychiatry. Consider, for example, Zilboorg, *History of Medical Psychology*, chap. 9, and Bromberg, *The Mind of Man*, chap. 8. It was Ellenberger's accomplishment to present this line of evolution in much greater detail than before and to highlight a large number of new historical figures and episodes in it.

[48] With the use of this phrase, Ellenberger is most likely playing off of Zilboorg's chapter "The First Psychiatric Revolution," in which Zilboorg described with high praise the work of Agrippa, Vives, and Weyer in the sixteenth and seventeenth centuries (see Zilboorg, *History of Medical Psychology*, chap. 7).

Elaborating on these points, Ellenberger reviews the range of techniques of hypnotization employed during the 1800s. He discusses as well a series of nineteenth-century cases of "ambulatory automatisms," or prolonged hysterical fugue states in which individuals in a post hypnotic state executed extraordinary activities.[49] Following this, in some of the most fascinating pages of the book, he narrates several semilegendary cases of multiple personality found in these writings, including the stories of Mary Reynolds (told by Dr. John Mitchell), "Estelle" (Despine), "Félida" (Azam), "Hélène Smith" (Flournoy), "Elena" (Morselli), Ansel Bourne (Hodgson and James), and "Miss Beauchamp" (Morton Prince).[50] Within this psychiatric literature, Ellenberger discriminates between the many types of multiple personality discovered at the time. He also describes the remarkable supranormal phenomena exhibited by these individuals, including suggestibility at a distance, enhanced mimetic abilities, sensory anesthesias and hyperesthesias, and anterograde and retrograde amnesia.

Psychotherapeutically, the first dynamic psychiatry, Ellenberger also shows, laid great emphasis on the "magnetic rapport" between doctor and patient. He reviews past theories of the origin and nature of the rapport (including electrical, astronomical, vitalistic, erotic, and psychological theories), and he exposes the range of effects (sedative, suggestive, authoritative, and cathartic) for which the rapport was employed. He estimates that the literature of Mesmerism and hypnosis investigated the emotional aspects of the patient-therapist relationship more deeply than anything preceding the psychoanalytic exploration of transference.[51] He closes with the decline of the first dynamic psychiatry around 1890, by which time certain dangers inherent in hypnotic research as well as its sensationalistic exploitation by popular demonstrators once again conspired to discredit the practice in official medical circles.

In the fourth chapter of his book, Ellenberger moves from textual analysis to historical contextualization. He contends that developments in the history of dynamic psychiatry become fully intelligible only against the background of social, political, and intellectual history. The Industrial Revolution, the great democratic political movements of Europe and America, and the fragmentation of the old hierarchical social structures were among the salient long-range historical developments during the period of the first dynamic psychiatry.[52] Culturally, this period was marked by the Enlightenment, the Romantic movement, and the era of positivism.

The most significant passages in this chapter consist of the four middle

[49] Ellenberger, *Discovery of the Unconscious*, 124–26.
[50] Ibid., 126–40.
[51] Ibid., 152–55.
[52] Ibid., 186–92.

sections devoted to the impact of the Romantic movement on psychological theorizing.[53] Following the interpretation of the German historian of medicine Werner Leibbrand, Ellenberger advances the concept of "Romantic medicine," which included, he proposes, a Romantic phase of psychiatric history.[54] German *Naturphilosophie* of 1800 to 1840, he observes, displayed a great interest in extreme and bizarre states of mind, including dreams, hallucinations, and many forms of mental illness. Ellenberger discusses in particular the ideas of Friedrich Wilhelm von Schelling, Gotthilf Heinrich von Schubert, Ignaz Paul Vital Troxler, and Carl Gustav Carus. Arthur Schopenhauer's *The World as Will and Representation* of 1819, which exerted an enormous influence on nineteenth-century German intellectuals, explored the irrational forces of the human mind and the dynamic character of human drives, including the sexual instincts. The German Romantic fascination with the unconscious culminated in Eduard von Hartmann's *Philosophy of the Unconscious* (1869).

Ellenberger then reviews the work of the "Romantic" psychiatrists proper, whose writings, he claims, contain many "modern" psychological insights. In *Rhapsodies on the Application for the Psychic Cure Method of Mental Disorders*, Johann Christian Reil expounded an entire program of psychotherapy for mental illness, including the use of "therapeutic theater." Johann Gottfried Langermann was a pioneer of occupational therapy. Johann Christian Heinroth studied the role of anxiety and guilt feelings in psychopathology. Karl Wilhelm Ideler emphasized the effects of frustrated sexual drives in the psychogenesis of mental diseases. And Heinrich Wilhelm Neumann devised an original system of psychology that emphasized the relationship between anxiety and masked sexual frustration in psychotic patients.[55] For many English-language readers, Ellenberger's discussion provided an introduction to these figures. Ellenberger finds that with the rise at mid-century of new scientific concepts, the study of brain anatomy became of prime importance in psychiatry and the work of the German *Psychikers* fell into disrepute. Nevertheless, Ellenberger evaluates their work highly and proposes that there was scarcely a single concept of Freud and Jung that was not anticipated by the German philosophies of nature and Romantic psychiatry.

In "On the Threshold of a New Dynamic Psychiatry," the fifth chapter of *The Discovery of the Unconscious*, Ellenberger abandons the longitudinal

[53] Ibid., 199–223.

[54] Werner Leibbrand, *Romantische Medizin* (Hamburg and Leipzig, H. Goverts Verlag, 1937), especially chap. 5. See as well Zilboorg, *History of Medical Psychology*, 464–78; Max Neuburger, "British and German Psychiatry in the Second Half of the Eighteenth and Early Nineteenth Century," *Bulletin of the History of Medicine*, 18 (1945), 121–45; and Leibbrand and Wettley, *Der Wahnsinn*, 465–508.

[55] Ellenberger, *Discovery of the Unconscious*, 210–15.

thematic evolution of dynamic psychiatry. He now focuses his historical microscope closely on the 1880s and 1890s. These were key transitional decades, bridging the old and new dynamic psychiatries; Ellenberger provides a detailed and searching analysis of the combined medical and cultural history of the period. He begins by reviewing the major characteristics of the closing quarter of the nineteenth century: the British Empire at the apex of its prestige and influence; Germany newly unified and growing rapidly in economic, political, and military power; Franco-German hostility continually at a high pitch; nationalistic unrest spreading across the Austro-Hungarian Empire; and so forth.[56] Within the sciences, he notes, the period witnessed the professionalization of one field after another. Increasingly, the loose collection of doctors, philosophers, quacks, and laypersons commenting in earlier times on matters of the mind gave way to "university psychiatry," situated institutionally in the major academic centers, dependent for clinical material on the new university clinics, and pursued in specialized scientific journals. He also highlights the new professional protocols of the period—the French patronal system and the *Korpsgeist* of the German and Austrian medical faculties—and considers the significance of these systems for the personal, professional, and theoretical behavior of doctors at the time.

Culturally, the *fin de siècle* brought a sharp reaction against the positivism and naturalism of the preceding generation. Ellenberger characterizes this as an age of "Neo-Romanticism."[57] As with the first Romantic period, there was again strong interest in the hidden depths of the human mind. The irrational, the occult, the primitive, and the mystical became choice subjects for novelists, poets, painters, philosophers, and physicians alike. A cult of decadence flourished in literary circles, and degenerationism, which had originated in the field of psychiatry in the 1840s and 1850s, became a major preoccupation of scientific intellectuals, as typified in Max Nordau's hugely influential *Degeneration* (1892). The neo-Romantic spirit flourished above all in Paris and Vienna, those quintessential capitals of the *belle époque*, which provided the two most important settings for the emergence of the new psychologies.[58]

Here, as elsewhere in his writings, Ellenberger highlights the anticipation of medicopsychological theories of the mind by philosophers and men and women of letters. In this regard, the most potent figure in late-nineteenth-century Europe was without a doubt Friedrich Nietzsche. Ellenberger adopts the interpretations of Ludwig Klages and Karl Jaspers

[56] Ibid., 254–62.
[57] He draws this term from Ika Thomese's *Romantik und Neu-Romantik* (The Hague, Martinus Nijhoff, 1923).
[58] Ellenberger, *Discovery of the Unconscious*, 278–84, 293–94.

and presents Nietzsche as an event equally in the histories of psychology and philosophy. In Ellenberger's view, Nietzsche was the great proponent of the "unmasking psychologies" of the day, which sought to reveal the hidden psychological functions of myths, religions, philosophies, and personal and social systems of secular morality. Nietzsche's exact influence on subsequent psychologists and psychiatrists is difficult to ascertain, Ellenberger concedes, but is nonetheless undeniable. Among the major theorists of the unconscious in the next century, only Jung, he writes, who engaged in a detailed exegesis of Nietzsche's writings, has acknowledged the great significance of the philosopher for his thinking.[59]

In other parts of this chapter, Ellenberger provides reviews of the European medical literature on several psychological themes prominent during the 1880s and 1890s. One characteristic of the final decades of the nineteenth century was the rapid expansion of investigations into sexual psychology and psychopathology. The literature of Catholic moral theory and the writings of authors such as Diderot, Rousseau, the Marquis de Sade, and Michelet had previously addressed with insight many aspects of human sexuality. However, beginning in the 1870s there emerged the idea of a *scientia sexualis*, including the psychiatric study of so-called sexual deviations. In 1870, Carl Westphal of the University of Berlin published the first "scientific" study of homosexuality or "contrary sexual instinct." In 1877, the French alienist Charles Lasègue coined the term *exhibitionism*, and ten years later the psychologist Alfred Binet provided a full clinical description of sexual fetishism. Ellenberger establishes that far and away the most influential early sexological text was Richard von Krafft-Ebing's *Psychopathia Sexualis*, the first edition of which appeared in 1886. A compendium of case histories of sexually "abnormal" individuals related in graphic narrative form, the *Psychopathia Sexualis* provided a comprehensive classificatory scheme for the full range of human sexual behaviors. Around the turn of the century, medical texts began to appear that were more sophisticated theoretically, including Albert Moll's *Inquiry into Libido Sexualis* (1897), Havelock Ellis's *Studies on the Psychology of Sex* (1897–1910), and Freud's *Three Essays on a Theory of Sexuality* (1905).[60]

In much the same vein, Ellenberger uncovers a rich European tradition of theorizing about dreams in the immediate pre-Freudian era. During the mid-nineteenth-century period of medical materialism, dreams had been viewed as meaningless by-products of uncoordinated cerebral activity. But during the last third of the century, they became the object of systematic interest. Again, the subject was addressed simultaneously in texts of philosophy, theology, imaginative literature, medicine, and popular folklore.

[59] Ibid., 271–78.
[60] Ibid., 291–303.

Ellenberger reviews the research on dreams of many French, German, and Dutch authors between 1860 and 1900 who speculated on the religious, psychological, physiological, and mythopoetic functions of dreaming. He centers his discussion on three texts from the 1860s that probed the subject most deeply, namely, Karl Albert Scherner's *The Life of the Dream* (1861), Alfred Maury's *Sleep and Dreams* (1861), and M.-J.-L. Hervey de Saint-Denis's *Dreams and the Means to Direct Them* (1867). Hervey de Saint-Denis, who taught Chinese languages and literature at the Collège de France, emerges as a particularly interesting figure who recorded his dreams on consecutive mornings for nearly his entire adult lifetime and learned to recall, examine, and even direct his own oneiric productions.[61] Ellenberger closes this chapter charmingly with an excursus on turn-of-the-century utopian literature, in which psychology and psychiatry figured with surprising prominence.[62] This is perhaps the richest chapter in the book.

Following this, we move to the second half of *The Discovery of the Unconscious*. Chapters 6 through 9 of the book offer extensive studies, monographic in length and detail, of the four figures Ellenberger judges to be the major theoreticians of modern dynamic psychiatry. Veritable micro-biographies in themselves, these chapters discuss the main events in the lives of the theorists, consider their personalities, delineate the intellectual development of their theories and practices, reconstruct the intellectual sources of their writings, discuss the contemporary reception of their ideas, and assess their scientific influence and cultural impact. Ellenberger unites these chapters with comparative references to the ideas and practices of other figures and by indicating numerous points of biographical contact between them.

The first of these chapters deals with Pierre Janet (1859–1947), the only Frenchman among the four. In 1970, Ellenberger's chapter represented the first detailed account of Janet's life to be given in any language, and it remains today the most comprehensive exposition of Janet's ideas in English. Later in this introductory essay, Janet's intellectual significance for Ellenberger will be assessed. It will be sufficient here to say that Ellenberger had great esteem for Janet and insisted throughout his lifetime on Janet's cardinal historical importance. In this chapter, Ellenberger surveys Janet's life, including his early academic career as a philosophy teacher in Le Havre during the 1880s, his work from 1893 to 1902 at the new Institut Psychologique at the Salpêtrière Hospital in Paris, and his long and distinguished later career at the Collège de France. In reconstructing Janet's biography, Ellenberger uses a large quantity of data from Janet's files lo-

[61] Ibid., 303–11.
[62] Ibid., 318–21.

cated at the Le Havre *lycée*, the École Normale Supérieure, and the Collège de France as well as from conversations with Janet's daughters, Hélène Pichon-Janet and Fanny Janet.[63] He fleshes out Janet's career by using the interesting French technique of providing brief parallel biographies of a number of his subject's contemporaries, in this case of the philosopher Henri Bergson and the experimental psychologist Alfred Binet.[64]

The bulk of this chapter is devoted to an in-depth presentation of the full evolution of Janetian psychology. Ellenberger canvasses Janet's early psychological ideas as they appeared in his doctoral thesis in philosophy, *L'automatisme psychologique* of 1889. This text, Ellenberger argues, is a classic of psychological science in which Janet studies with great acuity phenomena such as hysteria, catalepsy, amnesia, artificial somnambulism, and ambulatory automatisms.[65] Janet then pursued the clinical exploration of these subjects in his medical dissertation, published four years later under the title *L'état mental des hystériques*. Ellenberger considers at length a series of case histories of hysterical patients in this study, highlighting along the way Janet's superb clinical sensibility at this early stage of his career.[66] These early writings, he proposes, represent the first full psychologization of the neurosis concept following the neurological and gynecological theories of the preceding generation.

Ellenberger then explicates Janet's theory of "subconscious fixed ideas." According to this notion, neurotic illnesses originated in a frightening or traumatic experience remote in the emotional history of the individual that was then pushed into the patient's subconscious (a term Janet coined) and around which psychological delusions or physical symptoms formed. Through hypnotic suggestion returning the patient to the original scene of the trauma, as well as through other therapeutic techniques, Janet believed that an individual could regain control over these pathogenic memories. Ellenberger notes the affinity of these ideas of Janet with the Freudian therapy of catharsis and, through a close chronological review of texts, attempts to establish the priority of Janet.[67]

Ellenberger next turns to Janet's later studies. In *Névroses et idées fixes* of 1898, Janet elaborated on his ideas about neurotic psychogenesis. And in *Obsessions et psychasthénie* of 1903, he developed the important concept of "*désagrégation psychologique*—psychological dissociation."[68] After 1910, Ellenberger demonstrates, Janet moved from clinical case studies toward system and synthesis. In *Les médications psychologiques*,

[63] Ibid., 334–47, 354–56.
[64] Ibid., 353–56.
[65] Ibid., 356–64.
[66] Ibid., 361–74.
[67] Ibid., 361–64, 373–77, 406–7.
[68] Ibid., 177–86.

his masterwork published in two large volumes in 1919, he developed a vast and imaginative scheme of the five levels of mental functioning and the discontinuity between those levels that could lead to mental disease.[69] From the 1920s onward, he dedicated himself mainly to the psychology of religion, his major statement from this period being *From Anguish to Ecstasy* of 1926.[70]

Following this summary of Janet's lifework, Ellenberger attempts to elucidate the range of intellectual influences operating on Janet. He emphasizes the importance for the youthful Janet of his uncle, Paul Janet, a well-established academic philosopher. He considers the nearly lifelong friendship between Janet and Bergson, and he effectively places Janet's work in the context of the early French experimental psychological school of Binet, Théodule Ribot, and Charles Féré. He also points out that Janet was the first major figure in the history of European dynamic psychology to learn extensively from the Americans, in particular from Josiah Royce, James Mark Baldwin, and William James.[71] Conversely, Ellenberger emphasizes that Janet's influence on later psychological theorists, while often unacknowledged, was profound. He specifies the Janetian element in the work of Bleuler, Freud, Jung, and Adler as well as the importance of Janet for certain major French psychiatrists of the twentieth century, such as Henri Baruk, Jean Delay, and Henri Ey.[72] Ellenberger concludes with reflections on the posthumous decline of Janet's reputation, which he attributes to the rise to prominence of Freudian psychoanalysis and Watsonian behavioral psychology. In the closing lines of the chapter, he casts forward optimistically to a time when readers—physicians and historians alike—will unearth Janet's work, which is now submerged and out of sight like some enormous archeological structure from the past.

The seventh chapter of *The Discovery of the Unconscious* deals with Sigmund Freud. Running to 150 pages with over 540 notes of documentation, this is the longest section of the book. The chapter is very full factually, and despite the quantity of scholarly commentary on Freud in 1970, Ellenberger manages to bring forth numerous previously unknown facts about Freud's life as well as fresh, at times controversial, interpretations of his work. Ellenberger begins biographically by reconstructing Freud's family genealogy. One point emerging from this discussion is the diversity of social and cultural backgrounds among Austrian Jews in the nineteenth century and the variety in attitudes toward their social and professional lives held by their descendants in Freud's time.[73] Ellenberger also offers an

[69] Ibid., 386–94.
[70] Ibid., 394–400.
[71] Ibid., 400–406.
[72] Ibid., 406–7.
[73] Ibid., 418–27.

account of Freud's schooling, drawing in part on the recently discovered correspondence of Freud with his adolescent friend Eduard Silberstein. He discusses Freud's medical education, in part through an analysis of the official curriculum of the Vienna Medical School in the 1880s, which had been made available to him by the Viennese historian Renée Gicklhorn.

Concerning Freud's adult career, Ellenberger centers his presentation on a selection of biographical episodes that he believes have been misrecorded or misrepresented in the extant psychoanalytic literature. He offers revisionist readings of the reception of Freud's well-known lecture on hysterical disorders in male patients to the Vienna Gesellschaft der Ärzte in 1886; of the slow advancement of Freud through the academic hierarchy in Vienna; of the professional reception of Freud's early writings, including the *Studies on Hysteria* (1895) and *The Interpretation of Dreams* (1900); and of the role of Freud in the so-called Wagner-Jauregg Process of 1920 over the medical mistreatment of soldiers during the First World War. He also traces Freud's evolving and unstable relations with his many followers along with the history of Freud's involvement with various psychoanalytic organizations. Again, he provides parallel biographies of his subject's contemporaries, this time of the novelist Arthur Schnitzler and the psychiatrist and Nobel laureate Julius Wagner-Jauregg.[74] He also relates with poignancy the story of Freud's struggle against jaw and palate cancer during the last fifteen years of his life.[75]

Following this, Ellenberger offers a rather judgmental assessment of Freud's character. On the negative side, he presents a picture of Freud as self-absorbed, highly ambitious, and neurotically oversensitive to criticism, while on the positive he underscores Freud's hard work, high native intelligence, and passionate intellectual curiosity. In this evaluation, Ellenberger draws on many sources, including a highly interesting series of reminiscences about Freud by former patients. He praises Freud as a man of letters in the highest possible terms.[76]

The largest amount of space in this chapter is devoted to a copious intellectual-historical exposition of Freud's work. Ellenberger begins by placing a strong emphasis on Freud's first publications in the fields of neuroanatomy and neurophysiology. While historians of psychoanalysis had once ignored these early, nonpsychological statements, Ellenberger joins a growing number of scholars in believing that a knowledge of these writings is indispensable for understanding the origins of psychoanalysis. He then repeats the familiar account of Freud's scientific studies with Ernst Brücke, Sigmund Exner, and Theodor Meynert. As a part of this

[74] Ibid., 469–74.
[75] Ibid., 427–57.
[76] Ibid., 457–69.

discussion, he provides intelligent analyses of Freud's so-called "Project for a Scientific Psychology" (1895) and 1891 monograph on aphasia.[77] Ellenberger places these writings in the context of post-Griesingerian German-language neuropsychophysiology, with an accent on the *Hirnmythologie*, or "brain mythology," of Meynert. Following this, he uses Freud's published articles, the *Studies on Hysteria*, and the available portions of the Freud-Fliess correspondence to track Freud's intellectual movement over the years from 1886 to 1900, from neuroanatomy, to an anatomoclinical neurology, and finally to a dynamic conception of the neuroses.[78]

Ellenberger next supplies technically dense summations of the classic psychoanalytic concepts of repression and defense, the Oedipus complex, dream psychology, the parapraxes, and universal bisexuality. He observes that no psychological theorist before or after Freud had explored the unconscious mind so penetratingly. In his discussion, he stresses the period in the history of psychoanalysis from 1894 to 1899, during which time Freud's most momentous discoveries were inextricably caught up with his unprecedented, systematic self-analysis, a protracted period of personal neurosis, and an intimate intellectual dependency upon the physician Wilhelm Fliess. In his handling of *The Interpretation of Dreams* and *Jokes and Their Relation to the Unconscious*, Ellenberger follows the French critic Didier Anzieu in underscoring the masked autobiographical content of these books.[79]

Ellenberger then continues with his chronological review of Freud's work. He discusses the difficult and highly suggestive metapsychological essays of 1914 to 1924. He rehearses the dramatic shift in Freud's thinking following the First World War from a depth psychology to an ego psychology with a tripartite "structural" model of the psyche and from an emphasis on the global mechanism of repression to the notion of multiple defense mechanisms. Similarly, he summarizes Freud's movement during the 1920s from an exclusive stress on the role of the sexual instincts to a dualistic model of sexuality and aggression. He also reviews Freud's major texts dealing with anthropology (*Totem and Taboo*, 1912–1913), sociology (*Group Psychology and the Analysis of the Ego*, 1921), religion (*The Future of an Illusion*, 1927), and culture (*Civilization and Its Discontents*, 1930).[80] Lastly, he traces the development of Freud's therapeutic techniques during the 1880s and 1890s from suggestive hypnosis, to nonhypnotic suggestion, to the templar pressure technique, and finally to the free-

---

[77] Ibid., 476–80.

[78] Ibid., 474–80.

[79] Ibid., 444–49, 480–510. Didier Anzieu, *L'auto-analyse: Son rôle dans la découverte de la psychanalyse par Freud, sa fonction en psychanalyse* (Paris, Presses Universitaires de France, 1959).

[80] Ellenberger, *Discovery of the Unconscious*, 510–18, 525–34.

associative method, which, he states, provides a fundamentally new mode of exploring the unconscious. Ellenberger proposes interestingly that certain features of orthodox psychoanalytic procedure derived initially from the desire to avoid the dangers and excesses rampant in the treatment of flamboyant hysterical patients in the previous generation.[81] Ellenberger next moves in this wide-ranging chapter to the complex intellectual origins of psychoanalytic theory. Here, he expends considerable space and energy in an attempt to specify the intellectual influences operating on Freud during his lifetime. The dominant psychoanalytic historiographies, he polemicizes, portray a Freud that either emerged superhumanly from nowhere or existed in wholesale opposition to all preceding thinking about the human mind. Ellenberger, however—as we will see later on in greater detail—believed that Freud was in fact deeply and very complexly enmeshed in the Western cultural and intellectual tradition of the preceding two centuries.

To this end, Ellenberger considers the roles of German organicist psychiatry, Darwinian evolutionary theory, Charcot, Bernheim, and the French school, classical German literature (especially Goethe and Schiller), and the ancient Greek tragedians in the formation of Freudian doctrine. More controversially, he underscores the influence of figures and movements that were largely ignored or downplayed by Freud himself and by Freud's subsequent biographers. Fliess's significance in Freud's intellectual biography was much greater than currently believed, Ellenberger maintains. He also argues that in the formulation of specific concepts and practices, Freud owed a direct debt to Janet. And despite the fact that Freud remained officially scornful of philosophy, Nietzschean and Schopenhauerian themes pervade Freud's thinking. Furthermore, Ellenberger insists that Freud's work on dreams and sexual psychopathology must be viewed against the background of medical writing on these topics from the preceding generation that he discussed in the fifth chapter of the book. In Ellenberger's final view, the achievement of Freud to a large extent took the form of a powerful crystallization of ideas and observations previously in existence but scattered in many different fields of inquiry and now applied directly to psychology.[82]

Ellenberger ends his survey of psychoanalytic psychology with reflections on cultural influence. While it is too early, he concludes, to judge definitively the scientific status of psychoanalysis, Freudian theory has beyond doubt generated a potent tradition of psychological research as

[81] Ibid., 518–25.

[82] For more on Ellenberger's attitudes toward Freud and the historical literature on psychoanalysis, see "Revisionist Psychoanalytic History," below.

well as a cultural revolution still in progress. This revolution is comparable in scope to the revolutions unleashed by Newton and Darwin.

Chapter 8 of *The Discovery of the Unconscious* treats the life and work of Alfred Adler. Since the late 1940s, when an Adlerian study group existed in Zurich, Ellenberger has been interested in Adlerian psychology. However, the scholarship on Adler thus far, he observes, had been produced almost entirely either by Adlerians, who have been defensive and uncritically admiring of their hero, or by psychoanalysts, who have dwelt with disapproval on what they deemed Adler's defective discipleship with Freud. Ellenberger notes that in much of the existing literature, Adler is categorized only as a "neo-Freudian" or "psychoanalytic deviant."[83] In contrast, Ellenberger believes strongly that Adler merited historical consideration in his own right. In this chapter, then, he seeks to rise above previous sectarian perspectives and to provide a full and objective account of Adler's life and work.[84]

Adler lived from 1870 to 1937. In his biographical presentation about Adler, Ellenberger draws on primary materials from the Archives of the Jewish Community of Vienna and the libraries of the University of Vienna Medical School and the University of Zurich. Furthermore, a certain Hans Beckh-Widmanstetter, a physician and scholar in Vienna who for years had painstakingly collected information for a major biography of Adler, placed his materials at Ellenberger's disposal shortly before his own death. As a result, Ellenberger is able to relate in substantial detail the stories of Adler's large Jewish family, which originated in Burgenland, Hungary, of his childhood years in a Vienna suburb, and of his undergraduate and medical education during the 1890s. He also discusses Adler's developing socialist sympathies as a young man and his reformist writings about occupational health conditions among underprivileged laborers. He charts the history of the Adler-Freud relationship, including Adler's role as one of the earliest members of the so-called Wednesday evening discussion group and his activities as the first editor of the *Zentralblatt für Psychoanalyse*. He also rehearses the story of Adler's tense but inevitable parting from Freud in May 1911, when along with several other members Adler formed the independent Society for Free Psychoanalysis.

Ellenberger places the next stage of Adler's career against the back-

---

[83] See the treatments of Adler, for instance, in Bromberg, *The Mind of Man*, 208–15; Dieter Wyss, *Depth Psychology: A Critical History* [1961], translated from the German by Gerald Onn (New York, Norton, 1966), 256–64; and Franz G. Alexander and Sheldon T. Selesnick, *The History of Psychiatry: An Evaluation of Psychiatric Thought and Practice from Prehistoric Times to the Present* (New York, Harper and Row, 1966), 226–34.

[84] For a fair-minded appraisal of this chapter of the book, consult Paul Stepansky, *In Freud's Shadow: Adler in Context* (Hillsdale, N.J., Analytic Press, 1983), 1–7.

ground of Austro-Hungarian political history, including discussions of
Adler's activities in military medicine during the First World War and of his
political commentaries on the Bolshevik Revolution in Russia. He shows
that during the 1920s and 1930s, Adler increasingly devoted himself to
developing an independent school of psychology with its own theories,
journals, organizations, and membership. However, owing to political developments in central Europe in the 1930s, Adler's leftist sympathies were
increasingly unwelcome, so he began to spend more time at academic
locations in Britain and the United States. In 1937, shortly before his death,
he settled in the United States, where he believed the future of his psychology lay.[85]

Ellenberger appraises Adler as a major figure in the history of twentieth-
century psychology. Characteristically, he brings to light Adler's early pre-
psychoanalytic work in the field of social medicine, including a short but
previously unknown monograph, *Health Book for the Tailor Trade* of
1898.[86] He then analyzes Adler's mature psychological system. Adler's
ideas regarding psychology began to emerge around 1905, first in a number of papers delivered at the Wednesday evening sessions and later, after
the departure from Freud, in several monographs. Adler's system, which
Ellenberger strives to demarcate from Freudian psychoanalysis, experimental psychology, and traditional faculty psychology, was called Individual Psychology. Adler's initial perception involved the idea of "organ inferiority." From his general medical practice in the 1890s, Adler had been
struck by the prevalence of organ or organ-system defects in individuals
who went on to develop elaborate organic and psychological compensa-
tions for these internal deficiencies. Failure to adapt to organic weakness,
Adler believed, led to emotional disturbance. Adler theorized that these
defects often produced from childhood onward feelings of inferiority that
over time gave rise, in Adler's well-known phrase, to an "inferiority complex." Adler discussed many of the family constellations and situational
stresses that nourish such psychological formations.

Deeply read in Nietzschean philosophy, Adler, Ellenberger explains,
came to believe that the aggressive instinct represented the primary means
by which individuals strive to master their organic inferiorities. In a paper
presented to the Vienna Psychoanalytic Society in 1910, Adler identified
the aggressive drive and the will to overcome inferiority as a "masculine
protest" and a resignation or acceptance of this condition as a feminine
feature. In *The Neurotic Constitution* of 1912, Adler proposed that the
character traits, symptoms, and even the dreams of the neurotic operate as
means by which individuals attempt to compensate for feelings of insignifi-

[85] Ellenberger, *Discovery of the Unconscious*, 580–94.
[86] Ibid., 599–603.

cance and to assert their power over other people and life situations.[87]
Adler's later writings increasingly embraced a practical sociological and
educational perspective, and texts such as *Understanding Human Nature*
(1927) and *The Meaning of Life* (1933) are addressed equally to parents,
teachers, counselors, group therapists, and physicians.[88]

In the final section of this chapter, Ellenberger assesses the influence of
Adler's teachings. He observes the widespread tendency to attribute to
other psychologists, especially Jung and Freud, terms and ideas that originated with Adler. He points out the similarity between Adler's concept of
psychological inferiority and Janet's *sentiment d'incomplétitude*, and he
notes that Adler was the first clinician (preceding Freud by over a decade) to
postulate a central and autonomous aggressive drive. He also comments
on the Adlerian elements in the writings of Harry Stack Sullivan, Karen
Horney, Erich Fromm, Victor Frankl, and Binswanger. Adler, with his
observations about organ vulnerability and the inner image of the individual, pioneered psychosomatic medicine, and with his theories of childhood
inferiority feelings and emotional resocialization, he exerted a widespread
influence on current-day social psychiatry and group psychotherapy.[89]

The ninth chapter of Ellenberger's book, the last of the chapters devoted
to a single figure, concerns Carl Gustav Jung (1875–1961). Jung is the only
one of the major theoreticians canvassed in the book with whom Ellenberger had a personal acquaintance. In preparation for writing the chapter,
Ellenberger interviewed Jung, and Jung then read and offered commentary
on the chapter in draft form shortly before his death. As with Janet, Ellenberger, who shared numerous personal and cultural affinities with Jung,
consistently treats Jung with sympathy and admiration. As with Adler, he
stresses Jung's intellectual independence from Freud.

In his opening biographical section, Ellenberger once more produces
much new information about his subject. He reconstructs the distinctive
social and cultural atmosphere of Basel in which the Jung family had lived
for generations. The Jungs, he points out, included on both the paternal and maternal sides a number of notable cultural figures, including
physicians, writers, and Protestant ministers. Jung's paternal grandfather,
after whom Jung was named and with whom he identified in many ways,
was a colorful civic-minded personality involved in the local Romantic
movement who provided a link between the older and newer dynamic
psychiatries.

Ellenberger then reviews Jung's childhood and adolescence as well as his
education in the humanities and the medical sciences at the University of

[87] Ibid., 606–19.
[88] Ibid., 619–23, 623–25.
[89] Ibid., 636–48.

Basel. In writing about Jung's early years, he draws on personal interviews with members of the Jung family as well as the recently published memoirs of Jung's schoolmate Gustav Steiner. While in medical school from 1895 to 1902, Jung became engrossed with spiritism and occult phenomena. Ellenberger relates the story of the mediumistic séances that Jung organized in his household from 1895 to 1899 with his young cousin Helene Preiswerk and other members of the Jung and Preiswerk circles. These experiments, Ellenberger alleges, introduced young Jung to the mysteries of the unconscious mind. Much to the consternation of his family, Jung later used the case of his cousin (cited pseudonymously as "Miss S.W.") as the subject of his medical dissertation, which appeared in 1902 under the title *On the Psychology and Pathology of So-Called Occult Phenomena*.[90] From this formative period, Ellenberger also brings to light Jung's activities in the Basel section of the Zofingia Students' Association, where Jung first became convinced of the inadequacy of the materialist psychologies of his day.

In 1900, Jung traveled to the Burghölzli, the famous psychiatric clinic at the University of Zurich, where he studied directly under Eugen Bleuler. Ellenberger reviews Jung's activities during the Burghölzli years from 1900 to 1909. With the assistance of Ackerknecht, he unearthed from the University of Zurich archives the syllabi of courses taught by Jung as a *Privatdozent* at the hospital.[91] Furthermore, he examines Jung's early research activities in Zurich in which Jung pioneered diagnostic projective testing techniques. He also considers Jung's major publication from this period, the *Psychology of Dementia Praecox*. Published in 1907, this work, which offers an ingenious synthesis of the ideas of Kraepelin, Janet, Bleuler, Forel, and Freud, was designed to establish the primacy of psychogenic factors in the etiology of schizophrenia. In Ellenberger's analysis, it is a classic text, which represents the first monograph of the depth-psychological investigation of a psychotic patient.

The psychoanalytic phase in Jung's life runs from 1906 to 1913. Ellenberger reviews the events of this period as closely and objectively as possible. Soon after reporting about *The Interpretation of Dreams* to a discussion group of medical residents at the Burghölzli in 1900, Jung developed an intense interest in Freud's work. In this well-known story, Jung for several years played a highly active organizational role in the budding psychoanalytic movement. He founded the Freud Society in Zurich, organized the First International Psychoanalytic Congress in Salzburg in 1908, and edited the *Jahrbuch für psychoanalytische und psychopathologische*

---

[90] Ellenberger was intrigued by this case and returned to it often in his writings. See Chapter 11, "C. G. Jung and the Story of Helene Preiswerk."

[91] Ellenberger, *Discovery of the Unconscious*, 739 n. 31.

Forschungen. Without the benefit of the Jung-Freud correspondence, Ellenberger does his best to piece together the historic personal and intellectual relationship between the two figures. On theoretical matters, he shows, Jung at first wrote a number of essays that hew closely to the lines of classic Freudian analysis. In his most important statement, a two-part essay in the *Jahrbuch* in 1911–1912, Jung highlighted the functional parallels between the processes of the dream work, the thinking of children, the psychology of neurotic fantasies and delusions, and the structure of myths and legends. Over the years, Ellenberger acknowledges, Jung and Freud learned substantially from one another. It was Jung who adopted the word *complex*, who first suggested that all psychoanalysts undergo training analyses, whose work on the psychology and anthropology of myth-making inspired Freud's *Totem and Taboo*, and who provoked Freud into formulating his theory of narcissism. The two men, however, were fated to drift apart. Ellenberger traces Jung's independent formulation of a libido concept in *Metamorphoses and Symbols of the Libido* (1911–1912) and outlines Jung's growing reservations about the universality of the Oedipus complex. For these doctrinal as well as personal reasons, the two split, painfully, at the end of 1913.

The following year, Jung resigned his post at the University of Zurich and retreated to a residence in the cozy town of Küsnacht on the shores of Lake Zurich. There, he quietly entered a self-imposed period of systematic introspection lasting for nearly six years. Ellenberger sees this experience as transformative in Jung's life and likens it to Freud's self-analysis during the later 1890s. During this long meditative period, Jung formulated the major concepts associated with his mature psychodynamic system, Analytical Psychology. With his customary clarity, Ellenberger reviews the meaning and elaboration of these concepts. The Jungian "anima" designates the autonomous feminine sub-personality in the male psyche while the "animus" represents the masculine aspect in the female constitution. "Individuation" is the process whereby a person across the course of a lifetime achieves unity of personality and higher levels of consciousness. The Jungian "Self" is at once the agency and the product of this process while the "persona" is the accumulation of conventional, conformist images presented in public circumstances. Jungian "archetypes," Ellenberger explains further, are universal, primordial images that recur in individual dreams and fantasies and, on the collective level, in works of art and literature, in religions, and in mythologies. And the collective unconscious in Jungian psychology operates as a repository of ancestral experiences of the species accumulated over many generations. Ellenberger also includes in his discussion a section on Jung's psychotherapeutic ideas, a topic ignored in previous presentations of Jungian psychology.

From the 1930s onward, Jung increasingly restricted his movements to his arcadian retreat in Küsnacht. Ellenberger explains, however, that Jung maintained a private practice and became a highly sought-after psychotherapist. In his advanced years, he received many professional recognitions and honorary academic appointments, and within Switzerland he became a revered figure. Attempting to situate Jung among his contemporaries during these mature years, Ellenberger juxtaposes to Jung's life brief biographies of Karl Barth the theologian, Paul Häberlin the philosopher, and Rudolf Steiner the anthroposophist. One matter, however, seriously compromised Jung's growing international reputation during his later years, and that was the charge of Jung's alleged sympathy with the Nazis during the 1930s.[92] Ellenberger traces the origins and history of this accusation and then attempts with some indignation to absolve Jung of complicity.[93] Like Janet, Jung in his later years became interested in the psychology of religion as well as the philosophical problem of evil, subjects he explored most notably in his controversial work of 1952, *Answer to Job*.

Finally, Ellenberger explores the complex intellectual origins of Jung's psychological system. Numerous hitherto unknown sources of Jung's ideas are brought to light. Ellenberger considers the roles played by Jung's grandfather, by Goethe, by Emmanuel Swedenborg, and by the Protestant humanistic tradition of Basel. No figure under consideration in his book, Ellenberger remarks, owed more intellectually to German *Naturphilosophie* than Jung. In particular, Ellenberger highlights the significance of Carus, Schopenhauer, and Hartmann, three philosophers of the unconscious, as well as two lesser-known figures, Ignaz Troxler and Friedrich Creuzer. Ellenberger also stresses the importance for Jung of Nietzsche, Basel's most erratic and brilliant personality from the generation preceding Jung. Using Jung's unpublished multivolume commentaries on Nietzsche's *Thus Spoke Zarathustra*, a source he was the first scholar to consult, Ellenberger documents Jung's long intellectual engagement with the philosopher. He considers, too, the role of Western and Eastern mystical and occult traditions. Among psychological and psychiatric figures, Ellenberger records the influence on Jung of Bleuler, Janet, Binet, Flournoy, Adler, and of course Freud. He closes with a review of the multifarious influences of Jung's thought on others.[94]

---

[92] This issue was the subject of an envenomed controversy among psychiatric historians during the 1960s. Compare E. A. Bennet, *C. G. Jung* (London, Barrie and Rockliff, 1961), 56–62; Harms, *Origins of Modern Psychiatry*, chap. 25; Ellenberger, *Discovery of the Unconscious*, 675–78; and "Jung and the National Socialists," in Alexander and Selesnick, *History of Psychiatry*, 407–9.

[93] Ellenberger, *Discovery of the Unconscious*, 675–78, 740 n. 55. See also Ellenberger's review of C. G. Jung, "Letters: Volume I, 1906–1950," *Journal of the History of the Behavioral Sciences*, 11 (1975), 96–97.

[94] Ellenberger offers further observations on Jung in "L'autobiographie de C. G. Jung," *Critique*, 20, nos. 207–8 (August–September 1964), 754–79.

The tenth and final chapter of *The Discovery of the Unconscious* is entitled "The Dawn and Rise of the New Dynamic Psychiatry." In this chapter, one of the most interesting in the book, Ellenberger moves from a synchronic to a diachronic account of his subject. After the in-depth biographical and theoretical studies of Janet, Freud, Adler, and Jung, Ellenberger now provides a detailed year-by-year chronicle of events in Western psychiatric history, beginning in the early 1880s and extending to 1945. With this medical chronology, he intermixes pertinent developments in the social, political, cultural, and intellectual history of Europe at the time. This unique presentational device permits Ellenberger to recapitulate from a different perspective much of the historical material he has discussed in the four preceding chapters, and it allows him to consider the complex interrelationship of these major psychological systems with one another and with other minor ones that developed at the same time.[95]

This section of the book is a *tour de force* of descriptive detail that must be read through to achieve its effect. Much of its charm comes from the juxtaposition of figures, events, and texts not generally viewed together. At times, these juxtapositions are merely interesting. The year 1895, for example, brought publication of Breuer's and Freud's *Studies on Hysteria* and Gustave LeBon's influential *On the Psychology of Crowds*. It also witnessed the death of Pasteur, the beginnings of the Dreyfus Affair, the discovery of the x-ray, and the invention of cinematography. Other dates are noteworthy because they reveal divergent contemporaneous developments: Anna Freud's *The Ego and the Defense Mechanisms*, a key text in psychoanalytic ego psychology, and Egaz Moniz's first publication on the surgical treatment of the psychoses both appeared in 1936. In still other ways, Ellenberger's narrative yields insights into the history of the field that probably could be achieved only through such a diachronic perspective. Tracking the development of early popular and professional attitudes toward psychoanalysis, for instance, he discovers that it was only after around 1907 that an organized and hostile response to Freud developed and not much earlier, as had previously been believed. Moreover, this negative reaction, he finds, was aroused more by the organization of psychoanalysis into a school, with its own membership, conferences, and publications, than by Freudian ideas per se.

Another significant innovation of this final chapter is the use of new categories of primary source materials. For instance, Ellenberger reports on the medical and popular review literature about select psychiatric texts, such as Janet's early essays, Théodore Flournoy's *From India to the Planet Mars* (1900), and several psychoanalytic texts. This procedure allows him

---

[95] A possible model for Ellenberger's use of this device may be found in Edwin G. Boring, *A History of Experimental Psychology* (New York, D. Appleton, 1929), chap. 23.

to discuss not only the intellectual history of psychiatry but the critical contemporary reception surrounding key books and articles.

Ellenberger also makes extensive use of the proceedings of medical conferences. An outstanding feature of the history of the European sciences in the latter half of the nineteenth century was the holding of regular academic congresses. These conferences were major professional events, the participants in which often included philosophers, theologians, imaginative writers, and laymen as well as physicians. Moreover, the lectures delivered at the congresses as well as the subsequent discussions about them were often published in thick volumes. Throughout this chapter, then, Ellenberger examines the proceedings of over twenty such congresses, from the fields of general medicine, psychiatry, psychoanalysis, experimental psychology, neurology, hypnotism, and parapsychology, which took place between 1889 and 1914. Since many scientists presented their work first in conference papers, this proves an excellent way to study the cutting edge of thinking in the mental sciences.

Unfortunately, this final chapter of Ellenberger's book falls off noticeably in quality as it progresses. But the chapter retains its overall quality, above all because Ellenberger up to the end offers a steady flow of exceptionally interesting and suggestive historical data and ideas that were previously little known: a summary of the obituaries of Charcot from across the world in the summer of 1893; a review of the range of psychiatric therapies available to patients of different social classes in the 1890s; a sketch of the history of the term *libido*; an account of a long, perceptive review of *The Interpretation of Dreams* by Henri Bergson; an excursus on the similarities between Flournoy's *From India to the Planet Mars* and the science fiction of Jules Verne and H. G. Wells; a reference to Hermann Hesse's Jungian analysis in 1916–1917; a speculation on the impact of World War I on psychoanalytic theorizing; a lead about the unwritten early history of psychoanalysis in the Balkan countries; a citation of the first known history of psychiatry, written in Russia in 1929; a survey of theories of mass psychology accounting for the success of German and Italian fascism; a note on the origins of the term *group psychotherapy* in American medicine; a thought about the psychiatric significance of Jean-Paul Sartre's *Being and Nothingness* (1943).[96] This and much more awaits the reader of this final chapter.

Ellenberger ends the chapter powerfully, by conjuring up the two colossi of psychiatric medicine that dominated the world in 1945. On the one side, there was the psychoanalytic establishment, which originated in a central Europe that was now drained of its intellectual talent and which was

---

[96] Ellenberger, *The Discovery of the Unconscious*, 769–70, 765–67, 777–78, 757, 760, 778, 873 n. 143, 781–82, 880 n. 331, 826, 880 n. 346, 842, 844, 852, 884 n. 433.

entrenched doctrinally in the United States. On the other side, Pavlovian psychology and psychiatry, the official medical ideology of Soviet Russia, was now forcibly extended over most of eastern Europe to the exclusion of all other theories. The closing historical image is of a field of ideas and practices that remains active but sharply polarized—theoretically, politically, and geographically—and that has abandoned its native lands in western and middle Europe for the new superpowers of the East and West. Following a short conclusion, which recapitulates the main points and themes, Ellenberger's book comes to a close.

The Discovery of the Unconscious is a complex piece of empirical and interpretive work. Despite my enthusiastic presentation in the preceding pages, the book assuredly is not without its shortcomings. Methodologically, professional historians are most likely to be dissatisfied by Ellenberger's handling of the phenomenon of intellectual "influence." Like most historians of psychiatry at the time, Ellenberger's training was purely medical, and this becomes apparent in a number of ways. Throughout the work, Ellenberger is preoccupied with establishing the sources of thought of his four historical protagonists. He accomplishes this by locating two sources that are similar in descriptive idea content and then by designating the one that was written first as a "source" for the latter one. In this way, he ferrets out an impressive number of textual parallels. However, intellectual anteriority and priority are of course two different things, and the mere similarity of ideas, which often originated in wholly different periods, cultures, and fields of inquiry, is insufficient to establish a causal connection between them.[97] Ironically, at the moment Ellenberger was writing his book, professional historians of ideas were in the process of sophisticating themselves on this slippery methodological matter.[98] But Ellenberger had little interest in contemporary secondary literature, and his work suffers on this point as a consequence.

A second problem in *The Discovery of the Unconscious*, this one interpretive, concerns the lack of comparative evaluation among the historical materials presented. By the end of his chronicle, Ellenberger has presented a perfectly enormous number of ideas, observations, and theories about the dynamic unconscious mind from across the last two centuries. But at no point does he attempt to evaluate the intellectual merits, much less scientific truth value, of these ideas. Similarly, by granting, as it were, equal time

[97] Intellectual historians in America were most attuned to this problem in the book. See John C. Burnham, review of Ellenberger, *The Discovery of the Unconscious*, *Isis*, 62 (1971), 528; and Stepansky, *In Freud's Shadow*, 1–7.

[98] Quentin Skinner, "The Limits of Historical Explanations," *Philosophy*, 41 (1966), 199–215; idem, "Meaning and Understanding in the History of Ideas," *History and Theory*, 8 (1969), 3–53.

to the systems of Janet, Freud, Adler, and Jung, he imputes theoretical parity to them. Needless to say, all of these theories and practices, from Mesmer's earliest writings to Jung's final publications, cannot be of equal merit.[99] Many of the ideas that Ellenberger discusses are in fact mutually contradictory, and it is highly unlikely that posterity will judge equally the quality and significance of the work of even the four main figures. This feature of the book most likely results from Ellenberger's admirable attempt to avoid the factional polemics that marred so much previous historical commentary on psychiatry; but, in pursuit of the ideal of objectivity, his presentation at times appears uncritical.

A third and related problem concerns Ellenberger's Freudian revisionism. Ellenberger's attitudes toward Freud make for an interesting, complicated subject, which will be addressed in due course. Suffice it to say that, in reacting to what he perceived as excesses in the psychoanalytic historiography of his time, Ellenberger's writing in quite a few passages of *The Discovery of the Unconscious* comes off as tendentious. His biographical portrait of Freud is limited to those episodes for which he can offer revisionist accounts. To similar effect, in nearly every instance in the book involving a controversy with Freud—the priority debate between Janet and Freud, the Freud-Adler split, the quarrel between Freud and Jung—Freud is presented as the wrongdoer. Ellenberger's interpretations may or may not be correct, but the cumulative impression is that in these instances the author has strayed from his own ideal of nonpartisanship. Moreover, in pursuing his revisionist agenda, Ellenberger at times brings a different standard of evaluation to the historical evidence he adduces on Freud's behalf than for other figures.[100]

In the long run, however, these problems in Ellenberger's book only establish that no piece of work is beyond improvement and that Ellenberger too must be understood in ideological context. Ultimately, it would be misguided to dwell on the inadequacies of a work that in so many other ways represents an extraordinary achievement. In breadth and depth of coverage, *The Discovery of the Unconscious* was, and is, unmatched among histories of psychiatry. Across its nearly one thousand pages, the book draws together an immense quantity of raw primary source data,

[99] On this point, consult the thoughtful review of Erwin Ackerknecht in *Neue Zürcher Zeitung*, no. 496 (October 25, 1970), 53.

[100] To cite two examples: Ellenberger repeatedly criticizes Freud for forming around him a school, with a cult of the creator, closed membership, special institutions of study, and ritualized training methods, and he likens these practices to the religious and philosophical sects of earlier, prescientific times. However, the formation of the same phenomena around Jung and Adler fail to elicit his disapprobation. Similarly, Ellenberger discusses the voluminous European literature on dream psychology in the two generations preceding Freud's work, giving the impression that Freud borrowed surreptitiously from these earlier writings. Yet he fails to acknowledge the opening chapter of *The Interpretation of Dreams* in which Freud reviews conscientiously and in great detail the existing literature on dreams.

stretching across 175 years, written in half a dozen languages, and originating from twice as many fields of knowledge, and coordinates this mass into a coherent and compelling historical picture. On the factual level, the book abounds with fascinating detail while interpretively, it brims with interesting, important formulations. Throughout the work, Ellenberger's discovery of primary source materials is unceasingly impressive. In the second, third, and fourth chapters detailing the "first dynamic psychiatry," Ellenberger brings to light entire new episodes in the history of psychiatry. In his monographic studies of Janet, Adler, and Jung, he provides the most comprehensive studies available at the time of these figures. And the final chapter of the book represents an unprecedented attempt to write an *histoire totale* of psychiatry.

Moreover, Ellenberger demonstrates in *The Discovery of the Unconscious* a number of distinctive talents. He reveals a special awareness of the many minor, contributory figures in the history of psychiatry. To the delight of the specialist, he loads his footnotes with bibliographical esoterica. And he demonstrates repeatedly an outstanding ability to isolate from difficult texts those ideas, anecdotes, and bits of information that are historically telling. What is more, Ellenberger managed to accomplish all of these things in a volume that was written with great clarity and in a highly readable, almost novelistic, style accessible equally to readers medical and nonmedical, specialized and nonspecialized.

Ironically, perhaps the most significant accomplishment of *The Discovery of the Unconscious* has gone almost entirely unappreciated. To date, Ellenberger's book has been read overwhelmingly on the ideological and empirical levels. Because many topics in psychiatric history remain intensely controversial, one class of readers has been interested primarily in the positions taken by Ellenberger in the great political debates of the field, most notably those surrounding Freud and his rivals. Similarly, because *The Discovery of the Unconscious* is so rich factually, other readers have been content to mine the work as a kind of historical encyclopedia. However, as I mentioned above, limiting our approach to the book in these ways has the undesirable effect of obscuring the key thematic lines running throughout the volume. Even more importantly, these approaches ignore the fundamental *epistemological* nature of Ellenberger's enterprise.

In the preface to the French edition of *The Discovery of the Unconscious*, and in the single review of his book to which he responded, Ellenberger addressed this last issue.[101] In these two places, Ellenberger acknowledged the unfortunate tendency to approach his book mainly for its picturesque historical data. In reality, Ellenberger revealed, he had conceived of the

[101] Ellenberger, *A la découverte de l'inconscient: Histoire de la psychiatrie dynamique* (Villeurbanne, Simep-Éditions, 1974), vi–viii; Ellenberger, "Lettre à la rédaction de *Dialogue*," *Dialogue: Canadian Philosophical Review/Revue philosophique canadienne*, 10 (1971), 561–64.

work preeminently as a study in "historical epistemology," that is, as an epistemological analysis in the French sense of the historical development of a body of knowledge. From the very beginning of his reading on the subject as a young man, Ellenberger had been struck by the unique path of evolution followed by psychiatry as it developed into a mature and recognizable discipline. Other branches of medicine and science had followed more or less continuous and cumulative lines of development, usually growing incrementally from a single "prescientific" form into a modern science (i.e, from, say, alchemy to modern-day chemistry, or from astrology to astronomy). To a substantial extent, their histories remained internally cohesive. However, the historical structure of psychiatry, Ellenberger perceived, was strikingly different. Unlike any other field of organized inquiry that he knew of, psychiatry's historical origins were highly diverse and fragmented. Primitive medicine, ancient mythology, theology, philosophy, law, anthropology, literature, academic medicine, popular lay healing, and many other fields had all contributed at different times. The investigation of the unconscious in particular had been the collective accomplishment of a diversity of people, including shamans, exorcists, priests, philosophers, novelists, poets, doctors, magnetizers, hypnotists, spiritists, mediums, psychologists, psychiatrists, and psychoanalysts. Not until the final third of the nineteenth century had these scattered insights and observations come together to form the discipline known presently as medical psychology.

Furthermore, Ellenberger pointed out that the evolutionary pathway followed by the discipline was anything but clear and cumulative. Rather, psychiatric history had developed through a series of radical mutations and metamorphoses. It was riddled with ideas that had been discovered and published, then forgotten, and later rediscovered, with entire "obsolete knowledges," and with a dialectical dynamic between somatic and psychological theories of the mind that often required the repudiation of the teachings of preceding generations.

In a way, it is unfortunate that Ellenberger chose the title he did for his great work. "The discovery of the unconscious" sounds rather more Whiggish than the book in fact is. More accurately, the subject of Ellenberger's classic is the *constitution* of the unconscious.[102] In the broad perspective, *The Discovery of the Unconscious* investigates the remote and highly complex multidisciplinary origins of an entire field of medicine. Read on the *macroscopic* level, and from beginning to end, as it was intended to be, the book represents a study of the ways in which dynamic psychiatry came to be a unified, systematized, and self-conscious knowl-

---

[102] As Ellenberger once commented of his book, "Du point de vue philosophique ou plus exactement épistémiologique, il s'agissait d'étudier la façon dont s'était constituée cette connaissance du psychisme inconscient et de préciser la place de celle-ci dans l'ensemble général de la science" (*A la découverte de l'inconscient*, vi).

edge. Two decades after its appearance, Ellenberger's work on this score remains one of a kind.

The Historical Essays: Eight Themes

Generally speaking, Henri Ellenberger's *The Discovery of the Unconscious* was very well received upon publication. In 1970, when the book appeared under the impress of Basic Books, it was reviewed widely and enthusiastically in the United States and Britain. It was immediately accorded the status of a minor classic, which would long remain indispensable for scholars in psychiatric history.[103] As one reviewer remarked, *The Discovery of the Unconscious* established Ellenberger beyond doubt as "the premier historian of 'dynamic psychiatry.' "[104] In Continental Europe, reviews of the original English edition of the work were understandably fewer but included perceptive, detailed, and extremely positive commentaries by distinguished figures in psychiatry and medical history.[105] Beyond this, reactions to Ellenberger's book tended to differ according to the professional and ideological orientation of readers. Physicians in general medicine, psychiatrists, and psychologists found the book a useful compendium of historical material. Psychoanalysts were unhappy with many of Ellenberger's formulations about Freud, but grudgingly acknowledged the value of the work. Professional historians of medicine, including historians of psychiatry, hailed the book for its monumental scholarship.

Simultaneous with the American edition, *The Discovery of the Unconscious* was published in Britain by Penguin Books. In 1972, the work appeared in two volumes in an Italian translation. A year later, an excellent two-volume German translation was published by Hans Huber. And the same year, the book was printed in Spanish.[106] However, far and away the

---

[103] See the reviews by David Elkind, *Contemporary Psychology*, 17 (1972), 56–59; George Rosen, *Bulletin of the History of Medicine*, 46 (1972), 605–7; George Mora, *American Journal of Psychiatry*, 127 (1971), 156–57; Michael Shepherd, *Psychological Medicine*, 2 (1972), 438–39; "H.L.A.," *Journal of Individual Psychology*, 26 (1970), 178–82; Paul W. Pruyser, *Bulletin of the Menninger Clinic*, 35 (1971), 213–15; and Norman Reider, *Journal of the History of the Behavioral Sciences*, 7 (1971), 194–96.

[104] Review by Stanley Jackson in *Journal of the History of Medicine*, 26 (1971), 216.

[105] See above all the forty-page review by Henri Ey, "A propos de: *La Découverte de l'inconscient* de Henri F. Ellenberger," *L'évolution psychiatrique*, 47 (1972), 227–70; and Erwin Ackerknecht, review in *Neue Zürcher Zeitung*, 53.

[106] *The Discovery of the Unconscious: The History and Evolution of Dynamic Psychiatry* (London, Allen Lane, 1970); *La scoperta dell'inconscio: Storia della psichiatria dinamica*, 2 vols. (Turin, Boringhieri, 1972); *Die Entdeckung des Unbewussten*, 2 vols. (Bern, Hans Huber, 1973), with a reprint in Zurich by Diogenes Verlag in 1985; *El descubrimiento del inconsciente (Historia y evolución de la psiquiatría dinámica)* (Madrid, Editorial Gredos, 1974).

most dramatic reception occurred in the spring of 1974 when *The Discovery of the Unconscious* appeared in a long-awaited French edition.[107] With the assistance of the Fondation Européenne de la Culture, Ellenberger's book was uniquely and lavishly produced in France. The format of the volume is large, and the text is displayed in two vertical columns on each page with the documentation appearing in a third column, in the margins, directly alongside the text. The subheadings of each chapter are reproduced prominently, and the text is interlarded with illustrations, many more than in the American edition.

In France, Belgium, Swiss Romande, and French-speaking Canada, reviews of this edition of the book glowed without exception.[108] Critics repeatedly praised the author for his *ardeur investigatrice* and his stylistic clarity (which was seen to contrast refreshingly with the Lacanian and Althusserian obscurity just then hitting the Parisian intellectual world). Furthermore, French readers were enchanted by Ellenberger's rehabilitation of the work of Janet and his informed defense of the French psychological school. The appearance of the book in Paris was treated as a significant cultural event.[109] Despite the expense of the volume, sales were high. General newspapers and literary journals ran interviews of Ellenberger.[110] He was also interviewed on radio shows, and an hour-long roundtable discussion with the author and a group of Parisian illuminati aired on television in mid-December 1972.[111] This spirited reception culminated in an invitation for Ellenberger to spend the fall and winter semesters of 1975–1976 as a guest lecturer at the University of Paris.[112]

[107] Ellenberger, *A la découverte de l'inconscient*.

[108] M. Eck, *La nouvelle presse médicale*, 4 (June 14, 1975), 1817–22; S. Giudicelli, *L'encéphale*, n.s., 2 (1976), 187–88; Édouard Desjardins, *L'union médicale du Canada*, 54 (1975), 995–98; Jacques Dufresne, *Le devoir* (May 17, 1975), 32–36; and M. Schachter, *Annales médico-psychologiques* (1974), 354–55. See also the reviews of the earlier American and German editions of the book by Ey, *L'évolution psychiatrique*, 47 (1972), 227–70; Henri Vermorel, *L'information psychiatrique*, 47 (1971), 366–69; and Herbert Schaffer, *Annales de psychothérapie*, 3 (1972), 98–101.

[109] Gilbert Meyrat, "La capitale histoire de la psychiatrie du Suisse Ellenberger, parue aux États-Unis en 1970, enfin publiée en français!" *Journal de Genève* (July 5, 1975), "Samedi Littéraire," 3; and "I.S.," "Du sorcier au psychiatre: De l'exorcisme aux psychologies modernes," *Forum*, 4 (September 15, 1969), 4–5.

[110] "Freud en perspective," interview by Jacques Mousseau in *Psychologie*, 27 (1972), 35–42; interview in *L'express* (March 23–April 6, 1975); interview by Fernand Lot in *L'éducation* (May 1, 1975), 34–38; and interview by Gilbert Tarrab in *La presse* (May 24, 1975), E18-E20.

[111] "Un certain regard," December 16, 1972, Télévision ORTF.

[112] From mid-October to mid-January of 1975–1976, Ellenberger served as associate professor of psychopathology at the Laboratoire de Psychologie Pathologique de la Sorbonne of the University of Paris V (René Descartes). He lectured on the general history of dynamic

Nevertheless, despite this enthusiastic response among readers in France and elsewhere to the appearance of Ellenberger's book, the formal professional recognition that Ellenberger garnered from writing his history of psychiatry proved in the long run remarkably slight. In point of fact, soon after publication of *The Discovery of the Unconscious* Ellenberger began a process of withdrawal from public view that increased after his retirement in 1977 and that has continued until the present. Since the mid-1970s, Ellenberger has for all intents and purposes disappeared from sight, and, as mentioned in the Preface to this book, many people today have the impression that he is no longer alive. It is only a slight exaggeration to say that in the early 1970s Ellenberger was widely hailed as the leading historian of psychiatry who had produced a major, masterful contribution to the field—and was then effectively forgotten.

The reasons for this neglect are numerous and quite interesting. There is first the rather unorthodox course of the author's career. Ellenberger's movements during his lifetime, from South Africa to France to Switzerland to America and finally to English- and then French-speaking Canada, brought to him many cultural and linguistic advantages. But these peregrinations proved a hindrance to the professional aspects of his career, making it difficult for him to establish a secure and powerful institutional base of operation in any one location. In a similar way, over the years Ellenberger worked in a diversity of fields—including hospital neuropsychiatry, asylum administration, private-practice psychiatry, university psychiatric teaching, independent historical research, and academic criminology; this added to the difficulty in distinguishing himself in any one area.

Furthermore, in none of the professional positions that Ellenberger held throughout his career was he able properly to pursue his historical interests as a central activity. This seems particularly to have been a problem in Canada, where Ellenberger's professional peers were comparatively unappreciative of *The Discovery of the Unconscious*. Both at McGill University and the University of Montreal, his practical-minded colleagues remember Ellenberger as a quiet, gentle, even self-effacing man, who had strong but eccentric and somewhat irrelevant scholarly interests. Tragically, at no point in his career after leaving the Menninger Clinic (with the exception of the sabbatical term in Paris) has Ellenberger been able to teach the history of psychiatry. At no time has he supervised students conducting advanced research in psychiatric history. Even after 1970, he received few invitations to speak to medical or historical groups within Canada, and the conditions

psychiatry, taught a seminar on transcultural psychiatry, and provided medical consultations at the university psychiatric clinic of the Sainte Anne asylum.

of his appointment at the University of Montreal remained unaltered. More in frustration than anger, he recalls today that his requests for sabbatical leave to pursue new historical projects were again rejected.[113]

Other factors played a part as well. Within the field of psychological medicine, Ellenberger published extensively for over thirty years. However, his medical bibliography, which lists some 120 publications, lacks a center of gravity. Ellenberger wrote on topics ranging from child psychiatry to geriatric psychiatry, on nearly all of the major diagnostic categories of neurosis and psychosis, and in medical periodicals in Canada, America, and Europe. But there was no area in which he was perceived by his contemporaries as having made a decisive scientific contribution, a fact that perhaps made it easier for medical readers to overlook his historical work.[114] In the end, Ellenberger emerges as a scholar and an intellectual in an older European mold, who took a highly humanistic approach to the study of medicine, quietly resisting the demands for specialization and resenting (but conforming to) the imperative of the contemporary medical profession to publish or perish.

Moreover, a number of potential audiences for Ellenberger's work were for different reasons disinclined to pursue the path he set out so brilliantly in *The Discovery of the Unconscious*. Many members of the American psychoanalytic community, for instance, which in 1970 constituted a large and powerful sector within American psychiatry, disapproved of Ellenberger's book. (In manuscript form, the work had been rejected by three American publishing houses before finding harbor at Basic; Ellenberger attributes this rejection to his critical handling of certain psychoanalytic issues.) Not unnaturally, then, these readers had little interest in granting Ellenberger more attention than necessary. In a related development, *The Discovery of the Unconscious* appeared at a time when in other medical quarters a more biological perspective was emerging within North Ameri-

---

[113] To appreciate Ellenberger's circumstances at this point, we might contrast them with the careers of other major historians of psychiatry of his generation, such as Ackerknecht, George Rosen, and Jean Starobinski. In their later years, these men were (or are) fully integrated into their respective professional communities and received many academic honors and professional distinctions.

[114] This characterization of his medical writings should be contrasted with Ellenberger's historical and criminological work. Ellenberger is regarded today as an early leading figure in the study of the psychiatric aspects of criminology and a founding figure of the subdiscipline of victimology. See in particular his pioneering essay "Psychologishe Beziehungen zwischen Verbrecher und Opfer," *Zeitschrift für Psychotherapie und medizinische Psychologie*, 4 (1954), 261–80, subsequently reprinted as "Psychological Relationships between Criminal and Victim," *Archives of Criminal Psychodynamics*, 1 (1955), 257–90. In 1970, Ellenberger was awarded the Beccaria Prize by the German Society of Criminology, the highest international distinction in the field, and in May 1977 he was appointed professor emeritus at the University of Montreal specifically for his work in Canadian criminology.

can psychiatry. In Montreal in particular, where the prestigious Neurological Institute of McGill University was prominent, a neuropsychiatric approach to the mental sciences dominated. To many younger psychiatrists who might otherwise have drawn inspiration from his work, Ellenberger's preoccupation with dynamic psychiatry and with nonconscious models of cerebration may have appeared inadequate or old-fashioned. Generally speaking, Ellenberger's unwillingness to align himself with any single ideological orientation of his time, either within the medical world or within the academy, provided the crucial, critical distance for his history-writing, and it is unlikely that without this intellectual independence he would have written the type of book that he did. However, this strategy was not without its professional liabilities.

Still further, I believe there existed a connection between the reception of Ellenberger's writings in the 1970s and a number of ideological and methodological debates and developments during that decade. Professional historians of psychiatry praised Ellenberger's book more generously than any group of readers and were probably in the best position to appreciate the nature of his achievement. But *The Discovery of the Unconscious* was published at the peak of the controversies in Europe and North America over antipsychiatry. Many of the major antipsychiatric critiques of this period focused on the nature and validity of the mental hospital as a medical institution. In Britain and the United States, the movement was also linked to the dramatic process of "decarceration," or the moving of large numbers of previously hospitalized mental patients to so-called community health care centers. In addition, within professional historical studies the 1970s witnessed a turning away from traditional cultural and intellectual history and the rise of the "new social history." The combined historiographical effect of these developments was to rivet the attention of psychiatric historians for nearly a generation on the purely social and institutional aspects of psychiatry's past, subjects about which Ellenberger has had comparatively little to say. During the late 1960s and 1970s, the most absorbing debate within the field centered around "the birth of the asylum," and the most important writings of the period came from critics and historians such as Michel Foucault, Robert Castel, and Klaus Doerner in Europe, and Gerald Grob, David Rothman, and Andrew Scull in the United States. In contrast, the range of theoretical, cultural, and clinical aspects of psychiatry that Ellenberger addressed appeared at the time less interesting and urgent.

Finally, fate has played a not inconsiderable role in Ellenberger's later professional biography. In the spring of 1977, Ellenberger retired. Aged 72, he now intended quickly to gather and publish his miscellaneous historical papers and then to return to his old, original fascination with comparative cultural anthropology. Over the previous two decades, while engaged in historical research, he had continued to compile materials in this field, and during his final two years at the University of Montreal he had taught seminars on transcultural psychiatry. Freed now, at last, of his laborious academic duties, Ellenberger planned a major synthetic study—to be tentatively entitled *Études ethnopsychiatriques*—which would encompass the descriptive and theoretical aspects of the subject. However, four months after his retirement, Ellenberger was cruelly struck with the first signs of Parkinson's disease. The disorder progressed rapidly, and Ellenberger experienced a dramatic and depressing diminution of his physical and mental energies. By the late 1970s, he was unable to do sustained intellectual work. His final historical article based on original research dates from 1978, and his medical and criminological publications slowed to a trickle. He took his final trip to Europe in the summer of 1981.[115]

Among the casualties of this unhappy confluence of circumstances have been Ellenberger's historical essays. Between 1950 and the present, Ellenberger has written thirty-six essays of a historical nature (see Appendix C). Twenty of these essays appeared before 1970, and the other sixteen were written after publication of *The Discovery of the Unconscious*. The large majority of these essays first appeared in published form soon after they were written, in local French, Swiss, American, or Canadian medical, historical, or literary periodicals. Two essays (a study of psychiatric motifs in German literature and of the history of pre-Rorschachian visual testing techniques) were never published and exist today only in typescript. A number of the writings from the 1950s and 1960s were incorporated into *The Discovery of the Unconscious*, and four of the thirty-six take the form of article-length book reviews. Some of the essays are short and rather inconsequential statements—*écrits de circonstances*, Ellenberger calls them. Most of them, however, represent substantial pieces of scholarship based on extensive reading in the original sources and dealing with new and important subjects. Many exhibit the same outstanding qualities that characterize *The Discovery of the Unconscious*. All of them focus on European psychiatric history in the post-Enlightenment period.

The fourteen essays reprinted in this volume differ significantly in intellectual style and content. Several of them, such as the articles on Rorschach and Gustav Fechner, are polished scholarly performances. Other essays are primarily thought pieces, suggestive gatherings of ideas and sources awaiting further exploration. Still others serve as arguments that attempt to contribute to contemporary scholarly controversies, and one—"Pierre Janet, philosophe"—is a work of bibliographical reference. *The Discovery*

---

[115] Ellenberger, however, retains his acute powers of observation and his intellectual curiosity. See his most recent medical article, "Regards sur les institutions pour vieillards et malades chroniques," *L'union médicale du Canada*, 116 (1987), 195–200, a piece that is partly autobiographical.

of the Unconscious remains Ellenberger's magnum opus, a single, encyclopedic work coordinating a lifetime of reading. But the historical essays as a whole are of equal significance and, together with the big book, establish Ellenberger's place in the historiography of European psychiatry. Considering the nature of these writings, a point-by-point summation of their contents, as was given for *The Discovery of the Unconscious*, is inappropriate. However, a close reading of Ellenberger's essays reveals a series of themes, eight in total, that may be reviewed with profit.

The Swiss Contribution to the History of Psychiatry

When Ellenberger began writing historically in the 1950s, standard accounts of the history of psychiatry centered on events in Germany, Austria, France, Britain, and the United States. To a large extent, this remains true today. Ellenberger was deeply read in the psychiatric literatures of these countries; but in all of his work, medical and historical, he evinces a great interest in and familiarity with the work of physicians from countries that have traditionally been less well known, including the Netherlands, Belgium, Spain, Italy, and the Scandinavian countries. These countries, too, he demonstrates time and again, played decisive roles in the history of the psychological sciences. Given his personal and professional background, it is scarcely surprising that Ellenberger was particularly well informed about the Swiss contribution to psychiatry's history. In existing history books, he found that Swiss psychiatric theory and practice was routinely ignored or absorbed into French and German psychiatry. During the 1950s, he was further chagrined to encounter the vulgar American stereotype that the culture of Switzerland had produced over the years little more than chocolates and cuckoo clocks. As a result, Ellenberger was continually at pains in his writings to highlight the major figures, theories, texts, and institutions in what he regarded as a very substantial and distinctly Swiss psychiatric tradition.

Ellenberger's first historical publication consisted of a group of eight articles in which he detailed the history of psychiatry and psychology in Switzerland from the late nineteenth to the mid-twentieth centuries. These essays first appeared serially, between 1951 and 1953, in the French journal *L'évolution psychiatrique* and were later published as a monograph under the title *La psychiatrie suisse*.[116] It is an impressive little work of

---

[116] "La psychiatrie suisse," *L'évolution psychiatrique* (1951), 321–54, 619–44; (1952), 139–58, 369–79, 593–606; (1953), 298–319, 719–51; *La psychiatrie suisse* (Paris, Imprimerie Poirier-Bottreau, [1954]). As a monograph, this work is paginated nonconsecutively, as it appeared in its original periodical form.

which, unfortunately, only fifty copies were printed, and which remains today almost entirely unknown.

In *La psychiatrie suisse*, Ellenberger notes that for a long time Switzerland served as a kind of intellectual colony of German medicine. Through most of the nineteenth century, appointments to the major Swiss university medical faculties were invariably filled by German physicians. However, beginning with the work of Auguste Forel in the 1880s, Ellenberger shows, independent Swiss schools of psychology and psychiatry developed rapidly at numerous locations in the country and made original and durable contributions to the psychological sciences. Likening Switzerland in the twentieth century to Holland in the seventeenth, Ellenberger argues that the contributions of Swiss theoreticians and practitioners to the general psychological culture of the twentieth century have been exceptionally rich, greatly out of proportion to the political and geographical identity of the country. Ellenberger goes on in *La psychiatrie suisse* to review no fewer than six hundred texts, many written by unknown but significant Swiss figures who worked in every conceivable branch of psychological medicine from asylum psychiatry and psychoanalysis to child psychiatry and industrial job counseling. In Ellenberger's view, there exists no single school or theoretical program to Swiss psychology and psychiatry; but Swiss theory and practice since the late nineteenth century have tended to assume a broad humanistic approach, to favor psychological over organic approaches to the study of the mind, to encourage close and highly individualized doctor-patient relations, and to develop creative linkages with religion, philosophy, and pedagogy. One innovation of *La psychiatrie suisse* can be found in the second section of the work, in which Ellenberger portrays the unique, decentralized cantonal asylum system in the country.[117]

Ellenberger is fond of this early study and was disappointed that it failed to reach a larger audience. Therefore, in 1957, while at the Menninger Clinic, he wrote a shorter, compact survey of the subject. In "The Scope of Swiss Psychology," reproduced below, Ellenberger reviews the distinctive psychological and psychiatric traditions of Basel, Geneva, and Zurich, the three loci of activity in the Swiss psychological sciences.[118] Specifically, he discusses the classic asylum psychiatry of Forel and Bleuler as it developed at the Burghölzli after 1880; the Genevan traditions of experimental psychology, educational psychology, and parapsychology that emerged during the 1890s in the work of Théodore Flournoy, Édouard Claparède, Pierre Bovet, and Jean Piaget; and the so-called Swiss school of psychoanalysis that flourished between 1906 and 1913 in the work of Bleuler,

---

[117] "La psychiatrie suisse," 332–54.
[118] Ellenberger, "The Scope of Swiss Psychology," in Henry P. David and Helmut von Bracken, eds., *Perspectives in Personality Theory* (New York, Basic Books, 1957), 44–64.

Jung, Maeder, Pfister, Binswanger, and others. He also examines Jung's Analytical Psychology, the existential and phenomenological psychiatries of Ludwig Binswanger and Eugène Minkowski, and Rorschach's and Ludwig Klages's theories of characterology and graphology. From his years in Schaffhausen in the 1940s and 1950s, Ellenberger had an intimate knowledge of the writings of these figures as well as a personal acquaintance with many of them.

In other writings, Ellenberger focuses on individual Swiss authors or movements. His writings about Jung, for instance, should be viewed in part in this mildly nationalistic context. Jung was the best known of Swiss psychological authors and the only one who could boast international recognition and an extensive following outside the country. Accordingly, Ellenberger seized every opportunity to discuss Jung's work. He features Jung prominently in *La psychiatrie suisse* and "The Scope of Swiss Psychiatry,"[119] and in *The Discovery of the Unconscious*, we have seen, he treats Jung fully and sympathetically. In addition, he produced a perceptive critique of Jung's 1962 autobiographical memoir.[120] In 1978, Ellenberger published new biographical information about Jung's early years in Basel.[121] And in 1991, he revisited the case of Helene Preiswerk, Jung's clairvoyant medium–cousin who served as the subject of his medical dissertation. In this last essay, Ellenberger, drawing on several new primary sources including unpublished letters written in 1901 to 1902 between Jung and his college friend Andreas Vischer, relates in greater detail than before available the medical and biographical narrative of this case, which was so formative for Jung's psychological thought.[122]

A second figure in Swiss medicine that Ellenberger has studied closely is Rorschach, the subject of his most ambitious scholarly essay. As mentioned before, Ellenberger was surprised to find when he came to the United States a strong interest in the Rorschach inkblot test combined with an almost complete lack of familiarity with any other aspects of Rorschach's work. Ellenberger sought to rectify this situation in "The Life and Work of Hermann Rorschach (1884–1922)," a fifty-page study published in the autumn of 1954 in the *Bulletin of the Menninger Clinic*.[123]

Rorschach was born and brought up in Schaffhausen, received his psychiatric training at the Burghölzli from 1906 to 1909, and then worked as *Oberarzt* at a number of cantonal mental hospitals. Ellenberger was, there-

---

[119] *La psychiatrie suisse*, 151–58; "Scope of Swiss Psychology," 52–54.

[120] Ellenberger, "L'autobiographie de C. G. Jung." See also his review of the first volume of Jung's letters in *Journal of the History of the Behavioral Sciences*, 11 (1975), 96–97.

[121] Ellenberger, "Carl Gustav Jung: His Historical Setting," in Hertha Riese, ed., *Historical Explorations in Medicine and Psychiatry* (New York, Springer, 1978), 142–49.

[122] Ellenberger, "The Story of Helene Preiswerk: A Critical Study with New Documents," *History of Psychiatry*, 2, no. 5 (March 1991), 41–52.

[123] Ellenberger, "Life and Work of Hermann Rorschach."

fore, ideally suited to study him. With the type of scholarly industriousness that would become characteristic of him, Ellenberger returned to Switzerland in the summer of 1953 and assembled biographical material about Rorschach. He not only read all of Rorschach's articles and books but examined contemporary reviews of Rorschach's writings, located obituaries of him, and perused his case histories from the archives of the Waldau Hospital. He contacted Rorschach's wife, siblings, former schoolmates, and university comrades as well as colleagues from the Waldau and Münsterlingen asylums. He even located the death certificate and autopsy report for Rorschach, who had died suddenly and mysteriously in 1922 at the age of 37.[124]

In his article, Ellenberger explains that Rorschach at the time of his death had been a rising star in the Swiss psychiatric world. Ellenberger judges him a major scientific intelligence and a profound theorist of human nature whose work consists of much more than the single testing procedure bearing his name today. As a medical student, Rorschach had developed a strong interest in the artistic productions of schizophrenic patients. He later began to study patterned psychological responses to visual and auditory stimuli, which he believed offered a means to study the imagination and the unconscious and to diagnose certain behavioral, neurotic, and psychotic disorders.[125] Rorschach's research culminated in *Psychodiagnostics*, his masterwork, which appeared in 1922, just months before his death. Ellenberger reviews Rorschach's brief, eccentric, fitfully brilliant career, and he offers a detailed and technically recondite discussion of the contents of the *Psychodiagnostics*. He also speculates interestingly on the intellectual and psychobiographical origins of Rorschach's theories. Rorschach's book went largely unappreciated upon publication, but in later years it inspired an interest throughout Swiss psychiatry in visual and verbal psychodiagnostic testing while outside of Switzerland it anticipated German and American Gestalt psychology.[126]

Finally, Ellenberger's interest in phenomenological psychiatry and existential analysis should be noted. For Ellenberger, the most dramatic—and most indigenously European—developments in post–World War II psychology and psychiatry were not organic psychiatry or psychoanalytic ego psychology but phenomenological psychiatry and existential analysis. These two movements, which sought to reconstruct the lived subjective mental world of the suffering individual, brought a new sensibility to the practice of psychotherapy, Ellenberger believed. The philosophical foundations of phenomenological psychiatry and existential analysis derived from

[124] Ibid., 174–90.

[125] For the historical background to Rorschach's ideas on these matters, refer to Ellenberger, "From Justinus Kerner to Hermann Rorschach: The History of the Inkblots" (Lecture delivered at the Institut des Hautes Études de Bruxelles, January 9, 1976).

[126] Ellenberger, "Life and Work of Hermann Rorschach," 195–213.

Jaspers, Husserl, and Heidegger. But the key figures in the medical elaboration of their ideas were Eugène Minkowski, who had trained in Zurich under Bleuler and maintained many professional Swiss associations in Switzerland, and Ludwig Binswanger, another Bleuler progeny and a member of a distinguished Swiss-German medical family that for generations directed a private sanatorium in Switzerland. Both men were personal friends of Ellenberger. Not surprisingly, Ellenberger often comments in his historical writings on the work of Minkowski, Binswanger, and their followers.[127] In many publications, he argues for the psychotherapeutic significance of phenomenology and existentialism.[128] Most significantly, Ellenberger was instrumental in assembling an excellent anthology of writings in English translation by the major Continental theorists of these movements. Published in 1958 under the title *Existence*, this collection includes a dense, intelligent, and philosophically literate chapter by Ellenberger analyzing psychiatric phenomenology and existential analysis.[129] In concert with Rollo May, Ellenberger served as a conduit for the transmission of these two important central European movements into the United States, and many American and Canadian psychiatrists still associate him preeminently with his work in this area.[130]

The Importance of Pierre Janet

It was one of Ellenberger's most significant historical insights that the Paris and Nancy schools of psychology in the later half of the nineteenth century (i.e., the writings of Azam, Richet, Liébeault, Binet, Féré, Charcot, Luys, Dumontpallier, Bourru, Bernheim, Beaunis, and their followers) were fully

---

[127] *La psychiatrie suisse*, 308–11, 374–79; "Scope of Swiss Psychology," 55–56; *Discovery of the Unconscious*, 842, 843, 850, 853, 855, 863–65.

[128] Ellenberger, "Das menschliche Schicksal als wissenschaftliches Problem," *Psyche*, 4 (1950–1951), 576–610; "Analyse existentielle," *Encyclopédie médico-chirurgicale*, vol. 3, 37815 A 10, pp. 1–4; "Phenomenology and Existential Analysis," *Canadian Psychiatric Association Journal*, 2 (1957), 137–46; "The Psychology of Destiny," *Forum*, 3 (1959), 48–55; "L'existentialisme et son intérêt pour la psychiatrie," *L'union médicale du Canada*, 90 (1961), 939–47; "La psychopathologie d'Eugène Minkowski," *Dialogue: Canadian Philosophical Review/Revue philosophique canadienne*, 9 (1970), 93–100. See also Ellenberger, "Herméneutique et Psychanalyse: A propos du livre de M. Paul Ricoeur," *Dialogue: Canadian Philosophical Review/Revue philosophique canadienne*, 5 (1966), 256–66.

[129] Ellenberger, "A Clinical Introduction to Psychiatric Phenomenology and Existential Analysis," in Rollo May, Ernest Angel, and Henri F. Ellenberger, eds., *Existence: A New Dimension in Psychiatry and Psychology* (New York, Basic Books, 1958), 92–124.

[130] In *Phenomenology in Psychology and Psychiatry: A Historical Introduction* (Evanston, Ill., Northwestern University Press, 1972), Herbert Spiegelberg characterizes publication of *Existence* in 1958 as "the chief milestone in the development of American phenomenological and existential psychology" (p. 143). See Spiegelberg's further analysis of Ellenberger's book on pp. 163–64.

as important as the Vienna and Zurich schools. Throughout his writings, he strove to bring the main figures and writings of the French movement to attention. Most important in this regard was his work on Janet. Ellenberger's first piece of medical writing on one of the four major figures in *The Discovery of the Unconscious* was an essay on Janet's psychotherapeutic theories that appeared in 1950, just three years after Janet's death, in a commemorative volume of *L'évolution psychiatrique*.[131]

As we learned earlier, Ellenberger believed that Janet was a theorist of the first rank. His 1950 essay reveals that he formed this assessment very early in his career. By this date, Ellenberger had already come to the belief that a strong but subterranean Janetian current ran throughout twentieth-century dynamic psychiatry. He also followed many Frenchmen of his time in asserting that a portion of what Freud received credit for had previously been enunciated by Janet. Furthermore, from his years of medical education in Paris he knew that some of the most distinguished psychiatrists in France at mid-century, such as Ey, Baruk, and Delay, acknowledged the essential importance of Janet for their work. During the first half of his career, Janet had been seen throughout Europe and America as among the most important figures in medical psychology; but beginning around 1910, his work fell rapidly into eclipse. Moreover, Ellenberger observes that Janet, unlike Freud, Jung, and Adler, formed no school of followers to perpetuate his theories or to write commemorative biographies about him. As a result, Janet, to Ellenberger's continual astonishment, was often excluded almost entirely from historical accounts of psychiatry.[132]

To his regret, Ellenberger never met Janet personally during the 1930s when both men lived in Paris. Rather, he seems to have been introduced to Janet's *oeuvre* by one Leonhard Schwartz, a neuropsychiatrist in Basel. Swiss by birth, Schwartz had trained in Paris, where he befriended Janet and over time became a passionate devotee of Janet's psychotherapeutic ideas. During the 1940s, Schwartz worked toward a major study of Janet's thought, designed to bring Janet's psychological system to German-language audiences, where it was little known. The project, however, was cut short by Schwartz's death in 1948.[133] It was Schwartz, whom Ellen-

[131] Ellenberger, "La psychothérapie de Janet," *L'évolution psychiatrique*, special issue in commemoration of Pierre Janet, 15, no. 3 (July–September 1950), 465–84.

[132] For example, in Zilboorg's *History of Medical Psychology*, Janet's work is discussed on two pages (pp. 375–77). In the *History of Psychiatry* by Alexander and Selesnick, it receives two paragraphs (p. 173). In Wyss's *Depth Psychology*, Janet is dealt with in four sentences (pp. 52, 54, 329, 339), and in Leibbrand and Wettley's 670-page *Der Wahnsinn*, he gets one sentence (p. 173). Somewhat more satisfactory coverage is provided in Ackerknecht, *Short History of Psychiatry*, 78–80, and Harms, *Origins of Modern Psychiatry*, chap. 23.

[133] Schwartz's notes were later organized by his colleagues and published under the title *Die Neurosen und die dynamische Psychologie von Pierre Janet* (Basel, Benno Schwabe, 1951). A French translation of the book appeared in 1955.

berger met in Basel, who ignited in him "la flamme janétienne,"[134] and to an extent Ellenberger saw himself as continuing Schwartz's mission.[135]

Working virtually alone among psychiatric historians, Ellenberger attempted to rehabilitate Janet in a number of ways. He sought out Janet's daughters in Paris. He gained access to Janet's rich, voluminous private library, and he collected the complete corpus of Janet's writings. In "La psychothérapie de Janet," Ellenberger explored the therapeutic applications of Janet's theories. In *The Discovery of the Unconscious*, Janet is the first of the four main figures discussed, and it is unlikely that this placement is accidental. As we have seen, this chapter offers a detailed capsule biography of Janet as well as the first full exposition of Janet's lifework. Many reviewers of the book praised Ellenberger specifically for his rediscovery of Janet. In France, an excerpt of the chapter was printed separately before translation of the book as a whole,[136] and for a decade and a half, Ellenberger's chapter served as the most thorough presentation of Janet's life and work in any language.

In addition, one of Ellenberger's last historical essays was a short, suggestive study of Janet and the American psychological community.[137] From 1895 to 1910, Ellenberger shows here, American psychologists and psychiatrists followed Janet's work more closely than that of any European author. Ellenberger discusses Janet's six extended trips to the United States, his honorary degrees from American universities, the American editions of his books, and his scientific friendships with William James, Morton Prince, Stanley Hall, James Mark Baldwin, Adolf Meyer, and George Herbert Mead. He also demonstrates that the intellectual association between Janet and his American contemporaries ran in both directions, Janet being perhaps the first major European psychologist to learn extensively from the Americans. Ellenberger highlights in particular the significance of Janet for the Boston psychotherapeutic community.

In the present volume, Ellenberger's campaign on behalf of Janet is represented by "Pierre Janet, Philosopher," a meticulously detailed bibliography of Janet's writings.[138] At the end of his chapter on Janet in *The*

---

[134] Ellenberger, "Journal de voyage," entry for October 7, 1975.

[135] See Ellenberger's necrological notice about Schwartz in *L'évolution psychiatrique*, special issue in commemoration of Pierre Janet, 15, no. 3 (July–September 1950), 483, as well as his review of Schwartz's book in *Schweizerische Zeitschrift für Revue suisse de Psychologie*, 10 (1951), 260–61.

[136] Ellenberger, "Pierre Janet et 'La découverte de l'inconscient,'" *Annales de psychothérapie*, 4 (1973), 7–12.

[137] Ellenberger, "Pierre Janet and His American Friends" [1973], in George E. Gifford, Jr., ed., *Psychoanalysis, Psychotherapy and the New England Medical Scene, 1894–1944* (New York, Science History Publication, 1978), 63–72.

[138] Ellenberger, "Pierre Janet, philosophe," *Dialogue: Canadian Philosophical Review/Revue philosophique canadienne*, 12, no. 2 (June 1973), 254–87.

Discovery of the Unconscious, Ellenberger casts forward hopefully to a future revival of interest in Janet's work. However, he believed that for such a revival to occur, a full and accurate record of Janet's complete writings, many of which were unknown and widely scattered, was a desideratum. Ellenberger was especially concerned that the only publications of Janet that were familiar to physicians and historians were the clinical writings on hysteria from the 1890s. By providing a comprehensive bibliography, he hoped to underscore Janet's overall intellectual itinerary. In his introductory comments to the bibliography, Ellenberger also emphasizes Janet's pre-1890s writings, which he believes are important to understanding the philosophical underpinnings of the Janetian psychological system. Inexplicably, this article remains unknown today even to many Janet specialists.

The Intellectual Origins of Psychoanalysis

In the 1950s, when Ellenberger began contemplating psychiatric history, the literature on Freud was already very large. But the great majority of this writing consisted of interpretive and explicative commentary about psychoanalytic theory. What Ellenberger believed was badly needed at this stage was additional historical data about Freud and the world from which he had emerged and in which he had worked. In particular, Ellenberger was convinced that psychoanalytic theory had not emerged *ex nihilo* as many commentators suggested but rather was deeply implicated in Western cultural processes extending back over generations. Consequently, Ellenberger developed a strong interest in reconstructing the rich and complex intellectual universe around Freud, especially the young Freud.[139]

---

[139] In this endeavor, Ellenberger had several predecessors. See Maria Dorer, *Historische Grundlagen der Psychoanalyse* (Leipzig, Felix Meiner, 1932), especially pp. 71–106; Siegfried Bernfeld, "Freud's Earliest Theories and the School of Helmholtz," *Psychoanalytic Quarterly*, 13 (1944), 341–62; Ernest Jones, *The Life and Work of Sigmund Freud*, vol. 1, *The Formative Years and the Great Discoveries, 1856–1900* (New York: Basic Books, 1953), chaps. 4, 5, 10; Walther Riese, "The Pre-Freudian Origins of Psychoanalysis," in Jules Masserman, ed., *Science and Psychoanalysis* (New York: Grune and Stratton, 1958), 1:29–72; Ola Andersson, *Studies in the Prehistory of Psychoanalysis* (Stockholm, Norstedts, 1962); Juan Dalma, "La catarsis en Aristóteles, Bernays y Freud," *Revista de psiquiatría y psicología médica de Europa y América Latinas*, 6 (1963), 253–69; Paul Cranefield, "The Organic Physics of 1847 and the Biophysics of Today," *Journal of the History of Medicine and Allied Sciences*, 12 (1957), 407–23; and idem, "Freud and the 'School of Helmholtz,'" *Gesnerus*, 23 (1966), 35–39. Ellenberger knew the writings of these early Freud researchers well. See, for instance, his highly appreciative reviews of Andersson in *Journal of the History of the Behavioral Sciences*, 2 (1966), 98–100, as well as of Peter Amacher's *Freud's Neurological Education and Its Influence on Psychoanalytic Theory*, in *Journal of the History of the Behavioral Sciences*, 3 (1967), 100–103.

Ellenberger's interest in the intellectual, cultural, and scientific origins of psychoanalysis is most in evidence in *The Discovery of the Unconscious*. Indeed, on one level his entire book may be read as a massive contextualization of Freud's work.

In two of his historical essays, Ellenberger continues this line of research by investigating individual figures in the history of the nineteenth-century German-language sciences that exercised formative intellectual influences on Freud. Gustav Theodor Fechner (1801–1887) is widely known today as a founding figure of modern experimental psychology; Fechner's influence on Freud, however, is less familiar.[140] In 1956, Ellenberger wrote a short, straightforward study in science history exploring Fechner's place in the history of psychoanalysis.[141] After summarizing Fechner's biography, Ellenberger offers an analysis of his major work, the *Elements of Psychophysics* of 1860. It is a bizarre book, Ellenberger concedes, in which Fechner attempts to bridge the speculative mysticism of the Romantics and the new materialism of German physics and biology. We learn in Ellenberger's essay that it was essentially Fechner who imported the Helmholtzian biophysics of the mid-nineteenth century into the German mental sciences of the 1880s and 1890s. In a close, comparative reading of Fechner and Freud, Ellenberger specifies four themes in *Elements of Psychophysics* that were relevant for the constitution of psychoanalytic theory. These are the concept of mental energetics, including the notion of psychological constancy; a spatial or "topographical" model of the mind; the principle of pleasure and unpleasure in psychological functioning; and a theory of the repetition compulsion. Ellenberger then traces the creative transformations of these Fechnerian ideas through Freud's later work.[142]

In 1973, Ellenberger studied Freud and a second, lesser-known figure.[143] During the 1880s and 1890s, Moritz Benedikt was an associate professor of neuropathology at the University of Vienna and the director of outpatient services at the university clinic there. Ernest Jones's biography scarcely mentioned Benedikt. However, in his reading for the Freud chapter of *The Discovery of the Unconscious*, Ellenberger had noticed a footnote in the "Preliminary Communication" of 1893 in which Breuer and Freud commented, "We have found the nearest approach to what we have to say on the theoretical and therapeutic sides of the question [of hysteria]

---

[140] See the scattered remarks on Fechner in Jones, *Life and Work of Sigmund Freud* (1953), 1:374; vol. 3, *The Last Phase, 1919–1939* (1957), 258, 268, 305.

[141] Ellenberger, "Fechner and Freud," *Bulletin of the Menninger Clinic*, 20, no. 4 (July 1956), 201–14.

[142] See also Ellenberger, *Discovery of the Unconscious*, 215–18, 312–13, 479, 512–14, 542.

[143] Ellenberger, "Moritz Benedikt (1835–1920)," *Confrontations psychiatriques*, 11 (1973), 183–200.

in some remarks, published from time to time, by Benedikt."[144] Upon inquiries among his European contacts, Ellenberger found that Erna Lesky, director of the Institute of the History of Medicine in Vienna, shared his intuition about Benedikt's importance for Freud. Ellenberger traveled to Vienna and, using the excellent collection of Benedikt's writings at the Medical History Institute there, explored the subject.

Ellenberger finds that from the mid-1860s to the early 1890s, Benedikt published a number of statements about the etiology of hysteria and other neurotic disorders based on his observations of nervous and neurological patients at the Vienna clinic and that the contents of these writings are strikingly modern. At a time when hereditarian theories of nervous illness prevailed, and neurological and gynecological theories of hysteria were accepted unanimously, Benedikt argued for the psychogenesis of these disorders. In particular, he stressed the pathogenic role of repressed ambition, thwarted love, and functional sexual disturbances. Discussing sexual factors in the genesis of neurotic disorders, Benedikt repeatedly employed the term *libido*. And fully a decade before Charcot's work on the topic, Benedikt contended that males were as susceptible to hysterical disorders as females. Moreover, Benedikt developed with apparent success a number of short-term, nonhypnotic verbal psychotherapies to treat hysterical patients. Foremost among these techniques, Ellenberger finds, was the confession or catharsis-like release of concealed emotional and sexual secrets. In their clinical observations, causal explanations, and therapeutic prescriptions, Ellenberger concludes, no medical texts, including those of Janet, are closer to the *Studies on Hysteria* than Benedikt's writings. The psychological theories of Benedikt appeared over a thirty-year period and were scattered in unorthodox locations while Benedikt personally was despised by his colleagues because of his personal belligerence. As a result, his ideas failed to receive prominence in his own time. Ellenberger, however, makes a documented case for Benedikt as one of the most original scientific intellectuals of the late nineteenth century and a powerful, if unknown, influence on Freud.[145]

Revisionist Psychoanalytic History

It is characteristic of Ellenberger that he always refrained from direct polemics with other historians. However, in an interview in the French maga-

---

[144] Breuer and Freud, *Studies on Hysteria*, in *The Standard Edition of the Complete Psychological Works of Sigmund Freud*, translated from the German under the general editorship of James Strachey, 24 vols. (London, Hogarth Press, 1953–1974), 2:7 n. 3.

[145] Ellenberger also notes that Adler studied under Benedikt at the Vienna Polyclinic during the late 1890s and adds that "on comprendra mieux la psychothérapie d'Adler si on la

zine *Psychologie* in April 1972, Ellenberger revealed rather pointedly that his thinking and writing about Freud had been strongly influenced by the publication of Ernest Jones's three-volume biography during the 1950s.[146] The appearance of Jones's study corresponded chronologically exactly with Ellenberger's coming to America and the formation of his first ideas about psychiatric history. Ellenberger knew Jones slightly, found him personally agreeable, and acknowledged that his biography united invaluably a collection of primary materials about Freud. At the same time, many of Jones's interpretations did not square with Ellenberger's understanding of psychoanalytic history.

In particular, Jones in his first volume presented Freud's early psychoanalytic works as being received by the European medical community with either deafening silence or overt opposition. However, according to personal conversations Ellenberger remembered with members of the early Swiss psychoanalytic circle, and in particular with Oskar Pfister and Alphonse Maeder, this had not been true. In the summer of 1954, then, while in Europe, Ellenberger randomly selected one historical episode out of Jones's first volume—the contemporary reception of *The Interpretation of Dreams* in the medical and lay presses—and searched up as much documentation for this event as possible. Soberingly, Ellenberger states, he found that "80 percent" of Jones's facts about the subject were either "completely false or greatly exaggerated." "This incident was the starting point of my critical attitude [toward existing accounts of psychoanalytic history]."[147]

Ellenberger was not entirely alone at this time in responding skeptically to Jones's work and attempting to test it factually. In the late 1940s and early 1950s, Siegfried and Suzanne Bernfeld had conducted research on Freud's medical education and early professional activities and had compared their results to earlier "official" accounts of Freud's life.[148] Josef and Renée Gicklhorn had made important discoveries in the Vienna archives concerning Freud's academic career.[149] And Ilse Bry and Alfred Rifkin had

---

considère comme perfectionnement de la psychothérapie de Benedikt plutôt qu'une déformation de la psychanalyse de Freud" (p. 152).

[146] "Freud en perspective: Interview par Jacques Mousseau," *Psychologie*, 27 (1972), 35–43, translated and reprinted as "Freud in Perspective: A Conversation with Henri F. Ellenberger," *Psychology Today*, 6 (March 1973), 50–60.

[147] "Freud in Perspective," 54.

[148] Siegfried Bernfeld, "Freud's Scientific Beginnings," *American Imago*, 6 (1949), 163–96; idem, "Sigmund Freud, M.D., 1882–1885," *International Journal of Psychoanalysis*, 32 (1951), 204–17; Siegfried Bernfeld and Suzanne Cassirer Bernfeld, "Freud's First Year in Practice, 1886–1887," *Bulletin of the Menninger Clinic*, 16 (1952), 37–49.

[149] Josef Gicklhorn and Renée Gicklhorn, *Sigmund Freuds akademische Laufbahn im Lichte der Dokumente* (Vienna and Innsbruck, Urban & Schwarzenberg, 1960).

assembled a large number of reviews of early Freudian texts, which established conclusively that the contemporary reception of these works was varied, complicated, and by no means uniformly critical.[150]

The work of Bernfeld, the Gicklhorns, and Bry and Rifkin was important to Ellenberger; but these writings were specialized, and their message had failed to spread beyond a tiny circle of psychoanalytic historians.[151] Furthermore, during the 1960s a number of publications appeared that reinforced the Jonesian version of events. In 1961, Dieter Wyss, a German psychiatrist, published a lengthy history of dynamic psychiatry. Three years later, Marthe Robert in Paris published a new biographical study of Freud. In 1966, *The History of Psychiatry* by Franz Alexander and Sheldon Selesnick appeared, and in 1967 W. W. Norton reissued Zilboorg's *A History of Medical Psychology*. In addition, between 1959 and 1964, Jones's biography appeared in German, Spanish, and Italian translations and was met each time with acclaim. With the appearance in 1961 of a one-volume English abridgement of the biography, Jones reached a still wider North American and British audience.[152]

Collectively, these writings determined the popular and professional view of the history of psychoanalysis during the 1960s.[153] Without exception, these books were designed around the psychoanalytic historical teleology in which past psychiatric theory and practice were divided into pre- and post-Freudian periods and medical authors were interpreted primarily according to their relation to Freud. They presented Freud heroically, as a lone scientist of the truth who struggled in the first part of his career against ignorance, opposition, and incomprehension and in the second half against a succession of malicious professional enemies. Moreover, they routinely offered a radically decontextualized account of Freud's thinking

[150] Ilse Bry and Alfred H. Rifkin, "Freud and the History of Ideas: Primary Sources, 1886–1910," in Jules Masserman, ed., *Science and Psychoanalysis*, vol. 5, *Psychoanalytic Education* (New York, Grune and Stratton, 1962), 6–36.

[151] To the best of my knowledge, the only explicit general challenge to the Jonesian historiography of psychoanalysis by a historian of psychiatry during the period preceding Ellenberger's book was Harms, *Origins of Modern Psychiatry*, chap. 24.

[152] Dieter Wyss, *Die tiefenpsychologischen Schulen von den Anfängen bis zur Gegenwart* (Göttingen, Vandenhoeck & Ruprecht, 1961); idem, *Depth Psychology*; Marthe Robert, *La révolution psychanalytique* (Paris, Payot, 1964); idem, *The Psychoanalytic Revolution: Sigmund Freud's Life and Achievement*, translated from the French by Kenneth Morgan (London, George Allen and Unwin, 1966); Alexander and Selesnick, *The History of Psychiatry*; Zilboorg, *History of Medical Psychology*; Ernest Jones, *The Life and Work of Sigmund Freud*, edited and abridged by Lionel Trilling and Steven Marcus with an Introduction by Lionel Trilling (New York, Basic Books, 1961).

[153] David S. Werman has shown that the two most widely used texts of psychiatric history in medical schools during this period were Zilboorg and Alexander/Selesnick (Werman, "The Teaching of the History of Psychiatry," *Archives of General Psychiatry*, 26 [1972], 287–89).

in which the greatest part of the scientific and cultural setting out of which psychoanalysis emerged was blotted out.[154]

In retrospect, we can see that Ellenberger worked to revise the Freudian historiography of his day in three ways: by establishing in detail the rich and independent traditions of theorizing about the unconscious mind preceding Freud; by giving Freud's theoretical contemporaries equal space and interpretive weight in the history of psychiatry; and by verifying critically specific historical episodes from Freud's intellectual biography. We have already considered the first two strategies as they appear in *The Discovery of the Unconscious*; Ellenberger pursues the third approach in his historical essays.

In the middle of October 1886, Freud, recently returned from a period of study with Charcot in Paris, delivered a lecture on his experiences abroad to the Vienna Gesellschaft der Ärzte. The topic of his presentation was hysteria in the male. In this lecture, Freud rehearsed the basic Charcotian model of hysteria, including the contentions that hysteria had a neurological rather than genital etiology, that it occurred frequently and in clinically identical ways in both sexes, and that many instances of nervous disorders following physical traumas were hysterical in origin. According to Freud's *Autobiographical Study* (1925), his lecture was received by the conservative senior physicians in Vienna, including a number of his former teachers, with hostility and incomprehension. Members of the audience, Freud wrote, rejected the idea that hysteria, linked anatomically for centuries with the female, could occur in men. Furthermore, they challenged Freud to locate an example of masculine hysteria in one of the Vienna hospitals but then denied him access to their clinical wards to pursue his research. Based on the rude and incredulous response to his ideas, Freud wrote, he withdrew from the Society of Physicians, and gradually from academic medicine in general, thereby beginning the long period of "splendid isolation" of the 1890s during which he made his major psychoanalytic discoveries.[155]

The text of Freud's lecture to the Vienna Society of Physicians has unfortunately been lost. However, in 1968, in the French journal *L'information psychiatrique*, Ellenberger published his own study of this episode based

---

[154] Wyss's study, for instance, literally paints a picture of modern psychiatry without a past. Presenting itself as a general historical account of depth psychology, the book absorbs its subject entirely into the story of Freud and his followers and rivals. In contrast to Ellenberger, Wyss believed that the development of dynamic psychiatry began in 1892, with the publication of Freud's article on a case of successful treatment by hypnosis. The first sentence of *Depth Psychology* reads "Sigmund Freud was born on May 6, 1856, in Freiburg, a small town in Moravia, where his father was a business man."

[155] Freud, *Autobiography*, in *Standard Edition*, 20:15–16.

on extensive research in primary documents.[156] In the article, Ellenberger did the historian's hard work of contextualization. He began by rehearsing the history of the interpretation of this important event. He then studied the nature and development of the Vienna Gesellschaft der Ärzte as a professional organization, the biographical context of Freud's lecture, the state of European medical knowledge about male hysteria in the mid-1880s, and the contemporary controversy among physicians about the genesis of traumatic neurotic disorders. Most importantly, Ellenberger located six stenographical accounts of Freud's lecture in Austrian and German medical periodicals that recorded in detail the discussion following the lecture. From these sources, Ellenberger was able to verify that the reception accorded Freud's presentation was considerably less censorious than as described by Freud himself. He also found that the real source of criticism of Freud's talk had not been incredulity at the idea of male hysteria per se but rather the belief that the lecture offered little that was medically newsworthy coupled with the feeling that Freud's defense of the French position in the ongoing Franco-German debate over post-traumatic neuroses was impertinent and impolitic. Additionally, Ellenberger examined the membership records of the *Gesellschaft* and found that Freud had remained a member of the group, attending meetings of the organization intermittently for many years afterwards. In the end, Ellenberger argues, the traditional account of Freud's lecture of 1886 rests on a small kernel of fact, which had been amplified by Freud for subjective, psychological reasons, repeated for ideological purposes by latter-day psychoanalyst–historians, and then restated in a number of popular-cultural sources for dramatic effect.[157]

A second study by Ellenberger, probably the most controversial of his historical articles, concerns the case of Anna O. The *Studies on Hysteria* of 1895, which is often identified as the first distinctly psychoanalytic text, includes the famous story of the patient known pseudonymously as "Fräulein Anna. O." In the early 1880s, Josef Breuer, coauthor of the book, had treated Anna O. for a year and a half for a battery of bizarre and volatile hysterical symptoms that developed while the patient was nursing

---

[156] Ellenberger, "La conférence de Freud sur l'hystérie masculine (15 octobre 1886): Étude critique," *L'information psychiatrique*, 44, no. 10 (1968), 921–29. Ellenberger later summarized this article in *Discovery of the Unconscious*, 437–42.

[157] Ellenberger's evaluation of the evidence about this event has not gone unchallenged. See Jackson, review of *The Discovery of the Unconscious, Journal of the History of Medicine* (1971), 215; K. R. Eissler, *Talent and Genius: The Fictitious Case of Tausk Contra Freud* (New York, Quadrangle Books, 1971), 351–58; and Léon Chertok, "Sur l'objectivité dans l'histoire de la psychanalyse: Premiers ferments d'une découverte," *L'évolution psychiatrique*, 35 (1970), 537–61.

her beloved father through a long, terminal illness. In the course of his daily therapeutic sessions, Breuer discovered that he could relieve his patient's symptoms individually by having her recall in a self-induced state of hypnosis the precise painful moment in the past at which the symptom had initially appeared. Using this method—Anna O.'s well-known "talking cure"—each of the patient's symptoms proved to be rooted in a psychic conflict that had first arisen during the period of her nursing duties.

According to the case as presented in *Studies on Hysteria*, Anna O. enjoyed a full recovery after her treatment with this procedure and went on to lead a productive life. This rendition of events was then restated in Freud's *History of the Psychoanalytic Movement* (1914) and *Autobiography*. In a half-century of psychoanalytic literature, the case of Anna O. was cited as the prototypical instance of a cathartic cure and the originary case for psychoanalytic theory. Then in 1925, Jung reported informally in a seminar in Zurich that Freud once confided to him that Anna O. had in fact not recovered as claimed by Breuer but had required additional medical care. Furthermore, in 1953 Jones identified the patient in real life as Bertha Pappenheim and provided a number of new and titillating details about the case.[158] Here the story of this historic encounter between doctor and patient rested until 1972, when Ellenberger published "The Story of 'Anna O.': A Critical Review with New Data."[159]

Since the early 1950s, Ellenberger had noted factual inconsistencies in the accounts of Pappenheim's case as presented by Breuer, Freud, and Jones. Jones stated that Pappenheim, after her treatment in Vienna with Breuer, had at an unspecified later date required additional institutionalization at a medical establishment in Gross-Enzersdorf, a suburb to the east of the Austrian capital. Attempting to document this later stage of her illness, Ellenberger was unable to find evidence for the existence of a hospital in Gross-Enzersdorf. He speculated that Jones had confused this location with Inzersdorf, where a private sanatorium operated; but at Inzersdorf too he found no evidence that Pappenheim was ever treated there.

Then, pursuing a different line, Ellenberger obtained from Dora Edinger (the editor of a collection of Pappenheim's later writings) a photograph of young Pappenheim in 1882, the year in which she had allegedly completed her medical treatment. Embossed illegibly on the photograph was the name and location of the photographer. Ellenberger at the time was employed at the University of Montreal in the Department of Criminology. Examining the original copy of the photograph under the lights of the

158 Jones, *Life and Work of Sigmund Freud*, (1953) 1:223–26.
159 Ellenberger, "The Story of 'Anna O.': A Critical Review with New Data," *Journal of the History of the Behavioral Sciences*, 8 (July 1972), 267–79.

Montreal City Police forensic laboratory (!), he found that the picture bore the place name "Constanz," the small German city along Lake Constance on the border of Switzerland, hundreds of miles from Vienna.

This of course was familiar territory to Ellenberger. From his years in Schaffhausen, he knew that near Constanz was located the Bellevue Sanatorium in Kreuzlingen, one of the most exclusive private facilities in central Europe. He also remembered that public and private asylums in Switzerland preserved very thorough medical records. Ellenberger therefore immediately wrote to the director of the Bellevue Sanatorium in Kreuzlingen—who turned out to be Wolfgang Binswanger, the son of Ellenberger's old acquaintance, Ludwig Binswanger—for more information. He quickly gained access to the private medical archives of the hospital, and, in the summer of 1971, he located among the patient records in Kreuzlingen a file for Bertha Pappenheim. Inside, Ellenberger discovered a pharmacological report by a staff physician about the patient and the transcript of a twenty-one-page report, dating from 1882, in Breuer's own handwriting. The report reviewed the full course of Pappenheim's illness up to that date. Given the historical importance of the case, these were precious finds.[160]

In his article of 1972, Ellenberger offers a detailed, comparative reading of Anna O.'s case as it appeared in *Studies on Hysteria* and in the 1882 report of Breuer that he unearthed in Kreuzlingen.[161] In many respects, he finds, the information in the two documents is similar. On other points, however, the unpublished report diverges dramatically from the printed account of Breuer and Freud. Biographically, the report, from which Ellenberger reproduces extensive excerpts, provides a better sense of Pappenheim's intimate and dependent emotional relationship with her father and of her rivalry with her brother. Medically, the new document establishes at once that Pappenheim, far from recovering fully in June 1882, had been hospitalized from July to October of that year at a private clinic for nervous and mental disorders. This institutionalization had occurred at Breuer's recommendation. The patient's neurological symptomatology, the document reveals further, had been more elaborate than previously realized and had included muscular jerks and an acute facial neuralgia. It also indicated that Pappenheim's psychological symptoms had been severe and psychotic-like, often following a cyclical pattern and including at times suicidal behavior. Later, during her months at Bellevue, Pappenheim had

---

[160] It is possible to chart the course of Ellenberger's investigation of this matter by reading consecutively his "Report on My Study Trip to Europe," Appendix B of the present volume; review of Dora Edinger, ed., *Bertha Pappenheim: Leben und Schriften*, in *Journal of the History of the Behavioral Sciences*, 2 (1966), 94–96; *Discovery of the Unconscious*, 480–84; "The Story of 'Anna O.,'" 272–74; and *A la découverte de l'inconscient*, viii, 403–9.

[161] Ellenberger, "The Story of 'Anna O.,'" 274–78.

been heavily sedated with chloral and morphine, to which she developed an addiction. Most damagingly, Breuer's unpublished report of 1882 established that the official rendition of this crucial event in the history of psychoanalysis was highly inaccurate. As Ellenberger writes in his sharpest statement in the article, "the famed 'prototype of a cathartic cure' was neither a cure nor a catharsis." [162] Ellenberger does not pursue the matter further, allowing readers to draw their own conclusions; but the interpretive implications are seriously subversive. [163]

At this point, it is important for readers not to misconstrue the nature of Ellenberger's psychoanalytic revisionism. In essays such as the ones on male hysteria and Anna O., Ellenberger called directly into question the integrity of the psychoanalytic historiography of his time. However, at the same time, Ellenberger was very well versed in the medical literature of psychoanalysis. He reviewed favorably many psychoanalytic texts, [164] and he published in psychoanalytic periodicals. Nearly all of the Swiss medical intellectuals who influenced him in his youth, from Bleuler to Arthur Kielholz, maintained a deep interest in psychoanalytic ideas or were themselves psychoanalysts. His chapter on Freud in *The Discovery of the Unconscious* is nearly twice the length of any other chapter in the book. Several of his other articles in this collection are strongly pro-Freudian in orientation. Most importantly, at no point in either his historical or medical writings does Ellenberger criticize psychoanalytic theory proper. Ellenberger's revisionism, then, was directed specifically at the historical literature of psychoanalysis as it existed until the 1960s and to which he was exposed in strong doses during his years in the United States.

To psychoanalytic scholars whose understanding of Freud derived exclusively from Freud's autobiography and Jones's biography, and who believed that Freud's reputation was dependent upon the image of absolute and solitary creative genius struggling against a hostile external world, Ellenberger's work was profoundly unwelcome. [165] But in the final analysis, Ellenberger believes, those individuals who adhere inflexibly to an uncritical, hagiographical view did little honor to their subject. In his mind, to demystify a subject is neither to diminish it nor to denigrate it. Ellenberger

[162] Ibid., 279.

[163] Subsequent research into the case has revealed that Pappenheim was hospitalized three additional times from 1883 to 1888 for periods ranging from three weeks to five and a half months. See Albrecht Hirschmüller, *The Life and Work of Josef Breuer: Physiology and Psychoanalysis* (New York and London, New York University Press, 1989), 115.

[164] Characteristic are his reviews of Murray H. Sherman, ed., *Psychoanalysis in America: Historical Perspectives*, in *Psychoanalytic Review*, 53 (1967), 178–80; and Amacher, *Freud's Neurological Education, in Journal of the History of the Behavioral Sciences* (1967).

[165] In this regard, see above all Kurt Eissler's frantic forty-page defense of the traditional psychoanalytic historiography in the light of Ellenberger's book in Eissler, *Talent and Genius*, Appendix D, "Another Critical View of Freud," 342–80.

conceives of his scholarship on Freud as a clarification of the true nature of Freud's achievement.[166]

The Autobiographical Undercurrent in the History of Psychiatry

"Man can stretch himself as he may with his knowledge and appear to himself as objective as he may; in the last analysis, he gives nothing but his own biography."[167] This statement of Nietzsche's from *Human, All Too*

[166] Ellenberger's Freudian revisionism raises the additional question of his relation to the antipsychiatry movement, which was emerging just as he researched and wrote *The Discovery of the Unconscious*. The literature of antipsychiatry contains a strong historical component, and Ellenberger, by questioning powerfully the ways in which psychiatric history has been written by self-interested physician-historians in the past, might be seen as contributing to the movement. Yet, interestingly, Ellenberger was consistently hostile toward antipsychiatry.

His response to the movement was in character: at the height of the controversy, and after a systematic reading of works by R. D. Laing, Thomas Szasz, Erving Goffman, and Enrico Basaglia, Ellenberger traveled to Europe during the summer of 1971 and tried personally to meet a number of these authors. When this failed, he toured a dozen and a half French, British, Dutch, Danish, and Swedish mental-health facilities in order to test directly the ideas of these writers against contemporary institutional realities. The article that resulted from this investigation was an angry, uncomprehending, in places irrational statement in which Ellenberger relates in detail his observations on hospital conditions in Europe. He finds the new antipsychiatric critiques greatly lacking and charges that the movement is part of a wider "transient collective psychosis" marking the 1960s. (Ellenberger, "Psychiatrie ou antipsychiatrie? Enquête sur les courants de la psychiatrie institutionnelle actuelle en Europe," *L'union médicale du Canada*, 100 [1971], 1526–38; 1737–49).

Two years later, at the Hôtel-Dieu in Montreal, Ellenberger was one of four speakers (of whom Michel Foucault was another) at a conference addressing the question "Faut-il interner les psychiatres?" This time, Ellenberger strikes a more moderate note. He again rejects the analyses of Laing, Szasz, Goffman, and Basaglia and accounts for antipsychiatry as a fashionable form of "cultural nihilism." At the same time, he suggests that the movement may ultimately exert a favorable effect by causing certain psychiatric policies to be reassessed. (Ellenberger, "Les courants de la pensée antipsychiatrique," *L'union médicale du Canada*, 102 [1973], 2315–19). During an interview in *L'éducation* in 1975, the final question posed to Ellenberger was "Que pensez-vous de l'antipsychiatrie?" Ellenberger responded emphatically, "Je suis anti-anti-psychiatre. Comme deux négations valent une affirmation, je me considère donc comme psychiatre!"

These statements elucidate importantly the field of Ellenberger's radicalism. The goal of his historical work was not a critique of Freudian theory, nor an attack on the psychiatric profession as a whole, but rather *historiographical demythologization*. To the best of my knowledge, in no place does Ellenberger address himself to the ideas of Foucault—a striking omission given the years in which he wrote—and at no time did he perceive his own work as encouraging or contributing to the antipsychiatry movement. In short, he responded to antipsychiatry less as a historian with revisionist ideas and methods than as a lifelong practicing physician content with his chosen specialty.

[167] Friedrich Nietzsche, *Menschliches, Allzumenschliches*, I, no. 513; III, no. 369, in *Nietzsches Werke*, Taschen-Ausgabe (Leipzig, Nauman, 1906).

Human is a favorite of Ellenberger's. Nietzsche had in mind with this thought the work of academic philosophers; but Ellenberger felt strongly that this insight applied equally to the history of psychiatry. Numerous historians before had pointed out the relationship between the life and the work of a given psychologist or psychiatrist in the past. Ellenberger, however, from his panoramic reading in the field, came to believe that there was an autobiographical undercurrent that ran like an obscure but persistent and powerful subtext through the entire history of the psychological sciences.

In his essays, Ellenberger isolates a number of ways in which the subjective, experiential aspects of the lives of psychologists and psychiatrists have impinged upon their theorizing. First, there has been direct self-observation. Given the nature of the subject matter involved—the systematic exploration of the psyche—it has been inevitable, he believes, that scientists turned to the self as an intimate source of information. Nearly the entire literature on the psychology of dreams, he shows in *The Discovery of the Unconscious*, has derived from systematic introspection. In a similar way, Ellenberger notes in Freudian texts such as *The Interpretation of Dreams, The Psychopathology of Everyday Life*, and *Jokes and Their Relation to the Unconscious* the admixture of Freud's observations of himself and his patients.

The most memorable historical example of this phenomenon in Ellenberger's essays concerns Rorschach. In his 1954 article, Ellenberger traces the origin of Rorschach's interest in psychological matters to a dream Rorschach had as a medical student. One day during his clinical training in the pathology laboratory, Rorschach observed for the first time a dissection of the central nervous system. That night, he experienced an intensely vivid dream in which he perceived his own brain being sliced cross-sectionally with each cortical layer falling forward across his face, exactly as it happened in the autopsy theater earlier that day. It was a crucial experience for young Rorschach. Eight years later, the dream served as the nucleus of his medical dissertation on "Reflex Hallucinations and Kindred Manifestations" and subsequently for his lifelong fascination with delusional multisensory perceptions. "In that dream," comments Ellenberger, "we find nothing less than the germinal cell of the whole psychological concept underlying the *Psychodiagnostik* and the Rorschach Test."[168]

At other times in the history of the science, Ellenberger shows, psychological theory has functioned as a kind of objectification, by means of intellectualization, of a painful psychological situation in the life of the theorist. In "Psychiatry and Its Unknown History," written in 1961, Ellenberger reviews many such examples: Robert Burton, for instance, in his

---

[168] Ellenberger, "Life and Work of Hermann Rorschach," 178. See also pp. 199–200.

classic *Anatomy of Melancholy* (1628), described his own condition under the heading of "scholar's melancholy." A century later, George Cheyne in *The English Malady* (1735) offered a classic description of hypochondriasis based on several case histories, of which the longest and most realistic was his own. And in the 1850s, the French alienist Bénédict-Augustin Morel incorporated his own experience of phobias into his clinical description of "emotional delirium." Janet during his adolescence suffered from symptoms of "psychasthenia." Adler as a young man was painfully overshadowed by the accomplishments of his older brother, which may partly account for his theories of a family-based inferiority complex. And Pavlov, during a convalescence from surgery in 1927, suffered from a "cardiac neurosis," an experience that stimulated the evolution of his scientific interests from physiology to psychiatry.[169] In each of these instances, Ellenberger believes that individual neurotic experiences provided the prospective psychiatrist with an initial sensitivity to matters psychological, a subject of reflection and analysis, and a method of self-understanding and self-healing. Scientific psychological study here became a means of masking, and mastering, private psychological suffering.

The third, and most profound, form of autobiographical interaction found in the history of psychiatry, Ellenberger proposes, involves what he terms a full-scale "creative malady." This is one of Ellenberger's most interesting formulations and the subject of an essay published in the Canadian journal *Dialogue* in 1964.[170] From his knowledge of general cultural history, Ellenberger had long been struck by the diverse strategies of psychic organization that allowed for creativity of a high order. His interest in this subject extends equally to artistic, scientific, and spiritual creativity, which he believes often involve similar psychological operations.[171] In a small number of exceptional cases, he observes, the life and work of the psychological theorist followed a particularly complicated and distinctive pattern. In these cases, a person, usually at the beginning of his or her career, is engrossed with a certain idea or problem, to the growing exclusion of everything else. The problem proves intractable, and the theorist eventually enters a period of distress and depression, which sometimes brings with it neurotic, even psychotic, symptoms. This period of painful

[169] These examples appear in Ellenberger, "La psychiatrie et son histoire inconnue," *L'union médicale du Canada*, 90, no. 3 (March 1961), 281–83; and *Discovery of the Unconscious*, 79, 401, 889.

[170] Ellenberger, "La notion de maladie créatrice," *Dialogue: Canadian Philosophical Journal/Revue philosophique canadienne*, 3, no. 1 (1964), 25–41.

[171] Ellenberger also reflects on the role of "creative neuroses" in the lives of two major literary figures in his reviews of K. R. Eissler, *Goethe: A Psychoanalytic Study, 1775–1786*, in *Dialogue: Canadian Philosophical Journal/Revue philosophique canadienne*, 4 (1966), 540–45; and Jean Delay, *The Youth of André Gide*, in *American Journal of Psychiatry*, 120 (May 1964), 1139.

preoccupation can last for months or years. Eventually, however, the individual emerges spontaneously and with a sense of enlightenment in the form of a new insight or theory. Moreover, this insight is usually experienced epiphanously, as a sudden intellectual illumination. The new idea or theory represents a resolution at once of an intense and protracted inner conflict and a difficult artistic or scientific problem. From this point onward, Ellenberger continues, the individual devotes his lifework to the new theory and maintains an unshakable faith in its veracity. The experience of the creative malady permanently transforms the personality of the person and gives new meaning to his life.

Ellenberger was first attuned to the concept of creative neurosis by studying Fechner's biography in the 1950s;[172] but in time he identified the phenomenon in several other figures as well. In "The Concept of Creative Illness," a short and loosely suggestive piece, he explores the idea in the lives of a selection of people, including primitive shamans, Catholic mystics, the German Romantic poet and philosopher Novalis, Fechner, and Nietzsche. He speculates that Mesmer underwent such an experience in Vienna in the early 1780s, emerging with the theory of animal magnetism in hand. Among the major dynamic psychologists of the twentieth century, Freud and Jung, he projects, experienced these patterned *névroses créatrices*. The long training analyses of Freudian and Jungian analysts, he speculates further, represent ritualized repetitions of the creative illness of the theorist that are similar in function to the initiatory illnesses of ancient shamans. As such, they are required of all followers before they can share fully the psychological knowledge of the master and gain admittance to the inner circle of practitioners. "The history of dynamic psychiatry . . . ," Ellenberger concludes, "is inseparable from the history of the neuroses of its founders."[173]

The Concept of the Paradigmatic Patient

One of the most significant innovations in *The Discovery of the Unconscious* is the extensive citation of case-historical material. In virtually all of the histories of psychiatry and psychology written before 1970, the experience of the individual patient was overlooked. To an extent, this was due to the difficulty of documenting the subject satisfactorily; but it also resulted from the methodology in use at the time. Earlier descriptions of the field offered accounts of formal psychiatric ideas in which patients figured at

---

[172] Ellenberger, "Fechner and Freud," 202–3. Whether Ellenberger was previously sensitized to the idea because he may have suffered himself from a creative malady remains unknown.

[173] Ellenberger, "La psychiatrie et son histoire inconnue," 288.

most as the raw and inert "clinical material" from which medical scientists drew their observations and practiced their therapies. In contrast, Ellenberger believes that the case history is a highly important, if curiously underused, primary source and that the role of the patient is a major but greatly neglected factor in the history of psychiatry.

Ellenberger has attempted to integrate the experience of the patient into the narrative of psychiatric history in various ways. Intercalated through *The Discovery of the Unconscious* are over five dozen extended case histories. Among the most important sources in Ellenberger's discussion of the popular history of Mesmerism are compendia of cases of Alsatian patients published in Strasbourg. In his investigation of Puységur's work in eastern France, he expends as much time researching the life of Victor Race as reading Puységur's published writings. And some of the most memorable pages of *The Discovery of the Unconscious* narrate a succession of cases of multiple personality from the nineteenth century. Ellenberger, we have seen, spared no effort in reconstructing the biography of Bertha Pappenheim. Similarly, in his campaign to rehabilitate the work of Janet, he presents detailed summaries of Janet's early hysterical patients—such as Marie, Lucie, Marcelle, Madame D., Justine, Achille, and Irène—and he was instrumental in bringing to English-language audiences the subtlest piece of clinical writing in the literature of existential analysis, namely, Binswanger's case of Ellen West.[174] The intrinsic interest of these case histories is high, and their inclusion in Ellenberger's book and essays imparts a novelistic quality to his writing. In addition, they allow us to see the ways in which particular medical theories have emerged from specific clinical situations.

Moreover, Ellenberger has come to believe that the role of the patient in the history of psychiatry has been essentially creative in nature. In other branches of medical history, patients play a passive part, as the empirical subjects of analysis studied by physicians. However, in a number of key ways, Ellenberger knew, the structure of doctor-patient relations is fundamentally different in psychiatry.[175] In "Psychiatry and Its Unknown History" (1961), Ellenberger explores brilliantly the role of the individual patient in the production of past psychological theory.

As should be apparent by now, Ellenberger excels at detecting themes, which other scholars had perceived only in passing in the work of one figure or text, running throughout psychiatric history. Among the recur-

[174] Binswanger, "The Case of Ellen West" [1944], in May, Angel, and Ellenberger, *Existence*, 237–364. See also *Discovery of the Unconscious*, 864–65, where Ellen West is the final case history in the book.

[175] We find here a point on which Ellenberger's personal experience as a clinician informed his historical sensibility.

rent patterns that he finds in the long-term development of the field is "that of the psychiatrist who has for an object of study a certain patient, most often a female patient, generally a hysteric, with whom he establishes unconsciously a rather long, complicated, and ambiguous relationship, of which the final issue will turn out to be highly fruitful for science."[176] The hysterical women in these cases, Ellenberger elaborates, have usually been ill for only a single stage of their lives, most often during a vulnerable youthful period. They have tended to enter the practices of their physicians at important, intellectually formative periods of the doctors' careers, and they have often served as the clinical model—the founding case—of their theoretical work. These encounters between doctor and patient have typically been based on an emotional and psychological manipulation that was mutual, undeclared, and often unrecognized. Furthermore, after these early neurotic illnesses, the hysterical patients in question frequently went on to lead independent and self-expressive lives. Also, in many of these cases, Ellenberger believes, the patient's personality has been stronger than that of the therapist.[177]

Ellenberger proceeds to illustrate these important observations with a series of cases of female patients drawn from the practices of Mesmer, Kerner, Charcot, Janet, Breuer, Flournoy, and Jung.[178] In each of these instances, the "creative" psychiatric personality of the patient led to an intellectual creativity on the part of the physician. In each different clinical and cultural setting, a complex and unconsciously collaborative relationship evolved between neurotic patients and their physicians.

In the present selection of Ellenberger's essays, three articles in Part 3 take individual case histories as their subject.[179] We have already considered the case of Anna O. As Ellenberger and other historians have pointed out, it was Pappenheim herself who arrived at a method of removing symptoms through the exploration of past emotional experiences and who presented her "findings" to the doctor. "Frau Emmy von N.," another patient

---

[176] Ellenberger, "La psychiatrie et son histoire inconnue," 281.

[177] Ellenberger's first pronouncement on this subject appeared in "Discussion I," a response to a conference paper of Oskar Diethelm reprinted in the *Canadian Psychiatric Association Journal*, 6 (1961), 116–20.

[178] Ellenberger, "La psychiatrie et son histoire inconnue," 283–88. Elsewhere in his writings, Ellenberger discusses the creative role of a number of male patients. See *Discovery of the Unconscious*, 18–22, 73, 892, 893; and review of William G. Niederland, *The Schreber Case: Psychoanalytic Profile of a Paranoid Personality*, in *Bulletin of the Menninger Clinic*, 39 (1975), 598.

[179] The title of this section of the book—"The Great Patients"—is intended to recall the title of a classic study by a revered medical historian. See Henry E. Sigerist, *The Great Doctors: A Biographical History of Medicine*, translated from the German by Eden Paul and Cedar Paul (New York, Norton, 1933).

in the *Studies on Hysteria*, encouraged Freud to abandon the practice of hypnosis and pointed the way toward the technique of free association.[180] Similarly with Helene Preiswerk. Ellenberger's most recent historical essay, completed in 1991, returns to the case that Jung grappled with in his dissertation and that has fascinated Ellenberger since the beginning of his career.[181] He proposes that it was Jung's observations of this patient in the 1890s, struggling for emotional independence from her family, that provided the germ of Jung's later concept of individuation. Furthermore, he hypothesizes that Jung's personal emotional involvement with Preiswerk was revived many years later, when Jung projected his feelings about her onto Sabina Spielrein, his analysand and mistress, and emerged with the idea of the anima.[182] Ellenberger believes firmly that many discoveries in psychiatric history, in both the theoretical and therapeutic realms, owe as much to the patients as to their doctors. He points the way toward a historical account of psychiatry that integrates the achievements of the pioneering doctors and the prototypical patients.

The Cultural History of Psychiatry and the History of Psychiatric Ideas

In his reading, Ellenberger has ranged widely and comfortably across the humanities. During his undergraduate years at Strasbourg, it will be recalled, he studied philosophy and literature; he also maintained strong interests in languages, religion, and the visual arts. One result is that throughout his career Ellenberger has been highly attentive to the cultural history of psychiatry, a history that he believes is exceptionally rich but almost entirely unwritten. In *The Discovery of the Unconscious*, he interweaves a great deal of cultural information with the main historical narrative. Further, in presenting this material, he insists that it provides much more than simply background information. Rather, it is a matter of psychiatry *in* culture, with psychiatric theories and practices often deriving from, and in turn contributing to, larger cultural developments.

In particular, Ellenberger isolates several modes of interaction between psychiatry and its ambient cultural environments. There has been, for instance, direct popularization. In *The Discovery of the Unconscious*, he sketches the popular-cultural history of Mesmerism in Germany during the 1820s and 1830s and later reviews the spate of novels and plays dealing

---

[180] Ellenberger, "L'histoire d'"Emmy von N.': Étude critique avec documents nouveaux," *L'évolution psychiatrique*, 42, no. 3 (July–September 1977), 519–41.

[181] Ellenberger, "The Story of Helene Preiswerk."

[182] Ibid., 51–52.

with hypnotism, hysteria, and somnambulism that appeared in France during the late nineteenth century. In other places, he demonstrates that certain poets, novelists, and playwrights actually received their professional training in psychological medicine and then imported this knowledge into their artistic productions. During the 1880s, for example, the Austrian playwright Arthur Schnitzler was a physician in Vienna before becoming a writer. And André Breton, the Surrealist poet, worked as a medic at the French battlefront during the First World War. Breton later claimed that the painful and vivid experience of observing shell-shocked soldiers contributed to his formulation of a Surrealist aesthetic.

In other instances, Ellenberger brings to light important cultural representations of psychiatric figures, institutions, and theories. His most in-depth discussion along these lines is his article "Charcot and the Salpêtrière School," published in 1965.[183] With his usual resourcefulness, Ellenberger assembles over a dozen and a half texts—novels, literary memoirs, student reminiscences, newspaper editorials—pertaining to the popular and professional image of Charcot and the cultural reception of his work. The famous neurologist, he shows, read widely in the European literary classics and was highly interested in drawing, painting, sculpture, and architecture. In works such as *Les démoniaques dans l'art* (1887) and *Les difformes et les malades dans l'art* (1889), Charcot integrated medical and artistic materials, and during his famous Tuesday *soirées*, he surrounded himself with the cultural *beau monde* of Paris. In turn, many writers were engaged by Charcot personally and intrigued by his theories of hysteria, hypnotism, and ambulatory automatisms. Some of the most memorable contemporary portraits of Charcot, Ellenberger discovers, came from literary intellectuals, like Jules Claretie, the Goncourt brothers, Léon Daudet, and Axel Munthe. As late as 1928, the Surrealist poets christened Charcot's hysteria "the greatest poetical discovery of the end of the nineteenth century."[184]

The deepest forms of interaction between psyche and culture documented in Ellenberger's writings involve the literary construction of psychiatric syndromes or the incorporation of medical models of personality or consciousness into the style of narration or characterization developed in a work of art. In an unpublished lecture entitled "Psychiatric Problems as Reflected in German Literature" (1957), Ellenberger argues that psychiatry functions as an expression of the total culture of an epoch.[185] Culturally, he contends, history has displayed a cyclical pattern of attitudes,

[183] Ellenberger, "Charcot and the Salpêtrière School," *American Journal of Psychotherapy*, 19, no. 2 (April 1965), 253–67.

[184] Cited in ibid., 265.

[185] Ellenberger, "Psychiatric Problems as Reflected in German Literature," (Lecture presented to the Kansas Modern Language Association, Manhattan, Kansas, April 13, 1957).

alternating between periods of the stigmatization and repression of mental illness and the acceptance and exploration of it.

In the Romantic, *fin-de-siècle*, and Modernist periods, Ellenberger locates complex and culturally productive interactions between psychiatry, psychology, and imaginative literature. We have seen that he applied the term *Romantic* equally to poets, painters, and psychiatrists of the first half of the nineteenth century. And in *The Discovery of the Unconscious*, he explores the influence of medical writing about multiple personality on characterization in the stories and novels of E.T.A. Hoffmann, Edgar Allan Poe, Feodor Dostoevsky, Oscar Wilde, and Robert Louis Stevenson.[186] Similarly, in Charcot's work, he identifies "the starting point of a whole tradition of psychiatrically oriented writers, such as Daudet, Zola, Maupassant, Huysmans, Bourget, Claretie, Pirandello, Proust."[187] And in his essay on psychiatry and German literature, he reviews a sequence of texts (Goethe, Kant, Lessing, Hoffman, Kleist, Jenssen, Musil, Zweig, Hesse, Rilke) that analyze insanity, depict life in mental institutions, and present extreme psychological states of the author. In Franz Kafka's *The Trial*, he finds an illustration, more powerful than that in any medical text, of the subjective, innermost experience of a patient afflicted with delusions of persecution.[188] Ellenberger goes so far as to describe the complete writings of Daudet, Schnitzler, and Breton as "potential systems of dynamic psychiatry."[189] To Ellenberger, these artists form part of the cultural history of the unconscious.

Elsewhere, Ellenberger traces the history of a single psychological perception as expressed over many centuries in a diversity of cultural discourses. It is a belief of Ellenberger's that psychological insight over the generations has issued from many cultural domains, and that the exploration of depth-psychological themes in particular has often evolved from the religious, to the literary and the philosophical, to the medical and scientific. Goethe, Dostoevsky, Balzac, and Nietzsche, he affirms, are among the finest psychologists of modern times. And in *The Discovery of the Unconscious*, he proposes that the close systematic study of human sexuality began with Catholic "moral theology," continued in the autobiographical writings of Rousseau and de Sade, and was elaborated in nineteenth-century novels, short stories, and works of pornography before being picked up and developed by medical sexologists in the 1870s and 1880s.[190]

A beautiful example of Ellenberger's work in the cultural history of

[186] Ellenberger, *Discovery of the Unconscious*, 162–63.
[187] Ibid., 99–100.
[188] Ellenberger, "Psychiatric Problems as Reflected in German Literature," 15.
[189] Ellenberger, *Discovery of the Unconscious*, 898 n. 60.
[190] Ibid., 291–303.

psychiatric ideas is his essay "The Pathogenic Secret and Its Therapeutics."[191] Basically, the article studies the pre-Freudian history of the catharsis concept. The perception that an emotionally laden thought or experience may, if kept secret over a prolonged period of time, exert a deleterious psychiatric effect upon its bearer has found expression in many times and texts, Ellenberger demonstrates. In the body of the essay, he considers this idea in primitive psychotherapies, Catholic confessional literature, the Protestant theory of the "Cure of Souls," the novels and plays of Jeremias Gotthelf, Nathaniel Hawthorne, Henrik Ibsen, and Marcel Prévost, medical writings on magnetism and hypnotism, French and Austrian criminological writing of the late nineteenth century, and the theories of Benedikt, Janet, Freud, and Jung. For each body of writing, he examines the particular emotions suppressed, the clinical effects of the repression (ranging from depression to death), differences in the explanation of the pathogenic mechanism involved, and changes in the prescribed treatments. Illustrating his analysis with short case histories, he reflects in closing on differences in the structure of psychological relations between confessor and confessant, criminal and lawyer, analyst and analysand, and so forth.[192] It is a creative, effortlessly interdisciplinary piece of work.

The Study of the Historiography of Psychiatry

Finally, Ellenberger once commented that "it would be a great contribution to the secret history of science to analyze in detail those factors that bring fame to some scientists, oblivion to others."[193] From a lifetime of reading about the history of psychiatry, Ellenberger has come away struck by the subject of historical destinies. He is intrigued by the negative and positive mythologies that have grown up around particular historical figures, and by the inscrutable retrospective processes whereby certain individuals are granted premier status while others fall into obscurity. To some extent, obviously, this process involves the judgment of posterity on the intellectual achievement of past scientists. But Ellenberger has come to believe that historical reputations are determined to a notable degree by nonscientific factors that have relatively little to do with either the inherent intellectual merit of the work or its contemporary influence.[194] In a passage from *The Discovery of the Unconscious*, Ellenberger exemplifies this

---

[191] Ellenberger, "The Pathogenic Secret and Its Therapeutics," *Journal of the History of the Behavioral Sciences*, 2, no. 1 (January 1966), 29–42.

[192] Ibid., 40–41.

[193] Ellenberger, *Discovery of the Unconscious*, 270.

[194] Ellenberger may initially have been attuned to this phenomenon by Arnold Van Gennep's *La formation des légendes* (Paris, Flammarion, 1910).

phenomenon by contrasting the reputations of Jean-François Champollion
and Georg Friedrich Grotefend, the decoders, respectively, of the Egyptian
hieroglyphics and the ancient Persian cuneiform script. The two men lived
at the same time, and their achievements, Ellenberger asserts, were comparable; yet Champollion is hailed today as a genius while Grotefend is nearly
forgotten. Ellenberger then speculates on the factors responsible for these
divergent fates.[195]

In no branch of medical science, Ellenberger believes, has the process of
selective historiographical valorization been more conspicuous and curious and irrational than in the history of the mental sciences. The cultural
history of the avant-garde in modern times is replete with examples of
painters and poets, musicians and philosophers who did brilliant work,
languished in obscurity during their lifetimes, and were then recognized
posthumously. But psychiatric history, Ellenberger observes, evinces different patterns. Pinel, for instance, was lauded for generations as the founding
figure of modern psychiatry; but less a historical than a hagiographical
tradition grew up around him, which derived from a single symbolic action
at the beginning of his career—the unchaining of the insane in the 1790s—
and ignored his major later publications.[196] In Ellenberger's view,
Puységur is a figure equal in importance to Mesmer; and yet Mesmer is
widely known to readers while only specialists have heard of Puységur.
Charcot enjoyed international fame during his lifetime, but after his death
his reputation underwent a sudden eclipse in which his theories were dis-
mantled, his students abandoned his teachings, and the publication of his
collected works was terminated.[197] For many people today, he is little more
than a footnote in the prehistory of psychoanalysis. To Ellenberger, the
case of Janet was especially regrettable. Around 1900, there had been a
widespread feeling in French medical circles that the young Janet, with his
double doctorates in psychology and philosophy and his bold new psychological conceptualization of the neuroses, was a rising star. But by the end
of the First World War, Janet's work was followed by few physicians, and at
the time of his death he was largely forgotten outside of France. Pondering
these cases, Ellenberger proposes studying the inscrutable forces that determine the image and celebrity of figures in the history of psychiatry and then
comparing the results with those found in other sciences.

In the end, the formation of historical reputations has remained essentially an enigma to Ellenberger. (On this point, as on others, he would
benefit from a knowledge of contemporary literature on the sociology of

[195] Ellenberger, *Discovery of the Unconscious*, 270–71.
[196] Ellenberger, "Methodology in Writing the History of Dynamic Psychiatry," 27–28,
33–34; review of Walter Helmut Lechler, *Neue Ergebnisse in der Forschung über Philippe
Pinel*, in *Journal of the History of Medicine*, 19 (1964), 434–35.
[197] Ellenberger, "Charcot and the Salpêtrière School," 264–65.

science.) Nevertheless, Ellenberger, perhaps sensitized to this issue by the course of his own career, has been the first psychiatric historian to put his finger on this phenomenon. Moreover, he has highlighted a number of the factors that have contributed to the process. Through nearly all of its history, he notes, the scientific status of psychiatry has been less secure than that of other medical specialties, its history less neatly cumulative; as a result, there has been less of a stable and consensual vantage point from which to write the history of the discipline. Further, psychiatric history has been marked by great rivalries between figures and schools as well as by a dialectical movement between organic and psychological philosophies. As a consequence, writing about the subject has often entailed the negation of preceding or competing theories. Many figures of significance have fallen out of view or descended into marginal status. Entire bodies of knowledge have been obscured.

In addition, Ellenberger pinpoints a process whereby a certain author or theory can be rendered invisible for generations by another more prominent contemporaneous author or theory. This is especially possible if a theorist generates a school of followers with the intellectual and organizational resources to record its achievements in printed form. Pinel and Esquirol, for instance, fathered two generations of French *aliénistes* who then loyally erected legendary reputations about their mentors that endured throughout the nineteenth century while the similar work of others—for instance, the Italian Vicenzo Chiarugi—languished without a group of followers to memorialize it. In much the same way, as has been noted previously, one lamentable effect of the enormous success of psychoanalytic ideas has been to structure the twentieth-century historiography of the psychological sciences, dividing the field into precursors, disciples, and dissidents of Freud and ignoring nonpsychoanalytic dynamic psychiatries. In contrast, Janet did not form a school of students around him and was something of a loner intellectually and professionally. Ellenberger's writings demonstrate lastly that the history of psychiatry is intimately caught up with the history of the interpretation of psychiatry.

Ellenberger's Place and Significance Today

As I mentioned in the Preface, perhaps no area of study within the history of science and medicine today is expanding more energetically than psychiatric history. More books and articles are appearing on psychiatry's famous past all the time. Judging from academic dissertations either recently completed or in preparation, a generation of young scholars from a range of countries is entering the field. These scholars hail from many disciplinary backgrounds, including medicine; the history of science; social, cultural, and intellectual history; psychoanalytic studies; and women's studies. New collections of reprinted primary texts are bringing to prominence important writings by past psychiatric figures. Periodicals devoted specifically to the discipline have recently been established. Academic conferences on various aspects of the subject are being held at regular intervals in North America and abroad. And the European Association for the History of Psychiatry was founded in 1991. Furthermore, debates within the recent literature of psychiatric history have often had a considerable cultural resonance and have been followed closely in other fields within both the medical sciences and the humanities. What was once a rather antiquarian pastime of a small and uncoordinated group of practitioners has emerged in recent years as a new and thriving academic subdiscipline, one of the most active and controversial research sites in the humanities today.

The question to pose in the conclusion of this introductory essay is: What relationship does the work of Henri Ellenberger bear to this new historiography of psychiatry? Or, to adapt a formulation once used by Benedetto Croce, what is living and what is dead in Ellenberger's work? Hopefully, at this point the many ways in which Ellenberger's work remains exceptionally pertinent today will be evident to readers. It is not simply that Ellenberger wrote a general history of psychiatry that is still in wide use. Rather, his writings, with the eight features outlined above, anticipate to an impressive degree many of the most fertile areas of research in the field today. In other ways, the historical essays and *The Discovery of the Unconscious* point the way toward new and rich subject matter that remains unexplored. All in all, a remarkably large amount of Ellenberger's work remains alive today.

An accounting of recent scholarly writing in the Ellenbergerian tradition, with specific authors and titles, can be found in the bibliographical essay appended to this book. However, some basic connections may be made at this point. There is little doubt that Ellenberger was for many years one of the very few historians of psychiatry to immerse himself in original source materials. Today, the location and exploration of new bodies of primary sources, printed and archival, has become standard operating procedure among historians of the subject. Similarly, the notion of writing a less "iatrocentric" and more patient-centered medical history has of late become a major concern of scholars. Ellenberger provided a call for this approach as early as 1961. The exploration of the intellectual origins of psychoanalysis has in recent years generated a sizable volume of writing, and many of the principal figures involved in the formation of Freud's thought—Breuer, Meynert, Fliess, Krafft-Ebing, Charcot, Ellis, and others—have found, or are finding, their biographers. Equally, Ellenberger's revisionist view of Freud scholarship has proved highly influential.

The critical, if not hostile, reevaluation of psychoanalytic history as set down by the first-generation Freudians has in many quarters become a considerable preoccupation during the last fifteen years, and at this point a veritable counterliterature to the Jonesian version of events exists. A portion of this writing is indebted to Ellenberger's constructive historiographical iconoclasm. What is more, researching the personal and medical biographies of the major paradigmatic patients of the past, on the model of Ellenberger's essays, has become an absorbing pastime of many scholars.

Ellenberger has also pioneered important research strategies in the writing of the history of psychiatry. He has emphasized the significance of the earliest work of a theorist and the study of the contemporary reception of psychiatric texts. He has also led the way in the use by psychiatric historians of new categories of evidence, including local histories, family biographies, newspaper necrologies, case histories, contemporary book reviews, and academic conference proceedings.

At the same time, the study of certain figures and movements in psychiatric history undertaken by Ellenberger has developed apace. Mesmer and animal magnetism were once dismissed by historians as silly and charlantanish subjects while German Romantic psychism was viewed as mystical nonsense. Both subjects are currently attracting a great deal of scholarly attention. Likewise with the "French school" of psychology and psychiatry. Charcot studies, for instance, are developing rapidly today. Many of Janet's texts are being reprinted in both French and English, and a hearty revival of interest in Janetian psychology is under way. It would be possible to go on at length in this manner.

Clearly, the writings just referred to argue ideologically in many different directions, and it is not my intention here to attempt to adjudicate among them. The point is rather that, taken collectively, these trends define a large part of current-day psychiatric history-writing, and that time and again, Ellenberger was there first—discovering relevant primary sources, highlighting unknown figures and texts, challenging old ideas and methodologies, opening up new lines of inquiry, mapping out new subject matter. Indeed, the very rapid growth of psychiatric historiography in these directions makes it easy to forget how bold and original Ellenberger has really been. For this, it is necessary to envision him during the 1950s and 1960s, carrying the responsibilities of a full-time academic physician, lacking professional historical training and a supporting institutional environment (to say nothing of sabbaticals, research assistants, and word processors), and scything his way through masses of undigested primary source materials in an effort to master his subject factually and analytically.

To be sure, Ellenberger cannot be all things to all readers. Among historians of the human mind, Albert Deutsch was more reformist in his motivations, and Walther Riese was a superior medical scientist. Erwin Ackerknecht cut a more venerable academic figure and had many more students while Richard Hunter and Ida Macalpine integrated more successfully their medical and historical interests. Foucault has had a vastly greater influence upon academic intellectuals, and Jean Starobinski writes and thinks with greater elegance. Eric Carlson did more to maintain a network of professional contacts in the field, and George Mora has done more to bring important primary texts to attention. But, in many other ways, Ellenberger's position in the field today remains secure and singular. By any standard, his historical erudition is prodigious. His very broad, multidisciplinary perspective on psychiatric history has not been captured by any other historian. The chronological sweep of his work, and the trans-European scope of his reading, remain unsurpassed. His linguistic gifts are very considerable. It is also unlikely that we will again be privileged to know a historical commentator who has had such an extensive firsthand acquaintance with so many figures from twentieth-century European psychiatry. Above all, as the listing of themes above suggests, Ellenberger remains unmatched as a fertile source of ideas for future historical investigation.

Ellenberger's splendid, solitary achievement requires analysis on another level, too. It is important, I believe, to appreciate the degree to which the very subjects that Ellenberger chose for historical study represent interpretive acts. Given the fullness of Ellenberger's *oeuvre*, it seems churlish to criticize him for something he neglected to discuss. But one of the most revealing features of his historical work as a whole concerns what is missing, that is, the history of psychiatry that he chose *not* to write. In his thirty-six essays, and throughout *The Discovery of the Unconscious*, Ellenberger says almost nothing about organic psychiatry, descriptive clinical psychiatry, or behaviorial psychology—in other words, about *nondynamic* psychologies and psychiatries.

There are many conspicuous examples of these omissions: in *The Discovery of the Unconscious*, he discusses the coming of the German organicist tradition in the 1840s and 1850s under the chapter subheading "the mid-century crisis." Wilhelm Griesinger, arguably the most influential mental scientist of the century, receives one paragraph of analysis, and that paragraph examines the ignored psychodynamic element in his work. In the same vein, Ellenberger acknowledges the pathbreaking work of Griesinger's followers in the field of cerebral localization (Westphal, Wernicke, and Meynert) in only a single sentence. Morelian degeneration theory provided the primary etiological model for two generations of alienists in France and Italy; yet Ellenberger barely mentions the subject. And in the last chapter of *The Discovery of the Unconscious*, which purports to be a comprehensive chronological review of European psychiatry, Ellenberger fails to mention at all Kraepelin's formulation in the 1890s of the two great endogenous psychotic categories (manic depression and dementia prae-cox) while he cites Pavlov's Nobel Prize–winning research on psychologi-cal reflexology only in passing.[198] Similarly, medical events such as the isolation in the 1820s of general paresis as a distinct pathology with cere-bral lesions or the discovery of the syphilitic origins of general paresis of the insane in 1906 do not appear in the book. The pattern is unmistakable: however significant historically, those figures who related mental distur-bance to cerebral pathology and those therapies that applied chemical or physiological methods to the treatment of mental disease simply have not been incorporated into Ellenberger's historical vision.

In pointing out these omissions, I by no means intend to criticize Ellen-berger. After all, the psychological sciences themselves have not managed to achieve unity, so it is scarcely fair to demand that their histories do so. Rather, I make the point to clarify the nature of Ellenberger's reading of psychiatry. In a way that he is most likely unaware of himself, Ellenberger is the product of a time, and of a complex of cultures, in which it was possible effectively to equate the history of psychiatry as a whole with the develop-ment of the dynamic paradigm. Ellenberger was trained medically in France during the 1930s, when the first wave of Freudian ideas was infil-trating that country. He worked in German-speaking Switzerland during the 1940s and at the Menninger Clinic in the 1950s, two foci of profes-sional interest in psychological dynamism. His writings from the early 1950s onward reveal that he read very widely, almost comprehensively, in the contemporary literatures of depth psychology and psychiatry. In reac-tion against its German somaticist background, the Swiss psychological tradition has been overwhelmingly psychodynamic. And Ellenberger per-sonally knew many leading dynamic psychotherapists in Switzerland, France, Austria, Germany, Canada, and the United States. His one personal experience with psychotherapy involved a prominent lay psychoanalyst.

From this perspective, it is ironic that psychoanalytic readers a genera-tion ago first received Ellenberger's work critically. Since the 1950s, and particularly in the last twenty years, the theoretical pendulum that has characterized the history of psychiatric thought for two centuries has swung away from psychological dynamism. In the West today, biological psychiatry has found a much greater confidence than earlier in the century and has decisively taken the lead within the mental sciences. This change in orientation will undoubtedly over time prompt a rewriting of the history of psychiatry in which, one can well imagine, the story of "the discovery of the unconscious" will figure only in a relatively minor way. In Ellenberger's work, however, if the history of depth psychology is always larger than Freud, the history of psychology and psychiatry is no larger than the dy-

---

[198] Ellenberger, *Discovery of the Unconscious*, 222–28, 241, 242, 244, 787–88.

namic psychiatry of which Janet, Freud, Adler, and Jung were the major exponents. For Ellenberger, it seems self-evident that the conscious/unconscious duality is central to what psychiatry is about and that the exploration of the mysteries of unconscious cerebration represents the central intellectual drama in the history of the discipline. Ellenberger's approach to the study of the psyche has been a thoroughly humanistic one in which the most important allied fields are experimental psychology, philosophy, anthropology, religion, and the arts—not neuroanatomy, neurophysiology, endocrinology, pharmacology, and genetics. Whether the turn from Freud and the ascent of the biological and psychopharmacological models in recent years represent the end of depth psychology as it has been known earlier in the century, or only a temporary eclipse of it, or the beginnings of a new synthesis in the clinical human sciences, is a weighty question that remains to be settled. But we can see now that, in the broad view, Ellenberger's historical role has been to serve as the historian of the age of the pure dynamic psychiatries.

Nor is this quite all. Ellenberger, we have seen, believes that the early, at times obscure, publications of an author often hold important clues to that author's intellectual formation, that such writings represent the germs of a thinker's mature thought. In *La psychiatrie suisse*, written in 1951 to 1953, Ellenberger canvassed hundreds of publications on psychology and psychiatry in twentieth-century Switzerland. He concluded his study with several pages of reflections on the cultural impact of these fields in contemporary times.[199] The emergence and rapid development of the psychological sciences in Switzerland over the last three generations, he proposed, represents more than the growth of a single medical discipline. Psychoanalysis, child psychiatry, analytical psychology, neuropsychiatry, phenomenological psychiatry, existential analysis, forensic psychiatry, social psychiatry, psychiatric criminology, industrial psychology, characterology, graphology, the mental hygiene movement, and on and on: psychological modes of understanding were permeating Swiss culture and society. The psychological model of human nature was in the process of changing fundamentally the way in which Swiss people in the twentieth century thought about themselves and their society. Ellenberger even warned—although he was not really very worried about it—of the dangers of "overpsychologization—*surpsychologisation*." He labeled this pervasive development "the psychological revolution" and likened it, with only slight exaggeration, to the Industrial Revolution of the nineteenth century and the Scientific Revolution of the seventeenth.

The ideas in this passage from Ellenberger's early book, applied beyond

---

[199] Ellenberger, *La psychiatrie suisse*, 748–51.

the borders of one nation to the West in general, illuminate Ellenberger's work as a whole. In the eighteenth century, the most important new model of the natural world derived from the physical sciences, and its patron saint was Newton. In the latter half of the nineteenth century, the biological sciences provided the most powerful paradigm for understanding society and nature. It was "the Age of Darwin." We are in a position today to perceive that the twentieth century, the Freudian century, has been the heyday of the psychological sciences. The roots of this sea change lay in the late eighteenth century, and the key, transformative texts for the new age appeared from 1885 to 1910. The period running roughly from the final quarter of the nineteenth century to the end of the second third of the twentieth century witnessed an extraordinary burst of theoretical activity across the psychological sciences. Today, as a number of commentators have indicated, much of the most influential theorizing about human nature takes place in the psychological and psychiatric worlds. For better or worse, the mental-health professional replaced the priest, the judge, and the philosopher in the task of determining, diagnosing, and restoring "healthy" human behavior. Modern sensibility is preeminently a psychological sensibility. Given the volume of publications involved, the quality and innovativeness of the theories generated, the intensity of the debates aroused, and the number of cultural domains penetrated by these ideas, it is indeed appropriate to speak of a revolution in thought.[200]

Among the historians of our time, Henri Ellenberger has been alone in documenting this revolution. As mentioned earlier, a large quantity of the existing professional commentary about psychiatry and its history has been authored by either enemies or exegetes of individual psychological schools. Mired in the sectarian squabbles of its time, this literature has often succeeded valuably in organizing factual historical material. However, interpretively, time and again it has mainly served internecine ideological purposes. Ellenberger, it must be acknowledged, has not been wholly immune to these conflicts. But his reading has been sufficiently wide-ranging, his interests suitably catholic, and his theoretical and therapeutic allegiances eclectic enough that he has managed to achieve a broad, critical, *cultural* perspective on modern psychiatry. In the end, he has been able to write the history of psychiatry not simply as a defense of or attack on a single theory, figure, or school, or as a narrow disciplinary history. Rather, he has been able to conceptualize the subject as a study in modern cultural

---

[200] Many critics and historians have commented on this subject. For two well-known statements, see Philip Rieff, *Freud: The Mind of the Moralist* (Garden City, N.Y., Anchor, 1959), chap. 10, "The Emergence of Psychological Man"; and Martin L. Gross, *The Psychological Society: A Critical Analysis of Psychiatry, Psychotherapy, Psychoanalysis and the Psychological Revolution* (New York, Simon and Schuster, 1978).

and intellectual history. This, I believe, will emerge as Ellenberger's final identity, as the most intelligent and comprehensive chronicler to date of our psychological century. As professional scholars today explore the history of psychiatry and psychology with renewed interest and energy, and as the Institut Henri Ellenberger opens in Paris, it is well to recall the work of this remarkable man.

Part One _____

FREUD AND EARLY PSYCHOANALYSIS

1

Fechner and Freud

[1956]

THE GOAL of the present article is to attempt to define the ways in which G. T. Fechner, the nineteenth-century mystical philosopher and founder of experimental psychology, influenced Sigmund Freud, the empirical scientist and founder of psychoanalysis. In the course of the inquiry, we shall examine how Fechner's grandiose speculative ideas were utilized by Freud and integrated by him into the conceptual framework of psychoanalysis. In his *Autobiographical Study* of 1925, Freud in one place declared: "I was always open to the ideas of G. T. Fechner and have followed that thinker upon many important points."[1] Freud probably was introduced to Fechner's ideas when in high school in Vienna. He most likely then began systematically to read Fechner during the 1890s when studying dreams. At least he mentioned Fechner in 1898 in a letter to Wilhelm Fliess and quoted Fechner in the same connection two years later in *The Interpretation of Dreams*.[2] Freud also often referred in his writings to "the great Fechner" or more familiarly to "old Fechner."[3] Freud's increased interest in Fechner's theories is established in particular in his works *Jokes and Their Relation to the Unconscious* (1905) and *Beyond the Pleasure Principle* (1920).[4]

"Fechner and Freud," *Bulletin of the Menninger Clinic*, 20, no. 4 (July 1956), 201–14. The article also appeared in Japanese translation in *The Tokyo Journal of Psychoanalysis*, 15 (1957), 1–11.

[1] Sigmund Freud, *An Autobiographical Study* [1925], in *The Standard Edition of the Complete Psychological Works of Sigmund Freud*, translated from the German under the general editorship of James Strachey, 24 vols. (London, Hogarth Press, 1953–1974), 20:59.

[2] Sigmund Freud to Wilhelm Fliess, February 9, 1898, in *The Origins of Psychoanalysis: Letters to Wilhelm Fliess, Drafts and Notes: 1887–1902*, edited by Marie Bonaparte, Anna Freud, and Ernst Kris, translated by Eric Mosbacher and James Strachey (New York, Basic Books, 1954), 244. See also p. 376; *The Interpretation of Dreams*, in *Standard Edition*, 4:48.

[3] Freud, *Origins of Psychoanalysis*, 244; *Interpretation of Dreams*, in *Standard Edition*, 5:536.

[4] The influence of Fechner's theories on Freudian doctrine has previously been touched on by other scholars. See Imre Hermann, "Gustav Theodor Fechner," *Imago*, 2 (1925), 371–420; Siegfried Bernfeld, "Freud's Earliest Theories and the School of Helmholtz," *Psychoanalytic Quarterly*, 13 (1944), 341–62; Maria Dorer, *Historische Grundlagen der Psychoanalyse* (Leipzig, Felix Meiner, 1932); Rainer Spehlmann, *Sigmund Freuds neurologische Schriften* (Berlin, Springer, 1953); and Leopold Bellak and Rudolf Ekstein, "The Extension of

Fechner's Life and Personality

Gustav Theodor Fechner (1801–1887) was born in the village of Niederlausitz, Germany, where his father was a Protestant minister. He was the second of five children. At the age of 5 years, he lost his father, who died after a long sickness, a few days after the birth of his fifth child. The family was then dispersed and the young boy educated by an uncle, who was also a Protestant minister. At the age of 16, Gustav Theodor went to Leipzig, a town he did not leave for the next seventy years, that is, until his death in 1887. Why young Fechner decided to study medicine is not known. He was never interested in practicing it, and as soon as he received his medical diploma, he turned his interest toward experimental physics. In 1824, at the age of 23, Fechner was appointed as a lecturer in experimental physics at Leipzig University, where he started a series of experiments using the newly discovered laws of Ohm. This position was purely honorific, and to earn his living, Fechner worked for various scientific publishers. He did an enormous amount of work, translating texts of physics and chemistry from the French, compiling elementary textbooks for schools, and ghost-writing for a popular encyclopedia. He also published from time to time short literary pamphlets under the pseudonym of "Doktor Mises."

One of Fechner's earliest essays, *On the Comparative Anatomy of Angels* (1825), is particularly noteworthy.[5] Fechner alleged that the book was a joke, but admitted later that much of it had been written seriously. Under the cover of a fantasy, a mathematical way of thinking is applied to a problem of natural history: Fechner followed the curve of evolution of the animal kingdom from the amoeba to man and then, by extrapolation, attempted to construct the ideal form that a still higher being—an "angel"—should theoretically assume. He concluded that such futuristic beings must be spherical, that they must perceive universal gravitation in the same way human beings perceive light, and that they must communicate with each other by means of a language of luminous signs in the same way men converse with each other through an acoustic language. Eleven years later, in 1836, Fechner published under his own name a beautiful essay, *The Little Book of Life after Death*, in which a similar mode of thinking is applied.[6] Human life, Fechner now claimed, is divided into three periods: conception to birth, birth to death, and after death. Embry-

---

Basic Scientific Laws to Psychoanalysis and to Psychology," *Psychoanalytic Review*, 33 (1946), 306–13.

[5] Gustav Theodor Fechner (pseudo. Dr. Mises), *Vergleichende Anatomie der Engel: Eine Skizze* (Leipzig, Baumgartner, 1825). See also Fechner (Dr. Mises), *Räthselbüchlein* (Leipzig, G. Wigard, 1850).

[6] Fechner, *Das Büchlein vom Leben nach dem Tode* (Dresden, Grimmer, 1836).

onic life is a continuous sleep, present life is an oscillation between sleep and waking states, and life after death may be a continuous waking state.

In this same period of Fechner's life, two features deserve to be mentioned. One is his long and intimate friendship with a certain Martin Gottlieb Schulze, a man more remarkable for his brilliant ideas and poetical talent than for his character. The other is Fechner's three-month stay in Paris in 1827. Thanks to a scholarship, he was able to work with the famous French chemists Biot and Thénard and the physicist Arago. One of the results of his trip was his translations into German of the works of Biot and Thénard.

In 1833, at the age of 32, Fechner married Clara Volkmann after three years of engagement. Soon afterward, in 1834, he was urged by members of the faculty of Leipzig University to apply for the post of professor of physics there. Fechner reluctantly did so and was accepted. However, this seemingly happy event proved to be an instance of what Freud later called *Scheitern am Erfolg*, or "those who are wrecked by success." As one of his biographers wrote of Fechner: "From the instant he attained an independent position which would leave him freedom for his own work . . . his strength was broken. His excessive work had exhausted him. He had trouble finishing his lectures."[7]

This painful situation lasted for six years, from 1834 to 1840. During this period, while continuing research in the fields of physics and chemistry, the focus of Fechner's interest shifted toward experimental psychology. Fechner performed on himself observations and experiments on "postimages," on the perception of complementary colors, and on other subjective visual phenomena. These experiments resulted in a considerable strain on his eyes—possibly even a lesion of the retina from looking directly into the sun. The suffering from his eyes became intolerable, and in 1840, at the age of 39, Fechner collapsed emotionally and had to give up entirely his professional activity for three years.

An interesting account written by Fechner during this period, and fragments of his diary written at this time, were published in 1892 by his first biographer, Johannes Kuntze.[8] Fechner's illness might be diagnosed in modern psychiatric terminology as a severe neurotic depression with hypochondriacal symptoms. The real nature of the eye condition is not known, but during most of that time Fechner felt compelled to live in complete

[7] Wilhelm Wundt, *Gustav Theodor Fechner: Rede Zur Feier seines hundertjährigen Geburtstages* (Leipzig, W. Engelmann, 1901).

[8] Johannes E. Kuntze, *Gustav Theodor Fechner (Dr. Mises): Ein Deutsches Gelehrtenleben* (Leipzig, Breitkopf & Härtel, 1892). For other biographical statements, consult Kund Lasswitz, *Gustav Theodor Fechner* (Stuttgart, Fromanns, 1902), and Edwin G. Boring, *A History of Experimental Psychology* (New York, D. Appleton-Century, 1950), 265–87.

seclusion, remaining in a dark room or wearing a paper mask over his face. The walls of his rooms were painted black so as to minimize light stimuli. His mind, however, was not inactive, and in order to exercise it, he composed riddles and poems. Finally, in 1843, Fechner was able to open his eyes and to look at the light again. His ultimate recovery was ascribed by Wilhelm Wundt to the effect of autosuggestion.

This three-year period of depression was followed by a shorter one of elation. For a few months, Fechner expressed strange ideas of self-grandeur. He felt as if he had been chosen by God and that he was now able to solve all the mysteries of the world. He enjoyed an increased feeling of well-being and invulnerability. All this culminated in Fechner's conviction that he had discovered a universal principle, as basic for the spiritual world as Newton's principle of gravitation was for the physical world. Fechner called his discovery "*das Lustprinzip*—the principle of pleasure." This is a striking instance of what V. von Weizsäcker called a "logophania," or the metamorphosis of a bodily condition into an intellectual concept. In this instance, Fechner's hypomanic euphoria was transformed into a philosophical concept.

After this dramatic recovery, Fechner resigned as professor of physics at Leipzig University; however, he remained on the faculty but now as a professor of philosophy. Fechner's first course of lectures in this capacity was devoted to expounding his new pleasure principle, which also formed the basis of a new book, *On the Highest Good*, published in 1846.[9] After this date, and almost until the time of his death, Fechner never ceased to develop this concept and to apply it to new fields of knowledge.

During the second half of his life, not only was the physicist transformed into a philosopher but the feverish activity of the compiler gave way to calm elaboration of well-organized and highly original monographs and treatises. Fechner proved that, if he could discuss technical problems in a dry, matter-of-fact way, he could also be a master of German style. Many pages of his philosophical works are remarkable for their lyric beauty. In 1848, Fechner published *Nanna, or the Soul of Plants*, the first monograph in the history of Western science on the psychology of plants.[10] Three years later came his *Zend-Avesta*, a magnificent exposition of his own system of "philosophy of nature."[11] But by the time the book appeared, Fechner's mind was already working in yet another direction.

For many years, Fechner had been preoccupied with the relationship between the physical and the spiritual worlds. He felt that there must be a general law governing this relationship, and he strove to determine which mathematical formula would be the most probable for such a law. As he

[9] Fechner, *Über das höchste Gut* (Leipzig, Breitkopf & Härtel, 1846).

[10] Fechner, *Nanna oder über das Seelenleben der Pflanzen* (Leipzig, Voss, 1848).

[11] Fechner, *Zendavesta, oder über die Dinge des Himmels und des Jenseits* (Leipzig, Voss, 1851).

himself later related, the mathematical formula which he called the "psychophysical law" occurred to him suddenly, on the morning of October 22, 1850. After the "pleasure principle," this was the second great scientific intuition experienced by Fechner. He mentioned it briefly in *Zend-Avesta* the following year, and he devised a long series of experiments to discover whether this law was true. In the course of these experiments, Fechner elaborated several new principles, including the "differential threshold" and the "parallel law." Finally, in 1860, the findings of almost ten years of his work on these subjects were published in the two volumes of his magnum opus, *Elemente der Psychophysik*, or *Psychophysics*.[12] This work, nothing short of a milestone in the history of psychology, aroused considerable interest and was the starting point of modern experimental psychology. However, it would be erroneous to consider Fechner's *Psychophysics* a textbook of experimental psychology in the modern sense. A good part of it is devoted to "inner psychophysics" and is more metaphysical than psychological.

Among Fechner's later works was his criticism of Darwin's theory of the evolution of the species, titled *Some Ideas on the History of Creation and the Development of Organisms*.[13] Fechner's negative criticism of Darwinian evolutionary ideas was supplemented by the enunciation of his own, original concepts in the field. One of these concerned the "principle of the tendency to stability" or a universal, finalistic principle which Fechner proposed as complementary to the causal principle. After "the principle of pleasure" and the "psychophysical basic law," this was the third great universal principle enunciated by Fechner.

In 1876, at the age of 75, Fechner also published an important book on experimental aesthetics.[14] This was an attempt to base aesthetic theory on experimental research rather than deducing it from philosophical axioms. In this work, Fechner applied his earlier principle of pleasure–unpleasure to the theory of aesthetics and discussed also the psychology of wit and jokes. In 1879, he published an outline of his overall vision of the world, *Day Sight in Contrast to Night Sight*.[15] Fechner's own beautiful pantheistic vision of the world (the "day sight") is opposed to the dry, disconsolate conception of contemporary, materialistic scientism (the "night sight"). The same year, the first institute of experimental psychology was founded in Leipzig by Wundt.

In his last years, Fechner became interested in a new kind of research, the

---

[12] Fechner, *Elemente der Psychophysik* (Leipzig, Breitkopf & Härtel, 1860). See also Fechner, *Revision der Hauptpunkte der Psychophysik* (Leipzig, Breitkopf & Härtel, 1882).

[13] Fechner, *Einige Ideen zur Schöpfungs und Entwickelungsgeschichte der Organismen* (Leipzig, Breitkopf & Härtel, 1873).

[14] Fechner, *Vorschule der Äesthetik* (Leipzig, Breitkopf & Härtel, 1876).

[15] Fechner, *Die Tagesansicht gegenüber der Nachtansicht* (Leipzig, Breitkopf & Härtel, 1879).

experimental study of errors in measurements. His mind obviously had not lost the ability to search out new fields of activity. In spite of his inveterate suspicion of parapsychology, he had been persuaded at this time to attend meetings with the American medium "Slade." Fechner kept a diary of his observations of these meetings. Cautiously and reluctantly, he admitted that he had observed facts for which he could not think of any explanation by physical laws. When he died in 1887, at the age of 86 years, Fechner had won a belated fame as the father of experimental psychology. Leipzig, his adopted town, had become the center of this new science. Students came from all over the world to study the subject with Fechner's greatest follower, Wilhelm Wundt.

A Comparison between Fechner and Freud

In his 1901 biography of Fechner, Wundt ascribed to his master the following characteristics: a great gift for objective, methodical, scientific observation, which led him to develop the most appropriate means of investigation for each type of research; an acute capacity for sensory, particularly visual, observation, with an exquisite sensitivity to the world of light and colors; a deep religious feeling; and an absolutely unbiased and unprejudiced attitude in thinking.[16] "I am careful in believing and careful in not believing," declared Fechner. He was also absolutely serene in discussion and abstained from any kind of polemics.

A number of Wundt's characteristics of Fechner could also be ascribed to Freud, without much modification. Freud's gift for objective, methodical observation was surpassed only by his exquisite sensitivity and intuition for psychological manifestations. His earnest attitude toward the great enigmas of the universe amounted to Fechner's mystic feeling. Many other similarities could be added. Fechner and Freud were also men of absolute integrity, assiduous, and with a wide range of interests. Both wrote a great deal and were excellent stylists. Both were interested in art and discussed famous cultural works from the psychological point of view: Fechner the Madonna of Holbein, Freud the Moses of Michelangelo. Freud's interests, however, focused more on history and archeology, Fechner's on physical and natural sciences. Both were much concerned with the relation of body and mind.

Although Fechner's psychological crisis was much more severe, its similarities with Freud's "neurasthenia" during the 1890s are unmistakable. Not less striking is the attempt at self-healing, by means of autosuggestion with Fechner and of self-analysis with Freud. When the crisis was over, each

[16] Wundt, *Gustav Theodor Fechner.*

one was born to a new life. In both cases the crisis was connected with a great discovery: Freud had his historical "Irma dream" at the age of 39, Fechner his intuition of the pleasure principle at the age of 42. Both of these discoveries also resulted in a major creative work: for Fechner, *On the Highest Good*, at the age of 45; for Freud, *The Interpretation of Dreams*, at the age of 44. This turning point also brought a shift of scientific and professional interests—in Fechner from physics to philosophy and psychology, and in Freud from neurology to psychology and the study of the neuroses.

Fechner's Influence on Psychoanalysis

The preceding considerations explain in part why Fechner's influence on Freud, although indubitable, is very difficult to measure. When reading their works, one is often struck by similarities, not only in the content of thought, but in the style and in the way of thinking. To what extent is it a question, then, of the same culture, of similar personalities, of indirect influence, or of direct influence? Many similarities could be ascribed to the fact that Fechner and Freud had similar types of creative personality. In the life histories of many men of genius, one finds that they had only a period of one or two years of true inspiration and creative activity. In Fechner and Freud, however, there was a recurrence of such outbursts of inspiration and creativity. Each one of these periods of creativity resulted in the elaboration of a new system of thought, different from the preceding ones, but integrated into them so that the total construction became always more complex and comprehensive.

In this way, Freud elaborated first his "depth psychology" as a key for the deciphering of the unconscious operations of the mind; then a few years later, the theory of the libido, with its stages of development and its various vicissitudes; and still later his threefold system of ego–id–superego, with its manifold dynamic implications. Each one of these systems was integrated with the preceding one into the vast edifice of psychoanalysis. Fechner's system belonged to the same type of progressively growing construction and became a complex framework, whose study is fascinating but requires much time and thought.

Another feature common to Fechner and Freud was their propensity to enunciate "general principles" ruling the whole functioning of the mind (if not of the universe). Fechner propounded the pleasure–unpleasure principle, the "psychophysical basic law," the principle of stability, and several others. Freud took over from Fechner the pleasure–unpleasure principle, adding to it the principle of reality, the principle of repetition, and the principle of economy. This kind of approach was unknown to the classical faculty psychologists and to J. F. Herbart's dynamic associationism as well as to later psychological theorists. It is probable that Freud in this regard followed the example of Fechner, but it is doubtful whether he would have done so without a deep-seated affinity with Fechner.

It seems that when Fechner inaugurated his search for general principles, he was himself inspired by the example of the physicists of his generation in their formulation of the principle of the conservation of energy. However, it was not a physicist but a physician, Robert Mayer, who first formulated, in 1842, the principle of the conservation of energy as a universal law; it was a physicist-physician, Hermann von Helmholtz, who then developed the principle further, and finally another physicist-physician, Fechner, who introduced it into psychology. We will now consider at what points the influence of Fechner on Freud was the most certain and the most direct.

The Concept of Mental Energy

In his dynamic system of psychology, based on the assumption of ideal, purely psychological forces, Herbart computed the mathematical relations of these forces in their interplay and competition with each other. Fechner's approach was quite different. Fechner took as the starting point of his *Psychophysics* the principle of the conservation of energy. Energy exists in the universe under two aspects—potential and actual—and their sum in any closed system is constant.

Fechner contended that "psychophysical activity" is one among the various aspects of universal energy. Every human being is endowed with a certain quantity of physical energy, of which a part can be transformed into psychophysical energy. The nervous system is where this transformation, the mechanism of which is unknown, takes place. Potential energy can become psychophysical energy in two ways: under the effect of inner stimuli ("inner psychophysics"), or under the effect of external stimuli ("external psychophysics"). Fechner's experiments concerned only the latter, because only external stimuli, such as light, weight, or sound, can be measured. Fechner's "psychophysical basic law" is the mathematical formulation of the relation between stimulus and sensation. This law, however, is valid only within two limits: the "threshold" and the "summit." The threshold is the lower border of stimulus below which there would be no sensation, or below which, as Fechner put it, the "psychophysical movement" would be unconscious. The summit is the upper boundary of stimulus, beyond which an increase of sensation would be impossible. The sensation begins with the threshold value of the stimulus and its growth ceases at the summit of the stimulus. Between both limits, the intensity of the sensation increases with the intensity of the stimulus, according to a "psychophysical curve"; however, the increase of stimulus must reach a certain degree, the "threshold of distinction," in order to be noticeable. Fechner's experiments dealt chiefly with the threshold of sensation and with the threshold of distinction. He does not seem to have been much concerned with the summit, whereas Freud was very interested in what he called the *Reizschutz*, that is, the self-protection of the organism against excessive stimuli.

After Fechner, the concept of "mental energy" was adopted by many authors, and by the end of the nineteenth century it was quite common in European psychology and neuropsychiatry. In its various vicissitudes, three forms of the theory developed: (1) a properly "psychophysical" theory of mental energy, involving one specific form of physical energy and ruled by the same physical laws (in this respect, Wilhelm Ostwald remained closest to Fechner's original concept)[17]; (2) a neuropsychiatric theory, that is, an attempt to synthesize the concept of mental energy with the anatomy and physiology of the brain (Ernst Fleischl, Heinrich Sachs, and several other late-nineteenth-century German neurologists elaborated such theories)[18]; and (3) a purely psychological theory, postulating the existence of a "mental energy" of unknown nature and seeking to describe its manifestations without regard to its physical and physiological correlations (such were the theories of Pierre Janet and Carl Gustav Jung).[19]

Freud was for a time preoccupied with the establishment of a theory of the second type, reconciling the concept of energy, the theory of the neurone, and the data of normal psychology and of the neuroses. His "Project for a Scientific Psychology," which he wrote in 1895 and then sent to Fliess, is a curious attempt of this kind.[20] It was not long before Freud understood the artificial character of such constructions, and he did not retain brain anatomy and physiology in his later framework. Nevertheless, many theoretical discussions in *The Interpretation of Dreams*, and elsewhere, become more intelligible if one takes into consideration Freud's earlier attempts of this type and the whole background of Fechner's psychophysical theory.

The "Topographical" Concept of the Mind

While Freud was working on his book on dreams during the later 1890s, he complained in a letter to Fliess about the great deal of scientific literature he

[17] Wilhelm Ostwald, *Lebenslinien* (Berlin, Klasing, 1926).

[18] Ernst Fleischl, *Gesammelte Abhandlungen* (Leipzig, Barth, 1893); Heinrich Sachs, *Vorträge über Bau und Thätigkeit des Grosshirns und die Lehre von der Aphasie und Seelenblindheit für Aerzte und Studirende* (Breslau, Preuss & Junger, 1893).

[19] Pierre Janet, *La force et la faiblesse psychologique* (Paris, Maloine, 1932); C. G. Jung, *Über die Energetik der Seele* (Zurich, Rascher, 1928).

[20] Freud, "Project for a Scientific Psychology" [1895], reprinted in *Origins of Psychoanalysis*, 347–445.

was compelled to read. At one point he added that "the only sensible thing on the subject was said by old Fechner, in his sublime simplicity: that the psychical territory on which the dream process is played out is a different one. It has been left to me to draw a crude map of it."[21] In the first chapter of The Interpretation of Dreams, Freud quotes Fechner's assumption that "the scene of action [Schauplatz] of dreams is different from that of waking ideational life." He then remarks further that "it is not clear what Fechner had in mind in speaking of this change of location of mental activity," adding that it was not a matter of anatomical or physiological localization in the brain.[22] In the Introductory Lectures on Psychoanalysis (1916–1917), Freud declared of Fechner's Schauplatz that "though we do not understand this and do not know what to make of it, it does in fact reproduce the impression of strangeness which most dreams make on us."[23] And in his book Jokes and Their Relation to the Unconscious Freud extended the same spatial concept to wit.

Fechner had been led to this kind of formulation by his research on the so-called threshold of consciousness. He decided that the difference between the dream and the waking state could not be understood as the effect of a quantitative degree in the intensity of the psychological processes. The difference is too great, and one must admit, Fechner said, that mental activity is displayed alternatively on two "scenes." These two stages are close enough for the actors to go from one to the other. It might also happen that both theatricals play simultaneously, as occurs in a hallucinatory or somnambulic condition. Fechner added the following comparison: "In this way, a man may conduct a quite different kind of life in town than in the country, and when passing from one of his residences to the other he can always come back again to the same coherent way of life; but it would be impossible for him to change his way of life while staying in the same place. What is true for a man moving from one residence to the other is also true of the change of place within the psychophysical activity in man."[24] This spatial concept of Fechner must have been the more appealing for Freud because his own research led him to emphasize the radical difference between the conscious and the unconscious.

The Principle of Pleasure–Unpleasure

The Freudian principle of pleasure–unpleasure may be considered a late development of a very old concept, which under the name of hedonism

[21] Freud to Fliess, February 2, 1898, in Origins of Psychoanalysis, 244–45.
[22] Freud, Interpretation of Dreams, in Standard Edition, 4:48–49; 5:536.
[23] Freud, Introductory Lectures on Psychoanalysis, in Standard Edition, 15:90.
[24] Fechner, Elemente der Psychophysik, 2:515.

played an important role in the history of philosophy from Epicurus and Aristippus to Jeremy Bentham and Adam Smith. Psychological hedonism is the doctrine that all human acts are directed by the instinctive and permanent search for pleasure.

With Fechner, however, the hedonistic doctrine took a completely new form. At the end of his period of emotional illness, Fechner felt that he had discovered a general principle giving an explanation to psychological life as well as a sound basis for morals. He called it "the principle of pleasure." In his book *On the Supreme Good* (1846) and several subsequent articles, Fechner argued that the search for pleasure and the avoidance of unpleasantness was one basic drive of human conduct and activity.[25] The newborn baby already seeks its mother's breast, he noted, the first manifestation of this universal drive for pleasure.

At this point comes Fechner's most original contribution to pleasure theory: Fechner contended that man does not search for pleasure as it is in reality but for what in his conscious or unconscious experience is associated with the representation of pleasure. Inborn instinct, such as in the case of the newborn baby, plays a relatively small role. By far the most important determinant is what experience once taught us to be pleasure or unpleasure. If a certain object, or a certain form of activity, is constantly associated in an individual's experience with punishment or with any other kind of unpleasantness, this object or form of activity is avoided, while another individual will seek it if it has been associated with pleasure in his own experience. In this way the principle of pleasure finds its limits— reality on one side, the voice of conscience on the other. Conscience, Fechner added, is inborn in the rudimentary form of a moral instinct which needs to be developed; but, for the greatest part, conscience is the sum and result of thousands of pleasant or unpleasant associations resulting from the warnings, rewards, and punishments received by the individual in the course of his education. (In contemporary language, we would call it our "conditioning.") Fechner also developed a doctrine of moral hedonism, not unlike that of Bentham, but enlarged, since for Fechner the moral principle is to act in order to increase the sum total of pleasure in the whole universe, not only in mankind, as Bentham contended.

An amusing instance of parallelism between Fechner's and Freud's thinking is their answer to the same kind of objection. Fechner wrote: "Suppose that someone wishes to refute the principle that man acts in accordance with the principle of pleasure. This man will zealously do something that is supposed to be indifferent to him, or against his pleasure. But the observer

---

[25] Fechner, *Über das höchste Gut* (Leipzig, Breitkopf & Härtel, 1846); Fechner, "Über das Lustprinzip des Handelns," *Fichtes-Zeitschrift für Philosophie und philosophische Kritik*, 19 (1848), 1–30, 163–94.

will at once notice that this man only contradicts himself. For without his interest in the refutation, he would not have acted against his pleasure. His interest that this happens and the representation of his pleasure taken in that happening, are inseparable."[26] The psychoanalytic counterpart to this line of argument will be found in Freud's description of the "counter-wish dreams." Freud stated that some of his analysands had dreams in which a wish was overtly frustrated and that the same happened to readers of his book on dreams, in both cases just after they heard of his theory. In fact, Freud said, such counter-wish dreams simply fulfill these individuals' wish to contradict him.

After writing *On the Highest Good*, Fechner developed in many additional ways his theory of the pleasure–unpleasure principle. One important extension was its application to the field of aesthetics and to the psychology of humor.[27] It would be tempting to follow Fechner into that field and to show how much he inspired Freud. In his book *Jokes and Their Relation to the Unconscious*, Freud not only referred to Fechner's theory, but even quoted some of the riddles Fechner had composed during his emotional illness.[28]

The Principle of Constancy

About 1915, Freud revised and extended the formulations of his system of psychology. He declared that one may call metapsychology a formulation comprehending three points of view: dynamic, topographical, and economical. The *dynamic* metapsychological aspect concerns mental energy, the *topographical* aspect the conscious and unconscious, and the *economical* aspect the distribution of mental energy and its regulation through the pleasure–unpleasure principle. As we have seen, this concept of mental energy was derived more or less indirectly from Fechner while the topographical concept was taken over from Fechner directly as well as the pleasure–unpleasure principle. It is remarkable that Freud's *economical* point of view can also be traced back to Fechner!

At the beginning of *Beyond the Pleasure Principle* (1920), Freud connected the principle of pleasure–unpleasure and the "principle of constancy." His investigations led him to assume that the pleasure–unpleasure principle is ruled by the tendency to keep the quantity of stimulation of the mind as low as possible or at least as constant as possible. Freud added that

---

[26] Fechner, "Über das Lustprinzip des Handelns," 8.

[27] Fechner, *Vorschule der Ästhetik*.

[28] Freud, *Jokes and Their Relation to the Unconscious*, in *Standard Edition*, 8:67 n. 1. See also pp. 124, 135, 176.

he found a similar concept in Fechner's writings: Fechner had connected the pleasure–unpleasure principle with the "principle of the tendency to stability." As Freud remarked, the "principle of constancy" is thus one particular case of Fechner's more general "principle of the tendency to stability."[29]

According to Fechner, the first person to formulate that principle had been the German astronomer J.C.F. Zöllner, who applied it to a theory of the sunspots and of the movements of the comets.[30] Fechner was enthusiastic about this principle and adopted and enlarged it considerably. He was in search of a universal principle with which he could supplement the principle of causality in order to give a satisfactory explanation of the universe. Fechner's most general formulation of the principle was the following: "In any material system, abandoned to itself, there is a tendency of the parts to group themselves in a regular external form."[31] Fechner then distinguished three forms of stability:

1. *Absolute stability*, being a state of permanent immobility of the parts of a whole. This is, Fechner said, an extreme and ideal state which could only be reached if the total energy of the universe were degraded to its lowest possible form.

2. *Full stability*, when the parts of a whole are animated with movements that are completely regular to the extent that each part of the whole, at regular intervals, comes back to the same place with the same speed or the same variation of the speed.

3. *Approximate stability*, in which the parts of the whole have the *tendency* to come back, at regular intervals, to the same place with the same speed or the same variation of speed but do not reach perfect regularity in doing so. There are numerous degrees of approximate stability. Fechner said further that our solar system is an instance of a system endowed with approximate stability, not very far from full stability. Systems of more imperfectly approximate stability are shown in the living organisms, with their movements of the heart, the circulation of blood, and other rhythmic physiological activities.

After having defined the aspects of the principle of the tendency toward stability in the planets and in living organisms, Fechner applied the same principle to the human mind. Our mental activity, Fechner thought, displays itself in waves and oscillations, which show a tendency toward approximate stability. At this point, Fechner connects the principle of the tendency to stability and the principle of pleasure–unpleasure. Further-

[29] Freud, *Beyond the Pleasure Principle*, in *Standard Edition*, vol. 18, especially pp. 9, 62.

[30] J.C.F. Zöllner, *Berichte der math. phys. Cl. der Sächs. Soc. d. Wiss.* (1870), 338; (1871), 100. Source quoted by Fechner.

[31] Fechner, *Einige Ideen zur Schöpfungs und Entwickelungsgeschichte der Organismen.*

more, he distinguishes qualitative and quantitative dimensions of the pleasure–unpleasure principle. From the qualitative point of view, pleasure ensues when the waves and oscillations of the mind follow a certain pattern of regular stability with rhythmic movements, such as occurs when one is listening to harmonious music. From the quantitative point of view, pleasure results when psychological energy is directed in such a way that it brings the mind nearer to a state of approximate stability. Unpleasure occurs when the mental activity is directed in the opposite way, that is, brought away from a state of approximate stability. Another aspect of the quantitative point of view is that pleasure is proportional to the amount displayed in this kind of activity. In other words, the more energetic the movement toward a state of approximate stability, the greater the pleasure, and vice versa. These concepts were developed by Fechner and applied principally to his aesthetic theories.

Freud's discussions in *Beyond the Pleasure Principle* and in the 1924 essay "The Economic Problem of Masochism" become much more intelligible when one has in mind Fechner's theories. One of the main differences is that where Fechner wrote of the tendency of the mind to keep a state of approximate stability, Freud spoke of the tendency to keep an approximately constant level of stimulation. From Freud's point of view, pleasure occurs when excessive stimulation decreases and unpleasure when the level of stimulation is increased above certain limits. Moreover, Freud, unlike Fechner, was preoccupied with the *Reizschutz*, that is, the tendency of the organism to protect itself against the noxious effects of excessive stimulation. This difference shows that Freud conceived more clearly than Fechner the self-protective function of the principle of tendency to stability—in other words, he formulated a concept of what is today called "homeostasis."

The Principle of Repetition and the Death Instinct

In *Beyond the Pleasure Principle*, Freud introduced the concept of the "repetition compulsion."[32] In its more philosophical aspect, this principle was not particularly new. The observation of the movements of the stars led ancient Babylonian and Greek thinkers to the idea of an "eternal return" of all things, of "cyclic palingenesis." However, Fechner seems to have been the first to extend this principle specifically to the domain of psychology. The regular movement of the stars, the rhythmic activity of the heart and lungs, the alternation of sleep and waking, the function of pleasure and unpleasure—all these he put together as manifestations of "approximate

---

[32] Freud, *Beyond the Pleasure Principle*, in *Standard Edition*, 18:7–64.

stability." Another manifestation, according to Fechner, was that in its
ontogenesis an animal repeats the developmental stages of its ancestors.[33]
   Freud's idea that death is an instance of the compulsion to repeat, the
tendency of the organism to come back to its former lifeless state, diverges
significantly from Fechner's original concept. For Fechner, the principle of
repetition meant not death, but the overcoming of death. Fechner contended that there was, in the inanimate part of the universe, a tendency of
systems to go from a state of approximate stability to a state of absolute
stability. Living organisms, he said, are systems of approximate stability
while death is the transition from approximate to absolute stability. This is
the part of Fechner's theory that, apparently, inspired Freud's "Nirvana"
principle. However, there is an important difference between Fechner's and
Freud's points of view. For Fechner, this shifting from approximate to
absolute stability was characteristic only of the physical world. He obviously did not think of it as an instinct of living beings.

Conclusion

We have learned that, directly and indirectly, Freud received from Fechner
the inspiration for several fundamental theoretical parts of psychoanalysis,
and particularly the concept of mental energy, the "topographical" model,
and the principles of pleasure–unpleasure, of constancy, and of repetition.
However, there are at the same time great differences between Fechner's
and Freud's viewpoints. A large number of Fechner's concepts were based
on speculation for its own sake while Freud introduced such concepts in
psychoanalysis only when he needed conceptual tools. This might be compared with the destiny of the non-Euclidean geometries and the imaginary
numbers, which, after being purely plays of mathematical imagination,
later proved to be practically useful. Genius consists not only in creating
new ideas but also in giving previous ones new meaning and function.

[33] Fechner, *Einige Ideen zur Schöpfungs und Entwickelungsgeschichte der Organismen.*

2

Moritz Benedikt (1835–1920): An Insufficiently Appreciated Pioneer of Psychoanalysis

[1973]

THERE ARE at least two basic ways in which to conceptualize medical history, as well as the history of thought in general. One way is related to the theory of "great men." From time to time, this theory goes, a powerful genius arises in culture and brings fundamentally original ideas. Such a genius makes great discoveries, revolutionizes science. A second conceptualization derives from the Romantic notion of "the genius of the people." In this view, intellectual and cultural progress results from an accumulation of the ideas and discoveries of thousands of people over time. In the field of medicine, this means that a major role belongs to the work of a large number of obscure practitioners and patients.

However, a third approach to medical history might combine elements of these two approaches by stressing the contributions of the intermediate level of figures. Between the obscure practitioners of the past and the great individual geniuses, we find that there have existed in the past many intelligent and creative men who contributed significant new ideas but who, for different reasons, have remained in the historical shadows. The history of medicine has tended to ignore the role—indeed, at times the very existence—of people in this category. Yet these people often contributed to the revolutionary geniuses a decisive impulse. And at times, a theory of one of the revolutionary figures actually represents the elaboration of an idea or ideas borrowed from these unknown intermediate figures. In the present essay, I want to evoke the case of one such man, the Austrian physician Moritz Benedikt.[1] [. . .]

"Moritz Benedikt (1835–1920)," *Confrontations psychiatriques*, 11 (1973), 183–200.

[1] I am grateful to Professor Erna Lesky, director of the Institute of the History of Medicine at the University of Vienna, for having brought to my attention this important character. My study of Benedikt has been made much easier since the Institute of the History of Medicine in Vienna owns an almost complete collection of Benedikt's writings, including both his books and articles.

Who Was Moritz Benedikt?

It is surprising that historians of psychoanalysis have not suspected the important historical role that Moritz Benedikt played. Benedikt is in fact mentioned by Freud himself in a footnote at the bottom of a page in Freud's and Breuer's "Preliminary Communication" of 1893. We read there that "we have found the nearest approach to what we have to say on the theoretical and therapeutic sides of the question [of hysterical neuroses] in some remarks published from time to time by Benedikt. These we shall deal with elsewhere."[2]* (This comment, incidentally, was later noticed by the French psychologist Pierre Janet, who said that he regretted that he was unable to obtain copies of Benedikt's publications.) In the *Studies on Hysteria*, written by Freud and Breuer in 1895, Freud does not mention Benedikt. However, he is mentioned in the long third chapter of the book, written by Breuer and dedicated to the theoretical aspects of hysteria. In one passage, Breuer talks about the pathogenic conflict between the sexual impulses and the moral conscience of an individual as "a matter of everyday experience" which constitutes a source of psychological anxiety. A footnote at the bottom of the page reads: "Cf. on this point some interesting observations and comments by Benedikt in *Hypnotismus und Suggestion* (1894)."[3]

In Freud's writings, we find only one other short mention of Benedikt, in 1900, in *The Interpretation of Dreams*, concerning the psychology of daydreaming: "The part played in our mental life by these structures," Freud wrote there, "has not yet been fully recognized and elucidated by psychiatrists, although M. Benedikt has made what seems to me a very promising start in that direction."[4] In addition, we know, according to Ernest Jones, that Freud's personal correspondence mentions Benedikt at least twice. Jones, who had the opportunity to read Freud's personal letters to his fiancée, Martha Bernays, states that Freud was quite talented at describing people, and Jones mentions further that Benedikt was among the persons described by Freud.[5] We learn in another letter of Freud's to his fiancée that

*[*Editor's note*: This footnote accompanies the well-known formulation of Breuer and Freud that "hysterics suffer mainly from reminiscences."]

[2] Breuer and Freud, "Preliminary Communication" (1893), in Freud, *Studies on Hysteria*, in *The Standard Edition of the Complete Psychological Works of Sigmund Freud*, translated from the German under the general editorship of James Strachey (London: Hogarth Press, 1953–), 2:7 n. 3.

[3] Ibid., 210, 210 n. 1.

[4] Freud, *The Interpretation of Dreams*, in *Standard Edition*, 5:491.

[5] Ernest Jones, *The Life and Work of Sigmund Freud*, vol. 1, *The Formative Years and the Great Discoveries, 1856–1900* (New York: Basic Books, 1953), 100. Jones, however, provides no textual citation for Freud's description.

it was Benedikt who provided for Freud a letter of recommendation to Jean-Martin Charcot in Paris. Freud's letter about this matter, dated October 21, 1885, was recently published in an anthology of his correspondence. Freud says there that Charcot recognized Benedikt's handwriting even before opening the letter up. This detail confirms what Benedikt later recorded in his memoirs, about the close friendship between Charcot and himself.[6]

Within the abundant scholarly literature devoted to Freud, it is surprising to realize that there is almost no mention of Benedikt. Maria Dorer, in her study of the historical foundations of psychoanalysis (1932), has noted that Benedikt underlined the importance and the pathogenic role of the sexual instinct and its repression in the genesis of the neuroses.[7] In his biography of Freud, Jones mentions Benedikt several times. He speaks of him as one of the early promoters of the use of hypnotherapeutics in Vienna, and he relates two other incidents concerning Benedikt, but again, without providing sources. Also, in one of these passages, Jones states that Benedikt was a former student of the famous Professor Joseph Skoda and that when Benedikt began to teach, his first student was Ernst Brücke. This is an error. In fact, Brücke was sixteen years older than Benedikt, and it was rather the contrary, that Benedikt was among Brücke's first students in Vienna.[8] Jones also relates that when Hansen, the popular itinerant stage hypnotist, gave a public demonstration of hypnosis in Vienna, Benedikt asked Hansen if he had ever in his travels found a patient able to speak under hypnosis a language that the person did not know when awake. Hansen answered affirmatively, that he had indeed once heard in South Africa a British officer expressing himself under hypnosis in an unknown language. Benedikt then reportedly declared that this language must have been Welsh. The astonished Hansen admitted that this remark was true and asked him how he could have known this fact. Benedikt then answered, "I have the gift of communicating across great distances, and I can easily reach South Africa."[9] This same incident is related by Benedikt in his memoirs, but in a slightly different way. Benedikt reports there that he had noticed that a great part of what patients revealed under hypnosis referred back to their early childhood. Therefore, if a Briton spoke an unknown language, it was very likely Welsh, since Wales is the only part of Britain whose native people can speak an entirely "unknown language" in their childhood and completely forget it later in life.

The early psychoanalytic historian Ola Andersson seems to be the only scholar who has thus far given serious attention to the intellectual relation-

---

[6] Freud, *Briefe* (Frankfurt am Main, Gustav Fischer, 1960), 170.

[7] Maria Dorer, *Historische Grundlagen der Psychoanalyse* (Leipzig, Felix Meiner, 1932).

[8] Jones, *Life and Work of Sigmund Freud*, 1:251. See also p. 144.

[9] Ibid., 252.

ship between Benedikt and Freud. In his study of the prehistory of psychoanalysis, Andersson wrote:

> Moritz Benedikt's presentation of his therapeutic experiences in cases of hysteria
> includes the use of the whole range of therapeutic measures of the neuropathol-
> ogy of his day, but what was apparently of specific interest for Freud and Breuer
> in 1892 was the account of his attitude towards his patients and his often drastic
> psychological interventions. Benedikt stressed the importance for the therapist
> to intrude into the life history of his patients and to unveil secrets connected with
> the genesis of their disorders; and, in several of his clinical examples, the critical
> point of the treatment was such a procedure. What may have been of special
> significance for Freud was that Benedikt did not advocate the use of hypnotic
> suggestions and that he did not hesitate to deal with secrets belonging to the
> sexual sphere. On the contrary, he stressed the value of patients facing the
> unmasking of their secrets in a waking state.
>
> Benedikt's points of view are of special interest with regard to the development
> of Freud's ideas. As early as the end of 1892, Freud had, according to the case
> histories of "Miss Lucy R." and "Fräulein Elisabeth v. R." in *Studien über
> Hysterie*, made his first attempts to treat hysterical patients in the waking state,
> and his experiences in that connection would lead him to a consideration of the
> value of "moral courage" very similar to that expressed by Benedikt in 1889.[10]

This passage from Andersson's book can only stimulate our historical
curiosity about the life and work of Moritz Benedikt.

Moritz Benedikt's Life

Several key primary sources exist for biographical information about Benedikt. They include necrological articles published in Austrian medical
reviews after his death in 1920; descriptions by people who knew him,
especially that of Adolph Strümpell in his memoirs; Benedikt's autobiography, a little-known source that is of considerable interest and reveals a man
of literary talents; Benedikt's medical writings, which often contain personal details; and the excellent study by Erna Lesky of the history of the
Vienna School of Medicine in the nineteenth century, which includes several informative pages on Benedikt's life and work.[11] The best way to begin
is with Benedikt's autobiography, published in 1906, when he was 71 years
of age. It is the work of an old man, deeply disenchanted with his life and

---

[10] Ola Andersson, *Studies in the Prehistory of Psychoanalysis* (Stockholm, Norstedts,
1962), 115–16.
[11] Erna Lesky, *Die Wiener medizinische Schule im 19. Jahrhundert* (Cologne, Bohlaus,
1965), 390–93.

career, who talks about himself and about others with complete
openness.[12]

Moritz Benedikt was born on July 4, 1835. His father was a Jewish
retailer in the small town of Eisenstadt, in the province of Burgenland.
Benedikt's autobiography shows clearly that he experienced his childhood
and youth as years of dramatic change. In 1835, the year of his birth, the
Austrian monarchy still had a feudal and autocratic government in which
Jewish people exercised only limited rights. When Benedikt was 13, the
revolution of 1848 shook the foundations of the Austrian Empire. This was
followed by a temporary but very severe conservative political reaction. In
1852—Benedikt was 17 at the time—a long period of political liberalism
began. Jews now obtained equality of political rights, first unofficially
and then in 1867 officially. This period in Austrian history was also characterized by dramatic economic developments and by the rapid expansion of
public education. It was a time of political liberalism when anti-Semitism
was at a minimum for several decades. Romantic and nationalist sentiments were developing among certain German-speaking populations,
which spread to many minorities in the empire so that the government had
to deal with nationalist agitation from the Slavic and other minorities.
Toward the end of the century, however, widespread reactionary forces in
the political world and anti-Semitism reappeared. Benedikt was very interested in Austro-Hungarian public life. He was an ardent patriot, and he
thought that the government should give to the minorities a large linguistic
and cultural autonomy while preserving the cohesion of the old monarchy
through a reinforced devotion to the emperor. The military struggle of the
monarchy during the First World War, and its permanent collapse in 1918,
contributed to the deep disillusionment that Benedikt experienced later in
life.

As Benedikt himself relates it, the story of his life was a continuous
succession of scientific discoveries and professional disappointments. This
process seems to have started early, when Benedikt was in college. Benedikt
was very good at learning Latin; but his teacher refused to acknowledge
this. One day, the teacher gave a German text to be translated by the
students into Latin. The teacher had failed to notice that the text was a
German translation of a passage in Cicero. The young Benedikt simply
copied Cicero's text. Then when the professor began to criticize Benedikt's
Latin, Benedikt in return ridiculed him by producing Cicero's book from
which he had copied the original text.

This experience, we find, emerges as a leitmotif in Benedikt's life as told
by himself. In 1857, when he was 22 years old, Benedikt presented to the

[12] Moritz Benedikt, *Aus meinem Leben: Erinnerungen und Erörterungen* (Vienna, Carl
Konegen, Vienna, 1906).

Academy of Science in Vienna two lectures about discoveries he had just made in the field of physics; but he met with disillusionment. Benedikt claims that he had discovered a new law concerning electricity; but the same discovery was very shortly afterwards published by Siemens, who neglected to cite Benedikt and who was henceforth considered the author of the discovery. At this point in his career, one of Benedikt's mentors, Professor Johann Oppolzer, advised him to combine his talents for medicine and the physical sciences by devoting himself to the study and practice of medical electrotherapeutics. At the time, this was a new branch of medical science inspired above all by Remak's discoveries. Benedikt then proceeded to devote several years of research to medical electrotherapy while he continued to practice medicine. In 1868, he set down the results of his research in a book entitled *Electrotherapeutics*, which remained for a full generation a classic work in this field.[13]

I have not been able to determine the precise year when Benedikt became chief physician of the Vienna Polyclinic, that is, of the medical service for external consultations attached to the medical infirmary of the General Vienna Hospital. At this facility, Benedikt had occasion to examine and treat a large pool of patients afflicted with nervous disorders and diseases, including hysterics and other neurotic patients. Here, he became increasingly attracted to the study of the neuroses. In the 1870s, certain European physicians began to become interested in the study of hypnotism, which in part followed the demonstrations performed on the public stage by men such as Hansen and Donato. Benedikt was among those who tried to use this method to treat the neuroses. Paradoxically, Joseph Breuer, Freud's later coauthor, warned Benedikt against the use of hypnosis; but Benedikt claims that his skepticism on this score vanished after a discussion that he had about the matter with Charcot in 1878. We also know, according to Benedikt, that after an initial period of enthusiasm, he became disappointed with the therapeutic applications of hypnotism and soon abandoned it for other techniques. Later in his career, he came to the conclusion that most patients responding to hypnosis only pretended to be hypnotized in order to please the physician. From experiences such as these, Benedikt over time in fact became an outspoken opponent of the medical use of hypnotism.

Returning to Benedikt's autobiographical study, it is somewhat surprising to find the importance that Benedikt gives to other perceived professional injustices that he received during his lifetime. Benedikt claims, for instance, that he was the first physician to describe a certain specialized form of phobic behavior, which he termed *Platzschwindel*. However, shortly after this, Carl Westphal in Berlin described the same psychological

---

[13] Moritz Benedikt, *Elektrotherapie* (Vienna, Tender & Company, 1868).

syndrome under the name *Agoraphobie* and went on to gain all the credit
for it. Benedikt then started to study criminology. He measured the skulls
of many criminals; but he was soon imitated by Cesare Lombroso in Italy,
to whom is attributed the merit of founding the field of criminal anthropology. In neurology, Benedikt described a syndrome that is marked by hemi-
plegia and ocular paralysis on the opposite side of the body. Charcot in
Paris recognized the veracity and the value of this discovery and termed the
disorder "Benedikt's syndrome," a name that was widely employed in
French medical textbooks of the time. However, in Vienna, when one of
Benedikt's colleagues presented a case of this very same illness as extraordinary and unknown, Benedikt was compelled to inform his colleagues that,
everywhere except in Vienna, this disease was designated by the name
"Benedikt's syndrome."

Benedikt's autobiography presents still other instances of what the author considers the stupidity and insincerity of his professional peers. Benedikt complained bitterly about the city of Vienna and the Viennese
people. He believed that hatred of any kind of intellectual creativity or
superiority was a specific Viennese mentality. This was the reason, he
stated, that Mozart, Hayden, and Schubert had been discredited in Vienna
and the poet Franz Grillparzer had been persecuted and was recognized
only after his death. Yet it must be noted that Benedikt passed virtually his
entire life in Vienna, without ever considering moving elsewhere. Such an
attitude toward the city seems in fact to have been quite common among
the Viennese at the time. Herman Bahr, for instance, once wrote that "the
Viennese is a man who hates and despises all other Viennese, but cannot
live outside Vienna."

Another characteristic of Benedikt is the way in which he identified
himself in his autobiography with other figures who had been frustrated in
the history of science. He speaks, for instance, with deep indignation of the
injustices suffered by Ignaz Semmelweis, Duchenne de Boulogne, Karl
Rokitansky, and the Russian physiologist Cyon. I might add that Benedikt's autobiography presents a great deal of information about the
medical history of his day and that it contains memorable pictures of many
well-known Viennese physicians, such as the anatomist Hyrtl, the physiologist Brücke, and the pathologist Rokitansky.

At first glance, we would expect that his was a happy career: Benedikt
was a pioneer in clinical neurology, electrology, criminology, and psychiatry. He had a prominent teaching position at the University of Vienna as
well as a very lucrative private practice. He published many works, and
traveled extensively abroad, where he was widely considered one of Austria's most eminent physicians. He benefited from Charcot's admiration
and close friendship, and he paid Charcot a visit every year. Yet Benedikt's
memoirs reveal a frustrated man who nearly suffocated with resentment. It

is interesting to attempt to verify Benedikt's assertions about his career with information from other sources. The only detailed contemporary description of Benedikt that I know of is located in the autobiography of Adolph Strümpell, the German neurologist.[14] Strümpell was an intern in a number of Viennese hospitals in 1877–1878, and he paints a lively picture of the medical world of Vienna of that time. He describes many of its main figures, including Benedikt:

> Benedikt was undoubtedly gifted with extraordinary talents, almost those of the genius. Unfortunately, he lacked a methodical education as well as a capacity for self-criticism. This is why he could never exercise a lasting influence, in accord with his talents, on his own scientific field. Benedikt was the chief of the Neurology Service of the General Polyclinic in Vienna. His clinical demonstrations and explanations had the effect of fascinating his audiences, especially those of the young generation. Benedikt's narrow face, his eyes half-closed as he spoke, showed traces of passion and internal fights. He suffered from not being recognized by his colleagues and was looking for a substitute among his students. His lectures were always impressive because of the abundance of original ideas in them and for the seeming confidence of his judgments; but on close look, we were often led to doubt the accuracy of his assertions. Because Benedikt always practiced in outpatient medical services he missed the possibility for laboratory anatomical-pathological control. This is why he did not realize the inaccurate aspects of many of his diagnoses. . . .
>
> Therapeutically, Benedikt also lacked critical perspective. He considerably underestimated[15] the efficiency of his methods of galvanic treatment.
>
> During the following years, Benedikt had to face many trials from his family. When I came to visit him in Vienna in 1910, he was living as an old man, with one of his daughters, lonely and almost forgotten. His private practice, which had been quite large at one time, had disappeared little by little. He was in poor health and faced financial difficulties.[16]

Concerning the latter years of his life, we might add that Benedikt became interested in the so-called occult sciences, which he had earlier opposed strongly. At the time of his death in 1920, he was largely a forgotten figure. It is unfortunate that no one recorded Benedikt's thoughts about various events in medical history during his lifetime, including the rise of psychoanalysis.

We should also inquire as to why Benedikt felt that his colleagues rejected him. Two reasons appear most immediately. First, Benedikt, a man of multiple gifts, had been interested in many subjects, and he brought to

---

[14] Adolph Strümpell, *Aus dem Leben eines deutschen Klinikers* (Leipzig, Vogel, 1925).

[15] I translate here textually the world *unterschätzte*, but this is obviously a slip; the sentence should read not "underestimated" but "overestimated."

[16] Strümpell, *Aus dem Leben eines deutschen Klinikers*, 108–10.

each one a consistent contribution; but he never made a contribution of really first rank. Erna Lesky has shown that, in spite of the fact that he received a solid scientific training, and began his career brilliantly, Benedikt allowed himself to be carried away by his imagination. It is largely for this reason, it seems, that his colleagues had difficulty in taking him seriously. Secondly, Benedikt was excessively polemical. He not only answered sharply those who criticized him; but he made spiteful criticisms of other authors whose work he did not approve of. In 1894, for instance, Benedikt published a small book in which he violently attacked Richard von Krafft-Ebing for his practice of hypnosis. Benedikt was not content with the claim that Krafft-Ebing had been fooled by his patients. Rather, he attacked him personally, announcing that he was going to subject him to "psychological analysis," to dissect his personality into its basic elements and then reassemble it in order to make it intelligible.[17] Similarly, when Fliess published his theories about the correspondence between parts of the nasal fossae and the sexual organs, Benedikt ridiculed him in an article entitled "Die Nasen-Messiade," or "the messianic poem about the nose." There doubtlessly exist other reasons for Benedikt's lack of popularity in Vienna, and for these, we need to consider more closely the ethnic and familial background of Benedikt.

Benedikt's Ethnic and Familial Origins

Benedikt issued from a Jewish family in the province of Burgenland. In 1835, when he was born, the Jews living in Austria belonged to one of several distinct groups, whose political, social, economic, and cultural conditions differed from one another. The main categories were as follows: (1) a privileged group of "tolerated families" in Vienna who played a great role in the economic life of the country; (2) a second privileged category, also centered in Vienna, known as the "Israelite-Turkish" community. These were Jews speaking a Judeo-Spanish language, originally from Constantinople, who had for a long time been protected by the Sultan; (3) other relatively privileged communities, like the Jewish families of the little towns in the province of Burgenland, such as Eisenstadt and Kittsee; (4) Jews from the ghettos within cities, such as Presbourg (in Presbourg, some five thousand Jews were packed into long and narrow streets where most of them owned shops, some of them with considerable success; they submitted themselves to very strict religious obedience and lived according to the rules of harsh commercial competition); (5) Jews from Galicia living in small towns and in villages, who were quite numerous and who constituted

---

[17] Moritz Benedikt, *Hypnotismus und Suggestion* (Leipzig and Vienna, Breitstein, 1894).

strongly linked communities among themselves and with their Polish countrymen; and (6) Jewish refugees from Russia, on whom everyone else looked down.

The mentality of these Jews at the time was very different in each of these groups, and it is understandable that, after the Jewish emancipation and the 1848 revolution, these differences in outlook were maintained among their descendants. This means, then, that in studying the Jewish professional generation of the 1880s, it is necessary to take into consideration the original social and cultural community from which they emerged. We know, for example, that Benedikt Obersteiner, a medical professor and wealthy patron of the arts, came from one of the so-called privileged families of Vienna, that Jacob Moreno came from a Judeo-Spanish community, Benedikt and Adler from relatively privileged communities in the Burgenland, Bertha Pappenheim [the patient "Anna O."] from the Presbourg ghetto, and, finally, Freud from the Jews of Galicia. Interestingly, Benedikt, although his autobiography is full of remarks about the injustices he had to suffer at the hands of his academic colleagues and more generally of the Viennese, never once complained of being subjected to anti-Semitism.

Dr. Hans Beckh-Widmanstetter of Vienna, who was deeply informed about the history of the Vienna School of Medicine, informs me that Benedikt was a practicing Jew who had the responsibility for numerous religious functions in one of the local Vienna Jewish communities. Benedikt was the follower of a liberal rabbi, and he insisted on his fiancée's converting to Judaism. In Burgenland, approximately 300,000 Jews lived in the mid-1830s, when Benedikt was born there. In the large mosaic that constituted the Austro-Hungarian Empire at the time, the Burgenland was a small but important province. It constituted for a long time a kind of buffer state between Austria and Hungary. The Hungarian magnates who owned a large part of the territory there tended to be loyal to Austria, which was rare among the Hungarian nobility. Most of the population was German-speaking; but there were also some Croatian immigrants, many Hungarian gypsies, and some prosperous Jewish communities. The Burgenland Jews enjoyed a much more liberal environment than in other parts of the empire. Many of them were retailers, and they had links with Jewish communities both in Presbourg and Vienna. [. . .]

Benedikt's Theoretical Contribution to the Study of the Neuroses

Setting aside Benedikt's work in other fields, let us now consider his contributions to the study of the neuroses. As early as 1864, Benedikt rejected the idea that hysterical neuroses originated in a physical defect or infirmity of the genital organs, which was widely believed at the time.[18] On this point, Benedikt relied heavily on the teachings of Pierre Briquet, whose major study, *Traité clinique et thérapeutique de l'hystérie*, had been published five years earlier and brought a major change in thinking about hysteria. However, unlike Briquet, Benedikt believed that the causes of hysteria lay rather in some *functional* trouble of the sexual life.

Four years later, in 1868, Benedikt's influential handbook of electrotherapeutics included a forty-two-page chapter on hysterical disorders.[19] Benedikt attributed symptoms of hysteria to an abnormal disposition and to hypersensitivity of the nervous system, arising from premature psychological stimulation, especially of the sexual instinct, and to sexual frustration. Benedikt also cited four cases of male hysteria, which he attributed to poor treatment in childhood and to early troubles of the "libido," a term that Benedikt used several times in his writings. Benedikt did not believe that electrotherapy was effective in these cases, since the real cause of hysteria lay in troubles of the sexual life, which the patient tended to keep secret.

In 1889, Benedikt published another series of clinical observations that he had gathered for a lecture at an international congress in Paris.[20] The Austrian review in which these observations was published originally had only a limited circulation, so Benedikt later included these observations in his autobiography, where they are more easily accessible. These short case histories are of considerable interest. Benedikt reports, for instance, that he was once summoned to examine a young woman who suffered from intolerable headaches. It was feared to be a case of meningitis. Benedikt, however, did not discover any physical illness in the woman. He then took the patient aside and asked her to speak confidentially to him about any secret amorous attachments that she might have, but this was not the situation. Rather, the patient told him that she was suffering because her parents had recently taken her out of school, in spite of her burning desire to pursue her studies. Benedikt claimed that he would solve this problem with her parents, under the condition that she would get out of bed, dress, and then join the family for dinner. He explained to the parents how important this academic study was to their daughter, and they agreed immediately, so that when she came to dinner, her so-called meningitis had disappeared, and from then on she was cured.

In most other cases, the origin of the hysterical neurosis lay more complexly in a secret about the individual's sexual life. There was, for instance, the story of a married woman who, it was feared, was also suffering from a

[18] Moritz Benedikt, *Beobachtungen über Hysterie*, reprinted from *Zeitschrift für praktische Heilkunde* (1864).

[19] Benedikt, *Elektrotherapie*, 413–45.

[20] Moritz Benedikt, "Aus der Pariser Kongresszeit," *Internationale Klinische Rundschau*, 3 (1889), 1531–33, 1573–76, 1611–14, 1657–59, 1699–1703, 1858–60.

meningitis. In truth, her husband was impotent, and the woman had good reason to fear an illegitimate pregnancy. However, as soon as the gynecologist was able to reassure her that she was not pregnant, her "meningitis" disappeared.

In another case, Benedikt was called in consultation for a woman who had developed coughing fits all day long. The patient received Benedikt with the pronouncement, "Herr Professor, you will not cure me!" Benedikt understood that the woman suffered from some secret, and he advised the family doctor to do his best to discover it. The family doctor failed to find anything, and the cough persisted. The parents then brought the patient to Benedikt's office. Benedikt said to the young woman's mother that he had learned from experience that in such cases, women often were withholding a painful secret which they failed to reveal even to their parents. Had their daughter, perhaps, he inquired, been the victim of some sexual abuse in the past? At first the mother became indignant at this idea; but when she privately talked to her daughter, she learned that, when the girl had been 10, she had submitted many times to the sexual advances of a man that the family knew and whom she still happened to meet in social gatherings in Vienna. When Benedikt came back to visit the patient, she told him: "Now, doctor, you will cure me," and the cure was in fact quickly effected. Later, the woman married and led an apparently happy existence.

In a similar vein, Benedikt relates other cases of hysterical women who were cured by discussing openly their emotional and sexual secrets and by finding a solution to the problematic circumstance related to them. Among these patients, a number of supposedly paralyzed women regained their ability to walk. However, rather than claiming of these patients that their cases were purely psychogenic, Benedikt discussed their neuroses with them as physical illnesses that had disappeared after an adequate physical treatment.

In 1891, Benedikt again enunciated his ideas about hysterogenesis.[21] The disorder, he now argued, is rooted in an innate or acquired vulnerability of the nervous system; but its direct cause lies either in a psychological trauma (which can occur equally in the male or female) or in a functional abnormality of the genital system or in a difficulty of the sexual life which a patient, most often female, keeps secret, even from her parents and her physician. In this essay, Benedikt also asserts the uselessness of treatment by hypnosis and the necessity of administering treatment in a waking, conscious state.

Then in 1894, Benedikt published an important article about what he termed, in English, "the Second Life," which is to say the inner secret

---

[21] Moritz Benedikt, "Über Neuralgien und neuralgische Affectionen und deren Behandlung," *Klinische Zeit- und Streitfragen*, 6, no. 3 (1891), 67–106.

psychological life led by the healthy individual as well as the sick patient.[22] The "Second Life" consists in representations, imaginations, and mental ruminations, which the individual keeps to himself or herself. Certain individuals are more prone than others to an especially elaborate "Second Life," for example, persons who have not been recognized in their work by their peers, whose personality contrasts greatly with their environment, or who have been frustrated in their opportunity to develop their abilities. Benedikt describes several forms of this "Second Life." For instance, he speaks of eccentrics, gamblers, criminals—and neurasthenics. The "Second Life," Benedikt writes, is much more frequent among women than men. Women in contemporary society are submitted to a higher level of pressures for social conformity, and they are compelled to conceal more, emotionally and psychologically, than men. This is also the reason, Benedikt continues, that hysteria is more frequent among women than men. The inner psychological life is a field of the human mind which scientific men have not considered closely enough, concludes Benedikt, and yet which is of the utmost importance for psychotherapy. The first care of the therapist should be to explore this field, especially when confronted with a depressed or hysterical female patient.

In 1895, Benedikt inserted in a general treatise about the human psyche his article from the preceding year about the concept of the "Second Life."[23] He insisted on the fundamental role that the idea plays not only in the etiology of hysteria and the other neuroses but also in more serious mental illnesses as well as in some physical disorders. He emphasized here also the importance of unrequited love and of sexual difficulties in the psychogenesis of the neuroses, especially hysteria. Finally, in his autobiography of 1906, Benedikt returns to the theme of the inner life, where he clearly considers it to be one of his most significant contributions to psychological medicine. After a new account of his theories about the neuroses, he reviews a selection of the most important cases that he has treated throughout his medical career.[24] [. . .]

Benedikt's Role in the History of Dynamic Psychiatry

I will conclude with an attempt to assess the role that Benedikt played in the making of dynamic psychiatry as we know it today. During the last decades of the nineteenth century, a wave of professional interest in hypnosis spread across the European medical world. Moritz Benedikt was

[22] Moritz Benedikt, "Second Life: Das Seelenbinnenleben des gesunden und kranken Menschen," *Wiener Klinik*, 20 (1894), 127–38.

[23] Moritz Benedikt, *Die Seelenkünde des Menschen als reine Erfahrungs-Wissenschaft* (Leipzig, O. R. Reisland, 1895).

[24] Benedikt, *Aus meinem Leben*, 127–46.

among the first medical men to adopt hypnosis in a therapeutic setting. Interestingly, he was also among the first physicians to admit its weaknesses and then to condemn its use openly.

Benedikt was also among the first to underline the role played by the individual's inner psychological existence. The "Second Life," as he called it, is not restricted to the realm of daydreams. Rather, it corresponds to a life filled with disappointed ambitions, frustrated loves, and "pathogenic secrets" of all kinds. In fact, Benedikt seems to have been the first person to have introduced into the medical field, and in secular form, the very old notion of the pathogenic secret. He also insisted on the role played by the "Second Life" in neurosis, psychosis, and criminality. Benedikt was no doubt also a pioneer in the field of sexology, with his stress on the pernicious role played by repressed sexual tendencies in the pathogenesis of neurosis, and in particular hysteria.

Benedikt seems also to have been a master in the art of short-term psychotherapies. Across the nineteenth century, there appeared many different methods of psychotherapy (even though the word itself did not yet exist). Apart from hypnosis, suggestion, and the "Cure of Souls" practiced by religious people, some physicians practiced what was still loosely called the "moral treatment." These treatments, however, were not systematically taught. Benedikt improved these methods, adding to them the notion of the pathogenic secret and of the inner "Second Life." One can only wonder to what extent Benedikt, in his capacity as director of the neurology polyclinic in Vienna, taught these new techniques to his many students.

Equally, it is interesting to speculate on Benedikt's significance for both Freud and Adler. It is certain that Freud personally knew Benedikt, and we have already mentioned a number of citations of Benedikt in Freud's writings. As Andersson has indicated, one can perceive Benedikt's influence in Freud's insistence on the role played by the hidden inner life of the individual and in the roles of past traumatic events and of sexual secrets in the etiology of neurosis. Furthermore, as Andersson adds, it is very likely that Benedikt inspired Freud to explore directly his patients' innermost lives without the unreliable and roundabout method of hypnosis. No medical literature of the late nineteenth century resembles more closely the clinical essays and observations of Benedikt's than the case histories of Breuer and Freud in the *Studies on Hysteria*. In passing, it is interesting to note that Benedikt in his autobiography explicitly criticized Breuer and Freud for their theory of hysteria. Clearly, Benedikt did not believe that a traumatic event in the patient's life was unconsciously repressed. Similarly, Benedikt, as we have learned, was opposed by this time to the use of hypnotic sleep, in which he believed that the patient often simulated a hypnotic state in order to please the physician.[25]

---

[25] Benedikt, *Hypnotismus und Suggestion*, 64–65.

Benedikt's influence on Adler and Adlerian Individual Psychology is even more difficult to specify. The two men had one thing in common: both came from the Jewish communities of the Burgenland. Benedikt was born in Eisenstadt, while Adler's father was from the nearby village of Kittsee. It is unknown if the two families knew one another. According to Dr. Beckh-Widmanstetter, Adler received his doctorate in medicine at the University of Vienna on November 22, 1895, and then worked for a year in Benedikt's polyclinic. This very year, Benedikt delivered a series of lectures entitled "Selected Aspects of the Psychology of Nervous Patients and Mental Degenerates, with Special Attention to Craniology."

It is remarkable that, to my knowledge, Adler never mentioned the name of Benedikt or referred to his writings. Perhaps there existed some competition between the two families, or between the Jewish communities of Eisenstadt and Kittsee, or a tension between the two men regarding religion, since Benedikt always remained a practicing Jew while Adler converted to Protestantism. Whatever the case, Benedikt's influence is apparent in Adler's unwillingness to accept the idea of the unconscious, in his emphasis on short-term psychotherapies, in his idea of a "directing fiction" as the motor of a patient's life of illusions, and finally, what is very probable, in Adler's general therapeutic optimism. All in all, Adlerian psychotherapeutics may be better understood as a variant and refinement of Benedikt's psychotherapy than as a deformation of Freudian psychoanalysis.

It is my hope that these few notes will encourage historians of medicine to devote increasing attention to those many obscure and forgotten men, such as Moritz Benedikt, whose role in the history of science has so often been essential for the advancement of their scientific field.

3

Freud's Lecture on Masculine Hysteria (October 15, 1886): A Critical Study

[1968]

THIS ESSAY attempts to apply the standard critical-historical method of professional historiography to a particular episode in the history of psychoanalysis. I have chosen this particular event for examination in part because it is usually seen as the crucial starting point of a lifelong struggle between Sigmund Freud and the Viennese medical world in which he lived and in part because the episode proves relatively easy to study historically.[1]

The standard account of the event under inspection runs roughly as follows: after studying under Jean-Martin Charcot in Paris from October 1885 to February 1886, Freud returned to Vienna, highly enthusiastic about what he had observed and learned at the Salpêtrière Hospital. After his return, he delivered a lecture on the theme of male hysteria to the Vienna Society of Physicians, or the Gesellschaft der Ärzte, on the evening of October 15, 1886. Freud's presentation on this subject met with incredulity and hostility. After the lecture, Freud was challenged by his listeners to produce a case of masculine hysteria to the Society. Even though Freud produced such a case a month later, the animosity toward him and his ideas persisted, and his disagreement with professional colleagues in Vienna thereafter became irremediable.

A close critical-historical study of this well-known event should consider a number of points: What was the nature and history of the Vienna Society of Physicians as a scientific body? What was the state of the medical debate about male hysteria in European medicine in the late nineteenth century? What is actually known to have occurred during this famous meeting of October 15, 1886? How can the ascertainable facts about the meeting be interpreted? And what were the consequences, both immediate and long-term, of this experience for Freud?

"La conférence de Freud sur l'hystérie masculine (15 octobre 1886): Étude critique," *L'information psychiatrique*, 44, no. 10 (1968), 921–29; "La conferenza di Freud sull'isteria maschile, 15 octobre 1886," in Ellenberger, *I movimenti di liberazione mitica* (Naples, Liguori, 1986), 131–47.

[1] For their assistance in my research on this topic, I am indebted to Professor Erna Lesky, director of the Institute of the History of Medicine in Vienna, and to Dr. Erich Menninger-Lerchenthal, also of Vienna.

The Vienna Society of Physicians

In 1886, several medical societies, specialized and general, existed in Vienna. Freud delivered his lecture in front of the most famous of these societies, whose full and official name was the Imperial Society of Viennese Physicians—Kaiserliche Gesellschaft der Ärzte zu Wien. This was easily among the best-known medical societies in Europe, its fame being, for example, in no way inferior to the Royal Society of Medicine in London. A number of features characterized the Society in the late nineteenth century.[2] First of all, the organization maintained a strong interest in public health issues, such as the struggle against epidemics of infectious diseases and the debate about canalization. Second, the Society tried to maintain in every branch of medical debate the highest scientific standards, and indeed, an impressive number of discoveries were first announced at the Society.[3] For instance, it was at the Vienna Society of Physicians in 1853 that Wilhelm Czermak demonstrated for the first time the laryngoscope which had been discovered three years earlier by Ludwig Türch. On May 15, 1850, Ignaz Semmelweis proclaimed his discovery that puerperal infection at the hospital's maternity ward came from the nearby autopsy rooms of the hospital. And in 1869, Maximilian Nitze and Josef Leiter demonstrated their new cystoscope in front of this same body. In October 1884, that is, just two years before Freud's lecture there, Leopold Königstein and Karl Koller had announced in front of the Society their discovery that the drug cocaine could be employed as a local anesthetic in ocular surgery. Another characteristic of meetings at the Vienna Society of Physicians was that anyone was entitled to present their findings to the group provided that this information represented new scientific work. Further, while the members of the Society always acted with courtesy and dignity, they regularly subjected the evening presentations to rigorous criticism. As an illustration of this last point, the surgeon Burghard Breitner relates in his autobiography that once when he gave a talk to the Society, Julius Wagner-Jauregg "smashed him like a fly on the wall."[4]

Meetings at the Society of Physicians were held weekly, on Friday evenings, at the Academy of Science building. The tone of each event was

[2] Erna Lesky, *Die Wiener medizinische Schule im 19. Jahrhundert* (Graz, Böhlau, 1965); idem, "Neues zur Geschichte der Ärzte in Wien," *Wiener klinische Wochenschrift*, 115 (1953), 944–48; Erich Menninger-Lerchenthal, "Jubiläum der Gesellschaft der Ärzte in Wien," *Österreichische Ärztezeitung* (1964); Isidor Fischer, *Geschichte der Gesellschaft der Ärzte in Wien* (Vienna, Springer, 1938).

[3] A long list of these scientific "firsts" at the Society has been assembled by Erna Lesky in "Medizinische Pioneertaten, mitgeteilt in der Gesellschaft der Ärzte," *Wiener klinische Wochenschrift*, 75 (1963), 534–36.

[4] Burghard Breitner, *Hand an zwei Pflügen* (Innsbruck, Inn-Verlag, n.d.), 222–24.

formal. Discussions following each presentation were recorded by a secretary, or *Schriftführer*, and were then printed in the Society bulletin, a biweekly publication. In addition, numerous medical journalists attended the meetings and published reports about them in their respective medical periodicals in Austria and elsewhere. In other words, when Freud spoke about masculine hysteria in the autumn of 1886, he was lecturing in front of a medical audience of a high professional standard, which was open to new scientific findings, but which had a tradition of close, vigorous critical evaluation.

The Theme of Freud's Lecture: Masculine Hysteria

It is impossible to understand the meeting at the Vienna Society of Physicians on the evening of October 15, 1886, without a clear definition of the concept of "male hysteria" as it existed at the time in European medicine. The discussion among physicians on this subject that evening was in fact part of a much wider controversy taking place in the field of neurology for several years in Germany, Austria, France, Britain, and the United States.

During the previous decade, a great increase had taken place in railway travel. This in turn had brought a steady rise in the number of railway accidents and in insurance company claims for such accidents, both in Europe and in America. As a result, a new branch of medicine developed. The major figures in this new development were British physicians, such as Herbert Page, who concentrated in their work on the distinction between the syndromes of "nervous shock" and "traumatic shock" and between "railway spine" and "railway brain." Page asserted that a notable proportion of cases of "railway spine" were less the result of structural lesions of the nervous system than of functional troubles, which he qualified as "hysterical" in nature. Proof of this, Page said, rested in the fact that many such patients often also exhibited sensory hemianesthesias as well as other symptoms widely regarded as stigmati of hysterical disorders.[5]

Generally speaking, French and German physicians at the time tended to adopt the British terminology for these cases. However, Page's assertions provoked widespread and sharp discussion among neurologists on two issues: the comparative frequency of "organic" and "dynamic" (i.e., "functional") causation in these cases; and the propriety of equating "dynamic" and nonorganic troubles with the disease of hysteria. For insurance companies involved in these cases, for the new medical experts providing

---

[5] Herbert Page, *Injuries of the Spine and Spinal Cord without Apparent Mechanical Lesions and Nervous Shock* (London, Churchill, 1883).

forensic testimony about them, and of course for the patients involved, these issues had great practical importance.

Not surprisingly, Page's opinions prevailed in the British medical community, and in the United States, his ideas were defended by G. L. Walton and James Putnam, among others.[6] However, in Germany, this line of thinking met strong opposition. Above all, two eminent neurologists, Robert Thomsen and Hermann Oppenheim, objected that the presence of hemianesthesia was inadequate proof of hysterical neurosis, because the symptom could be observed in many other illnesses as well. Furthermore, Thomsen and Oppenheim found that hemianesthesias tended to be graver in cases involving so-called railway spine than in those of genuine hysteria. The nervous breakdown was deeper, and the illness was more resistant to treatment. Thomsen and Oppenheim, then, considered the nonorganic instances of "railway spine" to be cases of what they termed "traumatic neurosis" rather than of hysteria.[7]

In France, Charcot had adopted yet another point of view on the matter. He denied altogether the existence of Thomsen's and Oppenheim's new category of "traumatic neurosis." He agreed that the nonorganic cases of railway spine exhibited certain clinical peculiarities described by the German school, including accentuated hemianesthesias, the existence of a severe nervous or mental breakdown, and therapeutic recalcitrance. Nonetheless, Charcot asserted that these cases still represented forms of hysteria, and he believed that he had found irrefutable proof of this fact. The traumatic paralyses found in many of these cases revealed a symptomatology identical to those that could be produced experimentally under hypnosis. At least one important consequence resulted from Charcot's interpretation of these cases. Because many of these injured nervous victims were men, the diagnosis of "male hysteria," previously attributed only very rarely to men with the classical symptoms of convulsive hysteria, was now extended to males with post-traumatic functional troubles. In this way, the frequency of male hysteria, or at any rate the diagnosis of male hysteria, increased dramatically in France. In Paris during the late nineteenth century, then, there existed two primary forms of hysteria in the male: the "classical" form of the disorder, in which heredity was considered the main etiological

[6] G. L. Walton, "Case of Typical Hysterical Hemianesthesia in a Man Following Injury," *Archives of Medicine*, 10 (1883), 88–95; idem, "Case of Hysterical Hemianesthesia, Convulsions and Motor Paralysis Brought On by a Fall," *Boston Medical and Surgical Journal*, 3 (1884), 558–59; James J. Putnam, "Recent Investigations into the Pathology of So-Called Concussion of the Spine," *Boston Medical and Surgical Journal*, 109 (1883), 217–20.

[7] R. Thomsen and H. Oppenheim, "Über das Vorkommen und die Bedeutung der sensorischen Anästhesie bei Erkrankungen des Zentralen Nervensystems," *Archiv für Psychiatrie*, 15 (1884), 559–83, 633–80, especially pp. 656–67.

factor; and the new "post-traumatic" variety, in which environmental trauma rather than heredity played the most important part.

In the contemporaneous Viennese medical world, few physicians doubted the existence of "classical" male hysteria, and it is absolutely wrong to suggest that Meynert, for instance, denied its existence outright. Precisely one month before the meeting of October 15, 1886, in fact, one of Meynert's students, A. V. Luzenberger, had published in a local medical journal a case found in Meynert's own medical wards of this variety of hysteria in a male patient.[8] Luzenberger had published the case not because he considered male hysteria exceptional but because the patient in question presented a particularly rare hysterical symptom.

To sum up, then, it is important to take into account a number of facts in order to analyze properly the discussion that followed Freud's lecture. In German and Austrian medicine during the late nineteenth century, "male hysteria" connoted two quite different things: "classical" male hysteria, which was commonly acknowledged by this time, and Charcot's new notion of "traumatic" male hysteria, which in contrast was sharply contested among neurologists. Furthermore, discussions about traumatic male hysteria constitute one of the aspects of a wider controversy raging at the time about the correct interpretation and the consequences of railway accidents, a controversy that had direct practical interests for a number of groups of people besides physicians.

The Meeting of October 15, 1886

Unfortunately, we do not possess the original text of Freud's lecture to the Vienna Society of Physicians.[9] Therefore, any critical analysis of what occurred that evening should rely on documents as close as possible to the event itself. In this regard, we have the official summary of Freud's lecture as well as of the discussion that followed. These were recorded by the Society's secretary and were published in the monthly bulletin of the Society.[10]

---

[8] A. V. Luzenberger, "Über einen Fall von Dyschromatopsie bei einem hysterischen Manne," *Wiener medizinische Blätter*, 9 (September 16, 1886), cols. 1113–26.

[9] It is likely that the text of the lecture was similar in content to the account of his stay at Charcot's hospital that Freud submitted to the *Professoren-Collegium* of the Faculty of Medicine after his return from Paris to Vienna. This document has been published in Josef Gicklhorn and Renée Gicklhorn, *Sigmund Freuds akademische Laufbahn im Lichte der Dokumente* (Vienna and Innsbruck, Urban & Schwarzenberg, 1960), 82–89.

[10] *Anzeiger der k. k. Gesellschaft der Ärzte in Wien*, no. 25 (1886), 149–52. I am very grateful to Dr. Erich Menninger-Lerchenthal, who provided me with a copy of the pages of this nearly unobtainable publication.

Furthermore, accounts of the event were also written independently from one another by at least five other medical journalists at the time.[11] One of these accounts was taken by the future novelist and playwright Arthur Schnitzler.[12] Although a comparison of these accounts still does not allow a reconstitution of the atmosphere of the meeting that evening, it at least offers a rendering of the contents of Freud's lecture and of the arguments put forward by the auditors during the discussion period.

According to these documents, the meeting opened with the president of the Society, Professor Heinrich von Bamberger. Bamberger first allowed a local otorhinolaryngologist, Dr. Michael Grossmann, to speak. Grossmann gave a short clinical demonstration of a case of larynx and palate lupus. After this prelude there came Freud's presentation, which seems to have taken up the largest part of the meeting that evening. Freud began by explaining that he had recently spent several months in Paris with Charcot. He then presented the basic Charcotian theories of hysteria. Charcot, Freud stated, made a distinction between "major hysteria," which was characterized by a specific type of epileptiform convulsion, sensory hemianesthesias, and diverse other stigmata, and "minor hysteria." Charcot, Freud added, had the merit of showing that hysterical persons were not simulators, as had so long been believed, that hysteria did not result from a disease of the genital organs, and that male hysteria was much more frequent than generally admitted. Freud then went on to describe in the body of his lecture a case of male hysteria that he had observed in one of Charcot's clinical demonstrations. This case involved a young man who, after an accident in the workplace, suffered from a paralysis of one of the arms as well as from a series of stigmata. Using this case and others that were similar to it, Charcot, according to Freud's account, classified most cases of "railway spine" and "railway brain" as hysterical in origin, diagnoses with which Freud agreed.

Professor Moritz Rosenthal, a neurologist, opened the general discussion following Freud's presentation. Rosenthal noted at the outset that male hysteria was by no means rare. In fact, sixteen years before, he stated, he had published two cases of the disorder.[13] Next, Professor Meynert

[11] These accounts appeared in the *Allgemeine Wiener medizinische Zeitung*, 31 (1886), 505–7; *Wiener medizinische Wochenschrift*, 36 (1886), 768; *Münchener medizinische Wochenschrift*, 33 (1886), 768; *Wiener medizinische Presse*, 27 (1886), 1407–9; and *Wiener medizinische Blätter*, 9 (1886), cols. 1292–93.

[12] Arthur Schnitzler, who at this time worked as a young physician with a strong interest in neuropsychiatric medicine, contributed the report that appeared in the *Wiener medizinische Presse*, a periodical that was published by his father, the well-known laryngologist Johann Schnitzler.

[13] See Moritz Rosenthal, *Klinik der Nervenkrankheiten* [1870], 2d ed. (Stuttgart, Enke, 1875), 466–67.

declared that he had often observed cases of epileptic convulsions accompanied by a disturbed consciousness resulting from physical trauma. Meynert commented that it would be interesting to verify whether or not these cases would always present the symptoms just described by Freud. Bamberger then said that he respected Charcot greatly but that he did not see anything new in Freud's presentation. He also questioned Charcot's distinction between "major" and "minor" hysterias. As for male hysteria in particular, it was a well-known affliction. On the basis of his own observations, Bamberger dissented from the idea of assimilating "railway spine" to male hysteria in spite of the acknowledged similarities in the clinical picture. Following this, Professor Leidesdorf mentioned that he often examined patients who, following a train accident or some other form of physical trauma, exhibited organic symptoms that had nothing in common with hysteria. He was not denying that certain cases occurred in which hysterical symptoms formed subsequent to a trauma; but he said that one should not conclude hastily that hysteria was a direct consequence of the trauma, because at this state it was still impossible to evaluate the extent and significance of a possible structural lesion.

After Freud's lecture and the discussion about it, a Professor Latschenberger spoke about the presence of biliary pigments in the tissues and about the action of the humors in certain severe animal diseases. Professor Bamberger also lodged some strong criticisms of Latschenberger's assertions, and the meeting thereupon came to a close.

We might complete our brief account of the meeting by observing that none of the six accounts of the lecture and discussion that evening indicate any hostile words directed at Freud. Also, Ernest Jones, in his influential account of this episode, notes, it is true, that the report of the presentation in the official Society records "does not depict the coldness of the reception" later described by Freud; however, Jones fails to mention that a critical reception was typical at the Society and that Latschenberger, following Freud, despite his status as a full titled professor, was not treated any less critically than Freud.[14] Moreover, none of the six accounts examined mentions that Meynert defied Freud or challenged him to produce a case of hysteria in a male.

Interpretation of the Lecture and the Discussion

Moving now from the historical facts as they are known to us to questions of interpretation, how is it, we should ask, that Freud believed that his

---

[14] Ernest Jones, *Sigmund Freud: Life and Work*, 3 vols. (London, Hogarth Press, 1953), 1:253.

performance at the October 15, 1886, meeting was received with belligerence and rejection? First, we should consider, and eliminate, three possible explanations, namely, personal animosity toward Freud, anti-Semitism, and hostility toward Charcot. As for the first point, let us remember that Bamberger was a member of the committee that had granted Freud his fellowship to study abroad the year before.[15] Similarly, Meynert had been Freud's mentor for a year and had even offered to have Freud take over a class of his in his place. Also, in 1885 Freud had served as a temporary substitute physician for three weeks in Leidesdorf's private clinic.[16] The accusation of anti-Semitism is equally untenable, since three out of Freud's four critics at the meeting—Rosenthal, Leidesdorf, and Bamberger—were themselves Jews.[17] Finally, the idea that the Viennese neurological community was hostile to Charcot is erroneous as well. Charcot was in fact very popular in Vienna at this time. Benedikt for one used to visit him every year. Contrary to Jones's assertion, Meynert had an excellent professional relationship with Charcot, even though the two men disagreed on the identification of traumatic paralysis with male hysteria.[18] Leidesdorf was also on good personal and professional terms with Charcot.[19]

It appears more likely that there occurred a fundamental misunderstanding between Freud and his contradictors at the meeting both about the subject of Freud's presentation and about the nature of the critical discussion that followed it. Clearly, the debate at the Society that evening was not about the existence or nonexistence of male hysteria. The purpose of the discussion was rather to debate the question of whether or not male hysteria was to be assimilated clinically with the concept of traumatic neurosis. No one in Vienna at this time rejected the idea that "classical" hysteria could occur in male patients. Of the four specialists who spoke at the meeting, two of them, in fact (Rosenthal and Bamberger), expressly asserted that male hysteria was a well-known phenomenon. A third member, Leidesdorf, talked about it as a common notion. As for Meynert, he necessarily shared the same opinion, since, as mentioned earlier, a case of hysteria in a male patient from his own service had been published only a month earlier under his auspices.

Rather, from the perspective of the neurologists in the Society in 1886, Freud's presentation had a different meaning: giving voice to Charcot's doctrines, Freud had entered into a complex and very controversial issue

[15] Gicklhorn and Gicklhorn, *Sigmund Freuds akademische Laufbahn*, 9, 10.

[16] Jones, *Sigmund Freud: Life and Work*, 1:83.

[17] Mrs. Erna Lesky has obligingly provided me with this information.

[18] Dora Stockert-Meynert, *Theodor Meynert und seine Zeit* (Vienna and Leipzig, Österreichischer Bundesverlag, 1930).

[19] Paul Richer, *Études cliniques sur l'hystéro-épilepsie ou grande hystérie* (Paris, Delahaye & Lecrosnier, 1881), 258.

that had been debated for several years. The Viennese neurological community, which was often called upon to offer professional testimony in legal cases of post-traumatic nervous disorders, had adopted the thesis of Thomsen and Oppenheim against that of Charcot and the British school. In other words, they were much more cautious than their French or British counterparts in applying the hysteria diagnosis. [. . .]

Most likely, then, what irritated the neurologists in the audience was to see Freud interject himself into this discussion only by means of citing the authority of Charcot. Freud would most likely have received a more favorable reception if he had described a case that he himself had studied, rather than simply relating observations of Charcot's from back in Paris. What probably further irritated Freud's former teachers was to hear Freud attribute to Charcot the discovery that hysteria was neither a simulation nor a consequence of urogenital pathology. These two facts had been recognized in Vienna for a long time, and it is difficult to understand how Freud could have ignored the fact that Moritz Benedikt, among other local figures, had been teaching these very notions for nearly twenty years.[20] As for Bamberger's remark that "all this is very interesting but does not bring anything new," this reflects directly the traditional guideline of the Society that every presentation should offer material that was scientifically original. To summarize, then, the neurologists in the Society could find at least three reasons in Freud's performance to respond negatively: (1) Freud did not comply with the Society's tradition of presenting original scientific work; (2) he intervened without personal authority in a sensitive and complex debate with practical implications; and (3) by citing only Charcot's authority on behalf of his ideas, and by attributing paternity to medical beliefs about hysteria that were already well established in Vienna, Freud seemed to be dealing patronizingly with the physicians in attendance.

On the other side of the issue, let us now attempt to understand Freud's subjective experience of disappointment at the meeting the evening of October 15, 1886, and to determine why the event remained such a bad memory for him throughout his lifetime. To understand this, we need to consider the point in his career that Freud had reached in 1886.

Since his childhood, Freud had been animated by a strong sense of ambition. His letters to his fiancée testify very well to this ambitiousness during the 1880s. But Freud was finding it difficult to fulfill his goals because of the intense competition prevailing at the University of Vienna and because of the failures he had suffered in recent years. By 1886, Freud was 30 years old. He had spent several years already searching for a voca-

---

[20] See, for instance, Moritz Benedikt, *Elektrotherapie* (Vienna, Tender & Company, 1868), 413–45.

tion. His medical studies had dragged on. He had spent eight years completing a regular five-year training cycle, and he had then spent another year working in the laboratory. Taking into account a year more for military service, he was in all now three years behind other students who had begun with him in his professional advancement. During his medical training, Freud had devoted himself passionately to the study of cerebral histology and histopathological work in the laboratory of Ernst Brücke. Some meritorious, but not exceptional, work resulted from this time in the laboratory, which could have served as the starting point for a gradual career as a specialist in neurophysiology in some provincial university, had Freud wished to orient himself in this direction. At the Physiological Institute of Vienna, he had already explored the opportunities for full-time scientific research, and, according to Freud himself, his own teacher, Brücke, advised him to move in another direction. This unexpected change may already be considered Freud's first partial career failure.

During the three years of medical internship that followed for Freud at the General Hospital, Freud, like other young men at the time, dreamed about the great discovery that would bring him fame. He started with some experiments about the medicinal usages of cocaine; but his researches in this area twice brought him disillusionment.[21] In the end, it was Freud's colleague, Koller, rather than Freud, who conceived of the application of cocaine in ocular surgery and who thereby acquired immediate celebrity. Furthermore, because Freud persisted in his clinical and therapeutic experiments with the drug, at a time when the dangers of cocaine addiction were just becoming apparent, Freud was accused, mainly by Albrecht Erlenmeyer, of having unleashed a new plague on humanity. This was a second, and deeper, failure for the young Freud.

At this point came what Freud was to consider the greatest chance of his life, a University of Vienna grant that would allow him to enhance his medical studies with six months in a foreign university. As we know, Freud chose to go to Paris to the Salpêtrière. Here, he was positively dazzled by Charcot and was willing for some time to declare himself one of Charcot's disciples. Freud actually spent only four months with Charcot, and from this period must be subtracted the time that Freud spent in Germany with his fiancée at Christmas as well as a period when Charcot was ill. In fact, his stay at the Salpêtrière was too short to allow him to really get to know Charcot very well. Freud seems to have idealized Charcot, as is clear, for instance, in the necrological article that he wrote for Charcot in 1893.[22] Freud attributed to Charcot a concept of hysteria that actually dated from

---

[21] Erna Lesky mentions that in 1862 Dr. C. D. Schroff had already undertaken some experiments with cocaine in Vienna but had then abandoned them. See Lesky, *Die Wiener medizinische Schule im 19. Jahrhundert*, 276.

[22] Freud, "Charcot," *Wiener medizinische Wochenschrift*, 43 (1893), 1513–20.

Briquet. Curiously, he also seems not to have been aware of some of Char-cot's most forward-looking ideas about hysteria, such as were presented in Paul Richer's book. (In Richer's encyclopedic study of hystero-epilepsy, hysteria was described as a revival of a psychic trauma that was often of a sexual nature.) Also, Freud seems to have been impressed by the prestige of this "prince of science" but to have ignored that Charcot was surrounded by a large number of professional enemies.[23] More seriously, Freud evi-dently did not suspect the strong element of psychic contagion, of con-scious and unconscious suggestion and deception, that prevailed among the hysterical patients at the Salpêtrière. Significantly, the young Belgian physician Joseph Delboeuf also studied at the Salpêtrière in 1886; but upon his return to Belgium, Delboeuf published a moderate but critical account of what he had seen in Paris whereas Freud returned to Vienna with the fervor of a convert.[24]

In the autumn of 1886, several months after his return from France, Freud began a new stage of his career. He had finished his three-year medical internship, had acquired the title of *Privatdozent*, and had undergone additional training in a foreign country. After a very long en-gagement, he was also now married. He had begun to build a new medical practice, with the difficulties that this implies for a young doctor with no fortune and many new debts. In the eyes of his colleagues, he was sim-ply a young specialist, the author of some estimable but fairly obscure writings, whose name had also unfortunately been implicated in the case of the origins of the *Cocainsucht*. This, then, is the context for Freud's lecture on Charcot and male hysteria, in which Freud somewhat quix-otically, and without seeming to realize it, clashed with the sentiments and opinions of his former teachers, who had previously been well dis-posed toward him and upon whom he now relied for referrals for patients in his new private practice. From this perspective, we can conjecture that the frosty reception that Freud's lecture received on October 15, 1886, was perceived by him as a new setback in his career. Fortunately, Freud could still count on his old friend and protector Josef Breuer to send him patients and, when he was freed from his fascination with Charcot, to receive from him the idea that would later become the starting point of psychoanalysis. But, in the meantime, Freud lived on the defensive toward the Viennese medical world. It is difficult to determine meaningfully to what extent these accumulated experiences contributed to his perception of a lonely atmosphere in which the birth and development of Freudian theory occurred.

[23] Ellenberger, "Charcot and the Salpêtrière School," *American Journal of Psychotherapy*, 19, no. 2 (April 1965), 253–67.

[24] Joseph Delboeuf, "De l'influence de l'imitation et de l'éducation dans le somnam-bulisme provoqué," *Revue philosophique*, 22 (1886), II, 146–71.

Consequences of the Meeting of October 15, 1886

According to the reports of the October 15, 1886, meeting, Meynert noted that he currently had in his clinic several patients afflicted with post-traumatic disorders. Meynert added that it would be interesting to verify whether or not these cases exhibited the classical hysterical stigmata described by Charcot. None of the stenographical reports of the meeting records that Meynert challenged Freud to demonstrate such a case to the Society. In any event, Freud felt compelled to demonstrate such a case of male hysteria at a later date.

Masculine hysteria did not seem to be rare in Vienna at the time, since Freud was able to find a case of it, with the assistance of a colleague, only a week after the meeting. Freud then had his friend Dr. Königstein submit the patient to an ophthalmological examination on October 24. On November 24, Freud presented the case to the Society of Physicians.[25] Freud states first in this lecture that he was accepting the invitation (*Aufforderung*) of Professor Meynert to present to the Society a case of male hysteria afflicted with the stigmata described by Charcot.[26] The patient in question was a 29-year-old working man who, after having been hit by a carriage when he was 8, had become deaf in one ear and for two years had also undergone convulsions of an undetermined nature. Now, following an emotional shock three years ago, the patient was suffering from hysterical symptoms. He exhibited a serious hemianesthesia as well as other stigmata similar to those described by Charcot. Freud's presentation aroused no discussion from the audience this time, most likely because the program that evening was full of other events.[27]

No document of the time expresses any dissatisfaction by Freud regarding the reception of this second presentation. In his autobiography many years later, Freud even states that he was applauded at the occasion. More-

[25] Sigmund Freud, "Beiträge zur Kasuistik der Hysterie. I. Beobachtung einer hochgradigen Hemianaesthesie bei einem hysterischen Manne," *Wiener medizinische Wochenschrift*, 36 (1886), cols. 1663–68.

[26] Freud's word *Aufforderung* has a stronger meaning in this context than "invitation" (*Einladung*) and a milder one than "challenge" (*Herausforderung*); we might translate it as "pressing invitation."

[27] We might note in passing that the patient Freud produced at this meeting had suffered two traumas, one of a physical nature during childhood and the other emotional in nature from three years before. This was therefore an ambiguous case that could be diagnosed as either classical male hysteria or traumatic hysteria in Charcot's sense. To a degree, then, Freud's second presentation was not a direct response to the issue criticized during the earlier meeting, which had concerned the clinical relationship of railway spine to traumatic male hysteria.

over, according to the usual and "official" historical legend about the
October 15, 1886, meeting, Freud was so badly received by the Physicians'
Society that he "retired himself," that is, he resigned or stopped coming to
the meetings, and soon broke off his relations with the Vienna medical
world. But here, too, if we apply the golden rule of factual verification
before all else, we observe something quite different from the legend. Dr.
Karl Sablik of Vienna, under the guidance of Professor Erna Lesky, has
conducted research on this very point in the archives of the Vienna Society
of Physicians.[28] According to Sablik's findings, Freud was not yet a member of the Vienna Society of Physicians at the date of his lecture on October
15, 1886. Shortly after this meeting, however, Freud applied to the Society
and was accepted. His nomination as a member of the Society was announced on March 18, 1887. It is impossible to determine how often he
attended the meetings of the Society (the official record does not list the
names of members in attendance for each meeting); but it is certain that he
attended at least occasionally during the years that followed. According to
Sablik's research, Freud in fact remained a member of the Society until his
departure from Vienna in 1938 and, among other things, punctually paid
his annual dues to the organization. He was nominated and elected an
"honorary member" of the group in 1931, after which time he was no
longer required to pay dues.[29]

Three months later, Arthur Schnitzler alluded to the October 15, 1886,
meeting in his analysis of Charcot's most recent book translated by
Freud.[30] Schnitzler spoke there of Charcot as an "ingenious doctor—
geistreicher Arzt,"[31] and he noted that the Frenchman's ideas on traumatic
male hysteria had been received with reservations in the medical community. "This was proven," Schnitzler said, "when Doctor Freud recently
spoke on this subject at the Vienna Society of Physicians and an animated
discussion ensued." Moreover, for several years after Freud's lecture, discussions in Europe about the clinical connections between male hysteria
and traumatic neurosis continued passionately.[32] Around 1900, however,
interest in hysteria in the medical world began to wane, and the frequency

[28] Karl Sablik, "Sigmund Freud und die Gesellschaft der Ärzte in Wien" (Unpublished
article obligingly communicated to the author by Professor Lesky).

[29] Ibid.

[30] Arthur Schnitzler, book review in *Internationale klinische Rundschau*, 1 (1887), 19–
20.

[31] The German adjective *geistreich*, which literally means "ingenious" or "clever," can
take on an ironical connotation when applied to a scientist. It implies that Charcot, according
to the speaker, might have more imagination than critical sense.

[32] See, for instance, the review of the literature on the subject in Georges Gilles de la
Tourette, *Traité clinique et thérapeutique de l'hystérie d'après l'enseignement de la
Salpêtrière*, 3 vols. (Paris, Plon, 1891), 1:76–88.

of this sort of illness declined considerably. Neurologists now doubted the existence of the classical hysterical stigmata altogether; discussions such as the one at the October 15, 1886, meeting in Vienna no longer seemed relevant.

Thirty-nine years after the meeting, Freud, in his autobiographical memoir, related the episode with all the inevitable inaccuracies and deformations produced in a person's memory after so many years.[33] Jones corrected some of these errors of memory while others slipped his attention. Freud declares in his *Autobiography* that he was at first very badly received at the Society of Physicians, that Bamberger declared that his propositions were "incredible," that Meynert defied him to present to the Society a case such as the one that he had described in Charcot's clinic, and that his colleagues refused to let him examine their own clinical wards for such cases. According to Freud, he then also spent a long time attempting to locate a case of male hysteria in a Vienna hospital, after which time he demonstrated the case to the Society again and was applauded but still rejected by the authorities. Following this, he claimed, he was effectively reduced to a member of the scientific opposition, so that he retired from academic life and ceased contributing to any scientific association. As for the historical anecdote about the old surgeon who asked Freud, "How could hysteria in a man exist, since the word 'hysteria' comes from the Greek '*hysteron*—uterus'?," it appears to be a traditional medical joke about old surgeons who, it was said, were both old-fashioned in their medical knowledge and ignorant of classical languages. (At this time, all physicians should have known that the word in Greek for "uterus" was in fact *hystera*.)

About fifty years after this memorable meeting, Julius Wagner-Jauregg, in his posthumously published autobiography, gave his own, simplified version of the event. "On his way back to Vienna [from Paris]," Wagner-Jauregg wrote, "Freud delivered a lecture to the Physicians' Society in which he exclusively talked about Charcot and congratulated him in the highest terms. But the Vienna bigwigs took very badly to this. In the discussion, Bamberger and Meynert brushed him off, and this is how he almost disgraced himself in front of the faculty."[34]* However, by the time that Wagner-Jauregg wrote these lines, the legend about Freud was already

---

*[*Editor's note*: The preceding quotations of Wagner-Jauregg and Schnitzler would seem to contradict, rather than support, Ellenberger's interpretation of this event; Ellenberger, however, does not address this point.]

[33] Sigmund Freud, *Selbstdarstellung*, in Louis Grote, ed., *Die Medizin der Gegenwart in Selbstdarstellungen* (Leipzig, Felix Meiner, 1925), 4:1–52.

[34] Julius Wagner-Jauregg, *Lebenserinnerungen*, edited by L. Schönbauer and M. Jentsch (Vienna, Springer, 1950), 72.

widespread and had replaced and changed in a thousand ways the real story.*

In conclusion, the structure of this historical myth may be illustrated in tabular form, comparing the known historical facts about the event with the subsequent legendary accounts of it in the psychoanalytic literature:

The Legend: The central point of Freud's lecture to the Vienna Society of Physicians was to establish the existence of hysteria in males. *The Facts*: The central point of Freud's lecture was to assimilate cases of so-called railway spine to male hysteria.

The Legend: The "big shots" in Viennese medicine were so ignorant and conservative that they had not heard of Charcot's most recent discoveries about hysteria. *The Facts*: Charcot was very well known and respected by Viennese neurologists, who, however, tended to reject his theory of traumatic male hysteria.

The Legend: Freud's lecture shocked the members of the Society because of the novelty of its ideas. *The Facts*: Freud's lecture was received skeptically because, contrary to the traditions of the Society, it contained little that was new at the time.

The Legend: The cold and critical attitude of the members of the audience toward Freud was a manifestation of their personal hostility toward him. *The Facts*: The traditional tone and approach of the Society of Physicians toward its lecturers was of a formal politeness combined with ruthless criticism.

The Legend: Irritated by his hostile reception, Freud retired from the Society of Physicians, failed to attend any more of its meetings, and broke all professional relations with the Viennese medical world. *The Facts*: Shortly after his presentations to the Society in the autumn of 1886, Freud applied to the organization for admission and was elected in March 1887. He remained a member of the group until 1938.

It might be noted finally that the subsequent embellishments and distortions of this story all work in a single direction, toward the image of the mythical hero working in isolation to bring to humanity a great discovery which is then rejected and scorned by it.

Finally, there have been many latter-day mythical versions of Freud's famous meeting of October 15, 1886. In closing, I shall limit myself to

---

*[*Editor's note*: The full passage in which Freud describes the event in 1925 may be found in *An Autobiographical Study*, in *The Standard Edition of the Complete Psychological Works of Sigmund Freud*, translated from the German under the general editorship of James Strachey, 24 vols. (London, Hogarth Press, 1953–1974), 20:15–16.]

citing at length only one such account, a popular exposition in English of Freud's life and work that dates from 1952 and in which the author was not attempting to write a historical novel:

"What? Hysteria in a male? Impossible!" cried blonde Professor Meynert, and he sprang up from his seat at a meeting of the Vienna Medical Society, where a number of physicians had gathered to hear Freud read a paper on the cases he had observed at the Salpêtrière.

It was the custom of members of the medical faculty to honor in this way those who had travelling scholarships. And Freud was reporting on the cases of real and hysterical paralysis he had studied under Charcot.

The first part of his paper was listened to respectfully, but when he reported Charcot's statement that hysteria, before thought only a disease of women, could occur also in men, he created such an uproar at the meeting that grave Professor Bamberger, the chairman, had to knock three times for order.

"But gentlemen," Freud pleaded, "I have seen such cases!"

"Perhaps in France," someone suggested, "where the men are more effeminate."

And Professor Meynert, rising again, said trenchantly, "No doubt then, Dr. Freud, you can produce such a case of male hysteria for us here in Vienna!"

Sarcastic laughter and cries of "Hear! Hear!" greeted this challenge.

Freud gathered his papers together. "Indeed, I will!" he cried.

He went immediately to the male wards of the Vienna General Hospital. He looked over every case diagnosed as actual paralysis, and very soon he found a case of male hysteria, a man paralyzed, but not as the result of a cerebral hemorrhage. He showed the typical symptoms of hysteria. Here was a case to show to the members of the Vienna Medical Society!

But by this time the reason for his search had become known to everyone in the hospital, and when he asked the doctor in charge of the ward if he might make use of the patient, the physician asked him with raised eyebrows, "Why?"

"So that I can present him to the members of the Vienna Medical Society as a perfect example of male hysteria!"

He was about to demonstrate the symptoms which proved to him why this case could be so classified, but before he could lift the covers from the sick man, the doctor interrupted him.

"My dear sir," he cried, "how can you talk such nonsense? How can a man possibly be subject to hysteria? Don't you know that the very word hysteria is drawn from the Greek word *hysteron*, meaning womb? This is a disease suffered only by women!"

Over the sick man's head Freud looked at the doctor with astonishment. "I don't ask you to approve my theory," he said hotly. "I am only asking you to put the patient at my disposal!"

"Out of the question," replied the physician, turning on his heel, "quite impossible!" And he left Freud standing stunned by this affront at the bedside of the patient. [. . .]

Finally after a long search Freud found a sick man who dragged his hip and leg in the typical manner which Charcot had taught Freud to recognize as male hysteria. He persuaded the sick man to go with him to a meeting of the Vienna Medical Society. He faced the physicians who had laughed at him before. "Gentlemen," he said, "Here is a case of male hysteria. Examine the patient at your leisure."

One by one they came up. One by one they examined the patient. One by one they noted the symptoms which Freud pointed out to them, the area of paralysis, in the inverse proportion of severity from the most distant parts.

But one by one they shook their heads. Hysteria, they said, could not occur in a male!

Freud left the hall disgusted.[35]

If we require a conclusion to this essay, it would simply be that the history of psychiatry urgently needs to engage in strict and impartial research based on all available documents and sources that are as close as possible to the historical events under question. Such an investigation requires much time, effort, and meticulous work. In the long run, however, this approach proves infinitely more fruitful than the production of works of history based on second-, third-, and fourth-hand materials, which accumulate historical anecdotes, repeat the same inaccuracies, and appearing, as they do, in print so often without examination, eventually acquire the fallacious appearance of truths.[36]

[35] Rachel Baker, *Sigmund Freud for Everybody* [1952] (New York, Popular Library Edition, 1963), 36–38. Other accounts of the event offer their own imaginary renditions of what took place at the two meetings, such as that the audience burst out laughing when Freud used the term *male hysteria*, that they demanded Freud's resignation from the organization after the first lecture, and that Freud hypnotized his male patient during the second lecture.

[36] For further remarks on this subject, see my article "Methodology in Writing the History of Dynamic Psychiatry," in George Mora and Jeanne L. Brand, eds., *Psychiatry and Its History: Methodological Problems in Research* (Springfield, Ill., Charles C. Thomas, forthcoming).

Part Two

FIGURES AND MOVEMENTS IN THE HISTORY OF THE MENTAL SCIENCES

4

Charcot and the Salpêtrière School

[1965]

THE SCHOOL of the Salpêtrière in the late nineteenth century was strongly organized and headed by a powerful figure, the great teacher Jean-Martin Charcot (1825–1893), a neurologist who late in his career came to the study of certain mental phenomena. During the years 1870 to 1893, Charcot was considered to be the greatest neurologist of his time. He was the consulting physician of kings and princes, and patients came to see him "from Samarkand and the West Indies." But celebrity had come to Charcot only after long years of obscure and incessant toil, and few of those who marveled at his extraordinary later success realized that it was a belated achievement reached after many years of strenuous and unnoticed work. No real biography of Charcot has as yet been written. Most accounts, such as Georges Guillain's book, are based on necrologies and depict for the most part only the Charcot of the brilliant years.[1] Valuable memoirs have been recorded by Charcot's disciple Alexandre Souques[2] and by the Russian physician Lyubimov, who had been acquainted with Charcot during the last twenty years of his life.[3]

Charcot was born in Paris, the son of a carriage builder who, it was said, made carriages of great beauty and who was reputed to be more of an artist than an artisan. Very little is known about Charcot's childhood and youth. It is said that he was a cold, silent, shy, and aloof young man who had a speech impediment. He wore a black moustache (the story goes that his first rich patient was referred to him on the condition that he shave off his moustache). As an *interne* (medical resident), the young Charcot was assigned for some time to the Salpêtrière, an old hospital which at that time was mainly a medical poorhouse for four or five thousand old women.

"Charcot and the Salpêtrière School," *American Journal of Psychotherapy*, 19, no. 2 (April 1965), 253–67.

[1] Georges Guillain, *J. M. Charcot (1825–1893): Sa vie, son oeuvre* (Paris, Masson, 1955).

[2] Alexandre Souques, "Charcot intime," *Presse médicale*, 33 (I) (May 27, 1925), 693–98.

[3] A. Lyubimov, *Profesor Sharko, Nautshno-biografitshesky etiud* (St. Petersburg, Suvorina, 1894). [*Editor's note*: A French translation of this rare but highly informative source is also available under the title A. Lubimoff, *Le professeur Charcot: Étude scientifico-biographique*, translated from the Russian by Comtesse Lydie Rostopchine (Paris, A. S. Souvorine, 1894)].

Charcot realized that this hospital sheltered numerous patients with rare or unknown neurological diseases and would be a gold mine for clinical research. He kept this point in mind while he was slowly pursuing his career as an anatomo-pathologist. As a young doctor, Charcot was asked by one of his teachers to be physician and companion to a rich banker traveling to Italy, which gave him an opportunity to get acquainted with Italy's artistic wealth.[4] His medical career was at first rather slow and laborious. The turning point came in 1862 when, at the age of 36, Charcot was appointed chief physician in one of the Salpêtrière's largest sections and took up his old plans with feverish activity. Case histories were taken, autopsies performed, and laboratories opened, while Charcot was building at the same time a team of devoted collaborators at the hospital. He was inspired above all by G.B.A. Duchenne (de Boulogne), a neurologist of outstanding genius who had no official position and whom Charcot was always to call his "Master in Neurology."[5] Within a single, concentrated eight-year period, running from 1862 to 1870, Charcot made the discoveries that gave him his position of eminence.

In 1870, Charcot took on the supplementary charge of a special ward that the hospital administration had reserved for a fairly large number of female patients suffering from "convulsions." Some of these patients were epileptics while others were hysterics who had learned in remarkable detail to imitate epileptic crises. Charcot strove to discover means of distinguishing between hysterical and epileptic convulsions. He also started at this time to investigate hysteria with the same method he used for organic neurological diseases and, with his student Paul Richer, gave a description of the full-blown hysterical crisis, or *grande hystérie*.[6]

In 1878, probably under the influence of Charles Richet, Charcot extended his interest to hypnotism, of which he undertook a purportedly scientific study, taking as his subjects several of the most gifted female hysterical patients at the hospital. He found that these subjects developed the hypnotic condition through three successive stages: "lethargy," "catalepsy," and "somnambulism," with each stage exhibiting very definite and characteristic symptoms. Charcot read his findings at the Académie des Sciences at the beginning of 1882;[7] it was, Pierre Janet later said, a *tour de*

[4] Fernand Levillain, "Charcot et l'École de la Salpêtrière," *Revue encyclopédique*, 10 (March 1, 1894), 108–15.

[5] Georges Guillain, "L'oeuvre de Duchenne (de Boulogne)," *Études neurologiques*, 3d ser. (Paris, Masson, 1929), 419–48. See also Paul Guilly, *Duchenne (de Boulogne)* (Paris, Thèse Médicale, 1936).

[6] Paul Richer, *Études cliniques sur l'hystéro-épilepsie ou grande hystérie* (Paris, Delahaye & Lecrosnier, 1881).

[7] J. M. Charcot, "Sur les divers états nerveux déterminés par l'hypnotisation chez les hystériques," *Comptes-rendus hebdomadaires des séances de l'Académie des Sciences*, 94 (1882), 403–5.

force to have hypnotism officially accepted by the same professional organization that thrice within the past century had condemned it under the name of animal magnetism. This resounding paper gave magnetism a new dignity, and the heretofore shunned subject now became the topic of innumerable publications and widespread fascination.

Among Charcot's most spectacular achievements were the investigations of traumatic paralysis that he conducted in 1883 and 1885.[8] At this time, paralysis was generally considered to result from lesions of the nervous system caused by an accident, although the existence of "psychic paralyses" had been postulated in England by Benjamin Brodie as early as 1837 and by Russel Reynolds in 1869.[9] But how could a purely psychological factor cause paralysis without the patient's awareness of that factor and excluding the possibility of simulation?

Charcot had already analyzed the differences between organic and hysterical paralysis. In 1884, three men afflicted with a monoplegia of one arm consecutive to a traumatism were admitted to the Salpêtrière. Charcot first demonstrated that the symptoms of these paralyses, while differing from those of organic paralysis, coincided exactly with the symptoms of hysterical paralysis. His second step was the experimental reproduction of similar states of paralysis under hypnosis. Charcot suggested to some hypnotized subjects that their arms would become paralyzed. The resulting hypnotic paralysis proved to have exactly the same features as the spontaneous hysterical paralysis and the post-traumatic paralysis of the three male patients. Charcot was able to reproduce these conditions segment by segment and, conversely, to suggest their disappearance in reverse order.

His next step was a demonstration of the effect of the trauma. Charcot chose easily hypnotizable subjects and suggested to them, for instance, that in their waking state, as soon as they were slapped on the back, their arm would become paralyzed. When awakened, these subjects showed the usual posthypnotic amnesia, and as soon as they were slapped on the back, they were instantly struck with a monoplegia of the arm of exactly the same type as the post-traumatic monoplegia. Finally, Charcot pointed out that in certain subjects living in a state of permanent somnambulism, hypnotic suggestion was not even necessary. Such patients developed paralyses of the arm after being slapped on the back, without special verbal suggestion. The mechanism of post-traumatic paralysis seemed thus to be demonstrated. Charcot assumed that the nervous shock following the trauma was

---

[8] J. M. Charcot, *Oeuvres complètes: Leçons sur les maladies du système nerveux* (Paris, Progrès Médical, 1890), 3:299–359.

[9] Benjamin C. Brodie, *Lectures Illustrative of Certain Local Nervous Affections* (London, Longmans and Company, 1837); Russel Reynolds, "Remarks on Paralyses and Other Disorders of Motion and Sensation, Dependent on Ideas," *British Medical Journal*, 2 (1869), 483–85.

a kind of hypnoid state analogous to hypnotism which therefore enabled the development of an autosuggestion of the individual. "I do not think that in any physiopathological research it would often be possible to reproduce more accurately the condition which one had set oneself the task to study," Charcot concluded.

Charcot ranged hysterical, post-traumatic, and hypnotic paralyses in the group of "dynamic paralyses," in contrast to "organic paralyses" resulting from an ascertainable lesion of the nervous system. He gave a similar demonstration in regard to hysterical mutism and hysterical coxalgia. Here, too, he reported experimentally, by means of hypnotism, clinical pictures identical with the hysterical conditions. In 1892, Charcot distinguished "dynamic amnesia," in which lost memories can be recovered under hypnosis, from "organic amnesia," where this is impossible.[10]

In the last years of his life, Charcot came to realize that a vast realm of mental activity existed between that of clear consciousness and organic brain physiology. His attention was drawn to "faith healing," and in one of his last articles, he stated that he had seen patients going to Lourdes and returning healed from their diseases.[11] He tried to elucidate the mechanism of such cures and anticipated that an increased knowledge of the laws of "faith healing" would result in great therapeutic progress.

There are many descriptions and pictures of Charcot, but all of them pertain almost without exception either to him at his zenith of influence around 1880 or to the declining Charcot of the last years. The liveliest accounts were provided by Léon Daudet, who as a young man had studied medicine at the Salpêtrière and whose father, the novelist Alphonse Daudet, had been Charcot's intimate friend. Here is a condensed excerpt of Léon Daudet's memoirs describing Charcot:

> Charcot was a small, stout, and vigorous man with a big head, a bull's neck, a low forehead, broad cheeks. The line of his mouth was hard and meditative. He was clean-shaven and kept his straight hair combed back. He somewhat resembled Napoleon and liked to cultivate this resemblance. His gait was heavy, his voice authoritative, somewhat low, often ironical and insisting, his expression extraordinarily fiery.
>
> A most learned man, he was familiar with the works of Dante, Shakespeare, and the great poets; he read English, German, Spanish, and Italian. He had a large library full of strange and unusual books.
>
> He was very humane; he showed a profound compassion for animals and forbade any mention of hunters and hunting in his presence.

[10] J. M. Charcot, "Sur un cas d'amnésie rétro-antérograde, probablement d'origine hystérique," Revue de médecine, 12 (1892), 81–96. For an elaboration of this article, see A. Souques, Revue de médecine, 12 (1892), 267–400, 867–81.

[11] J. M. Charcot, "La foi qui guérit," Archives de neurologie, 25 (1893), 72–87.

A more authoritarian man I have never known, nor one who could put such a despotic yoke on people around him. To realize this, one only had to see how he could, from his pulpit, throw a sweeping and suspicious glance at his students and hear him interrupt them with a brief, imperative word.

He could not stand contradiction, however small. If someone dared contradict his theories, he became ferocious and mean and did all he could to wreck the career of the imprudent man unless he retracted and apologized.

He could not stand stupidity. But his need for domination caused him to eliminate the more brilliant of his disciples, so that in the end he was surrounded by mediocre people. As a compensation, he maintained social relationships with artists and poets and gave magnificent receptions.

It was one of his favorite ideas that the share of dream-life in our waking state is much more than just "immense."[12]

Many similar references to Charcot can be found in the famous *Diary* of Edmond and Jules de Goncourt.[13] These two brothers were known for their biting descriptions of contemporaries and seem to have been particularly antagonistic to Charcot, whom they described as follows:

Charcot was an ambitious man, envious of any superiority, showing a ferocious resentment against those who declined invitations to his receptions, a despot at the university, hard with his patients to the point of telling them bluntly of their impending death, but cowardly when he himself was ill. He was a tyrant with his children and compelled, for instance, his son Jean, who wanted to be a seafarer, to become a physician. As a scientist, Charcot was a mixture of genius and charlatan. Most unpleasant was his indiscretion in talking of his patients' confidential matters.

The description of the great doctor given by the Russian physician Lyubimov is so vastly different from the negative assessments of Daudet and the Goncourts that one can hardly believe it concerns the same person:

Besides his extraordinary gift as a teacher, a scientist, and an artist, Charcot was extremely humane, devoted to his patients, and would not tolerate an unkind statement about anyone in his presence. He was a poised and sensible man, very circumspect in his judgments, with a quick eye for distinguishing people's value. His family life was a harmonious and happy one; his wife, who was a widow with a daughter when he married her, helped him with his work and was active in

[12] Léon Daudet, *Devant la douleur. Souvenirs des milieux littéraires, politiques, artistiques et médicaux de 1885 à 1905*, 2d ser. (Paris, Nouvelle Librairie Nationale, 1917), 4–15. See also, by the same author, *Les oeuvres et les hommes* (Paris, Nouvelle Librairie Nationale, 1922), 197–243; and *Quand mon père vivait. Souvenirs inédits sur Alphonse Daudet* (Paris, Grasset, 1940), 113–19.

[13] Edmond de Goncourt and Jules de Goncourt, *Journal: Mémoires de la vie littéraire*, 4 vols. (Paris, Fasquelle & Flammarion, 1956). See especially the third volume in the set.

charitable organizations. He gave great care to the education of his son Jean who had spontaneously chosen to be a physician and whose first scientific publications were a great joy for his father. He enjoyed the devotion of his students and of his patients, so that his patron saint's day, the Saint Martin on November 11th, was celebrated with entertainments and rejoicing at the Salpêtrière.[14]

We may also wonder how it was that Charcot gained the enormous prestige that he enjoyed in the years 1880 to 1890. Several reasons may be distinguished. First, the Salpêtrière was anything but an ordinary hospital. It was in a sense a city within a city in the seventeenth-century style, consisting of about forty-five buildings with streets, squares, gardens, and an old and beautiful church. It was also a place of historical fame: Saint Vincent de Paul had carried out there his charitable activities; it had later been converted by Louis XIV into an asylum for beggars, prostitutes, and the insane; it was also one of the places where the notorious September Massacres had taken place during the French Revolution and where Pinel had achieved his celebrated mental hospital reforms. The hospital was also known for an episode in the classic novel *Manon Lescaut* by the Abbé Prévost. Similarly, its thousands of old women had inspired a number of Baudelaire's poems. Before Charcot, the Salpêtrière had been little known to medical students, and physicians did not relish the thought of being appointed there. Charcot was now credited with being the scientific wizard who had turned this historical place into a "Temple of Science."

When he arrived, this old-fashioned hospital with its antiquated buildings had no laboratories, no examination rooms, no teaching facilities. However, with an iron will—and with the help of his political connections—Charcot built out of the Salpêtrière a treatment, research, and teaching center. He had carefully chosen his collaborators; he installed consulting rooms for ophthalmology and otolaryngology as well as research laboratories and a photographic service. Later, he added a museum for anatomo-pathological specimens, an outpatient service where men were also admitted, and a large lecture auditorium. Among Charcot's disciples were Bourneville, Pitres, Joffroy, Cotard, Gilles de la Tourette, Meige, Richer, Souques, Marie, Raymond, and Babinski. Indeed, there is hardly a major French neurologist of that time who had not been Charcot's student. Over that school, which was largely his personal creation, Charcot exerted an absolute domination. Each one of his lectures was carefully recorded by students and published in one or the other of several medical journals he himself had founded. There came a time during the 1880s when no candidate could be appointed at the Paris medical faculty without his sanction. Patriotic feeling also contributed to Charcot's fame, for he

[14] Lyubimov, *Profesor Sharko, Nautshno-biografitshesky etiud.*

and Pasteur were to the French a proof of France's enduring scientific genius, a challenge to Germany's new alleged scientific superiority.

Furthermore, Charcot personified what the French call a "prince de la science." He was not only a figure of high scientific reputation, but also a powerful and wealthy man. Through his marriage to a rich widow and the very high fees that he was able to charge his patients, he was able to lead the life of the wealthy classes. In addition to a villa in Neuilly-sur-Seine on the outskirts of Paris, he had acquired in 1884 a splendid residence on the Boulevard Saint-Germain that had been decorated according to his own plans. It was a kind of private museum with Renaissance furniture, stained-glass windows, tapestries, paintings, antiques, and rare books. Charcot was himself an artist of not inconsiderable talent who did excellent drawings and was an expert in painting on china and enamel. He was also a keen connoisseur of the history of art.[15] Moreover, he was a master of French prose with an exhaustive knowledge of French literature. An infrequent thing among Frenchmen at this time, he also read English, German, and Italian and showed a particular admiration for Shakespeare, whom he often quoted in English, and for Dante, whom he quoted in Italian. Every Tuesday night, Charcot gave sumptuous receptions in his splendid home to the *Tout-Paris* of scientists, politicians, artists, and writers. He was known to be the physician and sometimes the confidant of kings and princes. Emperor Pedro II of Brazil, it was said, came to his home, played billiards with him, and attended his lectures at the Salpêtrière.

Charcot was also a very influential figure in English medical circles. At an international congress that took place in London in 1881, his demonstration of the tabetic arthropathies was received with a storm of applause. He had many admirers in Germany, although he declined invitations to congresses in that country after the Franco-German war of 1870–1871. In Vienna, he was well acquainted with Theodor Meynert and Moritz Benedikt. Charcot was very popular, too, in Russia, where he had been called several times as consultant physician to the czar and his family. Russian physicians welcomed him because he relieved them from their strong dependence on German scientists. According to Guillain, Charcot arranged an unofficial encounter between Léon Gambetta, the French prime minister, and the Grand Duke Nikolai of Russia, from which the Franco-Russian alliance was to issue.[16] Charcot traveled extensively, every year making a carefully planned journey to a different European country, visiting the museums, making drawings, and writing detailed travelogues.

[15] Henri Meige, "Charcot artiste," *Nouvelle iconographie de la Salpêtrière*, 11 (1898), 489–516.
[16] Guillain, *J. M. Charcot: Sa vie, son oeuvre*, 26.

Enormous as it was, Charcot's prestige was still enhanced by a halo of mystery that surrounded him, which had slowly grown after 1870 and which reached its peak with his celebrated paper on hypnotism in 1882. Charcot now gained the reputation of being a great thaumaturgist. Instances of his quasi-miraculous cures are reported by Lyubimov:

> Many patients were brought to Charcot from all over the world, paralytics on stretchers or wearing complicated apparatuses. Charcot ordered the removal of these appliances and told the patients to walk. There was, for instance, a young lady who had been paralyzed for years. Charcot bade her stand up and walk, which she did under the astonished eyes of her parents and of the Mother Superior of the convent in which she had been staying. Another young lady was brought to Charcot with a paralysis of both legs. Charcot found no organic lesion; the consultation was not yet over when the patient stood up and walked back to the door, where the cabman, who was waiting for her, took off his hat in amazement and crossed himself.[17]

In the eyes of the French public of the 1880s and 1890s, Charcot was the man who had explored the hidden abysses of the human mind, hence his nickname "Napoleon of Neuroses." He had come to be identified with the discovery of hysteria, hypnotism, dual personality, catalepsy, and somnambulism. Strange things were said about his hold on the Salpêtrière's hysterical young women and about happenings there. Jules Claretie, the novelist and playwright, related that during one of the annual patients' balls at the Salpêtrière, it happened that a gong was inadvertently sounded, whereupon many hysterical women instantaneously fell into catalepsy and kept the poses in which they found themselves when the gong was sounded.[18] Charcot was also the man whose searching gaze penetrated the depths of the past and who retrospectively interpreted works of art, giving modern neurological diagnoses to cripples represented in the history of painting and sculpture.[19] He founded a journal, the *Iconographie photographique de la Salpêtrière*, followed by the *Nouvelle iconographie photographique de la Salpêtrière*, which were probably the first journals to combine art, photography, and medicine. Charcot was also considered to have found a scientific explanation for demoniac possession, which, he assumed, was nothing but a form of hysteria; he also interpreted this condition retrospectively in works of art.[20] He was known as well for his own collection of rare

[17] Lyubimov, *Profesor Sharko.*

[18] Jules Claretie, *La vie à Paris, 1881* (Paris, Harvard, 1882), 128–29.

[19] J. M. Charcot and Paul Richer, *Les difformes et les malades dans l'art* (Paris, Lecrosnier & Babé, 1889).

[20] J. M. Charcot and Paul Richer, *Les démoniaques dans l'art* (Paris, Delahaye & Lecrosnier, 1887).

old books on witchcraft and possession, some of which he had reprinted in a series titled the Bibliothèque Diabolique.

All of these features contributed to the incomparable fascination exerted on the Parisian imagination by Charcot's famous weekly séances at the Salpêtrière. Tuesday mornings were devoted to examining new, heretofore unseen patients in the presence of physicians and students who enjoyed seeing Charcot display his clinical acumen, the assurance and swiftness with which he was able to disentangle the most complicated case histories and arrive at a diagnosis, even of the rarest diseases. But the greatest attractions were his solemn formal lectures on Friday mornings, each of which had been prepared with the utmost care. The large auditorium was filled to capacity with physicians, students, writers, and an inquisitive crowd long before the beginning of the lecture. The podium was always decorated with pictures and anatomical schemata pertaining to the day's presentation. Charcot, with his stately bearing, entered promptly at ten o'clock, often accompanied by an illustrious foreign visitor and a group of assistants who sat down in the first row. Amidst the absolute silence of the audience, he started speaking in a low pitch and gradually raised his voice, giving sober explanations which he illustrated with skillful colored chalk drawings on the blackboard. With an inborn acting talent, he imitated the behavior, the mimicry, the gait, the voice of a patient afflicted with the disease he was discussing that day, after which the patient was brought in. The patient's entrance was sometimes also spectacular. When Charcot lectured on tremors, three or four women were introduced wearing hats with long feathers which by their quivering made it possible to distinguish the specific characteristics of tremors in various diseases.[21] The interrogation usually assumed the form of a dramatic dialogue between Charcot and the patient. Most spectacular were the lectures delivered about hysteria and hypnotism. Another of Charcot's innovations was the use of photographic projections, a procedure which at that time was unusual for medical teaching. Each lecture concluded with a discussion of the diagnosis and a recapitulation stating the lecture's main points, both of which were models of lucidity and concision. These lectures lasted for two hours, but the audience, it was said, never found them too long, even when they concerned rare organic brain diseases.[22] Lyubimov points to the difference between Charcot's lectures and those of Meynert, which he had also attended in Vienna and which left him exhausted and confused, whereas he departed Charcot's lectures with a feeling of exhilaration.

[21] Charles Féré, "J. M. Charcot et son oeuvre," *Revue des deux mondes*, 122 (1894), 410–24.

[22] Levillain, "Charcot et l'École de la Salpêtrière," 110.

It is easy to understand the spellbinding effect Charcot's teaching exerted on laymen, on many physicians, and especially on foreign visitors, such as the young Sigmund Freud, who spent four months at the Salpêtrière in 1885–1886. Other visitors were more skeptical. The Belgian physician Joseph Delboeuf, whose interest in Charcot's work had brought him to Paris the same year as Freud, was soon assailed by the strongest doubts when he saw how carelessly experiments with hysterical patients were carried out. On his return to Belgium, Delboeuf published a strongly critical account of Charcot's methods.[23]

Those visitors who came to see Charcot in Paris for a short visit and were envious of him were often unaware that he was surrounded by a host of powerful enemies. Charcot had been stamped as an atheist by the clergy and the Catholics (one of the reasons being that he had the nuns at the Salpêtrière replaced by lay nurses). At the same time, some atheists found him too spiritualistic. Increasingly, he was publicly accused of charlatanism by certain other medical figures interested in hypnotic research.[24] He also had fierce enemies in political and social circles, as is obvious from the *Diary* of the Goncourt brothers. Among neurologists, most of whom had been his admirers as long as he remained on the solid ground of neuropathology, many deserted him when he shifted to the study of hypnotism and to spectacular, sensationalistic experiments with hysterical patients. Lyubimov, for instance, tells how the German neurologist Carl Westphal expressed deep concern about the new turn taken by Charcot's research after visiting him in Paris.[25] Charcot was attacked on the same grounds by the British psychiatrist Sir John Bucknill. Nonetheless, George Beard, the formulator of the concept of neurasthenia, while admitting that Charcot had made "serious mistakes" later in his career, nonetheless proclaimed that he still respected him "as a man of genius and a man of honour."[26] Charcot also increasingly had to wage a continuous battle against the Nancy school, to which he was steadily losing ground to his opponents. Moreover, Hippolyte Bernheim, the leading figure among the Nanceans, sarcastically proclaimed that among thousands of patients he had hypnotized, only one displayed the classic three stages described by Charcot, and she was a woman who had spent three years at the Salpêtrière!

Charcot also met with undying hatred on the part of some of his medical

[23] Joseph Delboeuf, "De l'influence de l'imitation et de l'éducation dans le somnambulisme provoqué," *Revue philosophique*, 22 (1886), 146–71.

[24] Bué in *Le magnétisme humain: Congrès International de 1889* (Paris, Georges Carré, 1890), 333–34, 338–39.

[25] Lyubimov, *Profesor Sharko*.

[26] George M. Beard, *The Study of Trance, Muscle-Reading and Allied Nervous Phenomena in Europe and America, with a Letter on the Moral Character of Trance Subjects and a Defence of Dr. Charcot* (New York, 1882).

colleagues and particularly on the part of his former disciple Charles Bouchard, an ambitious man twelve years his junior. Perhaps worst of all, a few of Charcot's seemingly loyal students duped him by showing him more and more extraordinary manifestations which they had rehearsed with patients behind his back and then demonstrated to him. It is true that many of his disciples never participated in such activities, but no one apparently dared warn him. He had been extremely cautious for a long time, but eventually La Rochefoucauld's maxim, that "deception always goes further than suspicion," applied to him also. According to Guillain, toward the end of his life Charcot began to feel strong doubts about his earlier teachings and was thinking of taking up again the entire study of hypnotism and hysteria. Death, however, prevented him from doing so. The secret enemy, who was so well acquainted with his medical condition that he sent him anonymous letters depicting his angina pectoris and announcing his impending death, most likely belonged to the immediate medical circle around Charcot.[27]

The extremely divergent contemporary opinions prevailing about Charcot—the fascination he exerted on the one hand and the fierce enmities he aroused on the other—made it extremely difficult in his lifetime to make a true assessment of the value of his work. Contrary to expectations, the passing of time has not made this task much easier. It is therefore necessary to distinguish the various fields of his activity. It is often forgotten that first in his career Charcot was an internist and anatomical pathologist who made extremely valuable contributions to the knowledge of pulmonary and kidney diseases and that his lectures on diseases of old age were for a long time a classic of what is now called geriatrics.[28] Similarly, in neurology, which was his "second career," Charcot made outstanding discoveries upon which his lasting fame will indisputably rest: the delineation of disseminated or multiple sclerosis, of amyotrophic lateral sclerosis ("Charcot's disease"), and of locomotor ataxia, with its peculiar arthropathies ("Charcot's joints"), as well as his work on cerebral and medullary localizations, on aphasia, and on many other topics.

On the other hand, it is most difficult to evaluate objectively what could

[27] G. Hahn, "Charcot et son influence sur l'opinion publique," *Revue des questions scientifiques*, 2d ser., 6 (II) (1894), 230–61, 353–79. See also Féré, "J. M. Charcot et son oeuvre."

[28] Writings from this period of his career that are available in English include Jean-Martin Charcot, *Lectures on Bright's Disease of the Kidneys*, translated by Henry B. Millard (London, Baillière, 1879); idem, *Clinical Lectures on Senile and Chronic Diseases*, translated by William S. Tuke (London, New Sydenham Society, 1881); idem, *Lectures on the Pathological Anatomy of the Nervous System: Diseases of the Spinal Cord*, translated by Cornelius G. Comegys (Cincinnati, Thomson, 1881); and idem, *Clinical Lectures on the Diseases of Old Age* (London, Sampson and Low, 1882).

be called Charcot's "third career," that is, his exploration of hysteria and hypnotism. As happens with many scientists, Charcot lost control of the new ideas that he had formulated and was carried away by the doctrines and the movement he created. Pierre Janet has analyzed intelligently Charcot's methodological errors in this field.[29] The first error was Charcot's excessive concern with depicting specific disease entities, choosing as model types those cases that showed as many symptoms as possible while assuming that all other cases were incomplete forms of the disease. Since this method had proved fruitful for pure clinical neurology, Charcot took it for granted that the same would hold true for mental conditions as well. He thus gave arbitrary descriptions of *grande hystérie* and *grand hypnotisme*. A second methodological mistake was to oversimplify the description of these disease entities in order to make them more intelligible to his students. A third, and fatal, error was Charcot's lack of interest in his patients' backgrounds and in the conditions of ward life at the Salpêtrière. During the 1880s, Charcot hardly ever made clinical rounds himself; rather, he saw his patients in his hospital examination room while his students, who had examined them in the wards, reported to him. Charcot never suspected that his patients were often visited and magnetized repeatedly on the wards by incompetent people. Janet showed that the alleged "three stages of hypnosis" were nothing but the result of training which Charcot's patients underwent at the hands of magnetizers. Seeing that the early history of magnetism and hypnotism was forgotten, Charcot—even more than Bernheim—believed that all the manifestations he noted in his hypnotized patients were new discoveries.

Another fact that from the start distorted Charcot's investigations in the field of dynamic psychiatry was the peculiar collective spirit that pervaded the Salpêtrière at this time. This closed institutional community not only sheltered crowds of old women, but also comprised special wards for hysterical female patients, some of them young, attractive, and cunning. Nothing could be more eminently propitious to the development of mental contagion. Some of these women developed into star attractions who were utilized time and again to demonstrate certain dramatic cases to medical students and in Charcot's lectures to the Parisian public. Owing to Charcot's paternalistic attitude and his despotic treatment of students, his staff never dared contradict him; they therefore would show him what they believed he wanted to see. After rehearsing the demonstrations, they showed the subjects to Charcot, who, in turn, was careless enough to discuss their cases in the patients' presence. As a result, a highly distinctive atmosphere of mental suggestion developed between Charcot, his collab-

[29] Pierre Janet, "J. M. Charcot, son oeuvre psychologique," *Revue philosophique*, 39 (1895), 569–604.

orators, and his hysterical patients which would certainly be worthy of a full sociological analysis.

Janet also has pointed out that Charcot's descriptions of hysteria and hypnotism were based on a very limited number of patients. Blanche Wittmann, the *prima donna* of the hysterics, deserves more than anecdotal mention. The role of patients in the elaboration of dynamic psychiatry has been all too neglected and would also be worthy of intensive investigation. Unfortunately, it is often very difficult to gather relevant information in retrospect. We know nothing, for instance, of Blanche Wittmann's origins and biographical or medical background prior to her admission to the ward for hysterical patients at the Salpêtrière. According to A. Baudouin at the Salpêtrière, Wittmann was young when she arrived at the hospital and rapidly became one of Charcot's most renowned subjects. She was nicknamed "la reine des hystériques."[30] She was often exhibited in order to demonstrate Charcot's "three stages of hypnosis," of which she was not only an example, but the prototype, according to Frederick Myers, who had seen her perform.[31] Baudouin states that Wittmann is in fact the woman in full hysterical crisis, depicted between Charcot and Babinski in André Brouillet's famous painting. She can also be recognized in several pictures in the *Iconographie photographique de la Salpêtrière* and elsewhere. She was authoritarian, capricious, and unpleasant toward the other patients and toward the personnel.

For some unknown reason, Blanche Wittmann left the Salpêtrière in the late 1880s and was admitted to the Hôtel-Dieu, where she was investigated by Jules Janet, Pierre Janet's brother.[32] After achieving the "first stage of hypnosis," that is, lethargy, Jules Janet modified the usual technique and saw the patient in quite a new condition. Under these new circumstances, a new personality, "Blanche II," emerged, showing herself much more balanced than "Blanche I." The new personality disclosed that she had been permanently present and conscious, hidden behind "Blanche I," and that she was always aware of everything that occurred during the many clinical demonstrations when she had acted out the "three stages of hypnosis" and was supposed to be unconscious. Myers noted that "it is strange to reflect for how many years the dumbly raging Blanche II has thus assisted at experiments to which Blanche I submitted with easy complacence."

Jules Janet kept Blanche Wittmann in her second state for several months and found that she was remarkably (and apparently lastingly)

[30] A. Baudouin, "Quelques souvenirs de la Salpêtrière," *Paris-médical*, 15 (I) (May 23, 1925), x–xiii.

[31] Frederick Myers, *Human Personality and Its Survival of Bodily Death*, 2 vols. (London, Longmans, Green and Co., 1903), 1:447.

[32] Jules Janet, "L'hystérie et l'hypnotisme, d'après la théorie de la double personnalité," *Revue scientifique*, 3d ser., 15 (May 19, 1888), 616–23.

improved by his treatment. What later happened to Blanche Wittmann has been succinctly reported by Baudouin. In time, the patient returned to the Salpêtrière, where she was given a job in the photographic laboratory; later, when a laboratory of radiology was opened, she was employed there. She was still authoritarian and capricious; after Charcot's death, she denied her past history of hysteria and became angry when she was asked about that period of her life. Since the dangers of radiology were not yet known, Wittmann became one the first victims of the radiologist's cancer. Her last years were a calvary which she crossed without showing the least hysterical symptom. She had to suffer one amputation after another and died a martyr of science.

Coming back to Charcot's third career, it was this segment of his work more than anything else that contributed to his contemporary fame. The writer Teodor de Wyzewa, in an obituary he wrote on Charcot, said that in a few centuries Charcot's neurological work might be forgotten, but that he would stand in the memory of mankind as the man who had revealed to the world an unsuspected realm of the mind.[33] It is through his psychological work (and not owing to his literary works, which have remained unpublished) that Charcot exerted a powerful influence on literature. As stated by De Monzie, Charcot was the starting point of a whole tradition of psychiatrically oriented writers, such as Alphonse Daudet and his son Léon Daudet, Zola, Maupassant, Huysmans, Bourget, Claretie, and later Pirandello and Proust, not to speak of many authors of popular novels.[34] Charcot himself served as the model for a specific character type in many novels and plays in the 1890s: the great scientist of world renown impavidly pursuing his uncanny research into the darker mysteries of the human mind.

An American visitor who saw Charcot at the beginning of 1893, near to the time of his death, noticed that, while his intellectual energy was as great as ever, his physical health was greatly shaken.[35] Charcot kept working feverishly until August 15, 1893, when he left for a vacation with two of his favorite disciples, Georges Debove and Isador Straus, intending to visit the Vézelay churches in the department of the Nièvre in central France. Charcot died unexpectedly in his hotel room on the night of August 16 and was given a state funeral in Paris on August 19. In spite of the deluge of praise that was lavished on his memory, his fame soon waned. The publication of his complete works, which had been planned in fifteen volumes, was abandoned after the ninth volume appeared in 1894. According to Lyubimov,

[33] Teodor de Wyzema, Le figaro, August 17, 1893.
[34] A. de Monzie, "Discours au centenaire de Charcot," Revue neurologique, 32 (I) (1925), special issue for the centennial of Charcot's birth.
[35] C. F. Withington, "A Last Glimpse of Charcot at the Salpêtrière," Boston Medical and Surgical Journal, 129 (1893), 207.

Charcot had left a considerable number of literary works: memoirs, illustrated travelogues, and critical studies on literary and philosophical works, all of which he did not want published in his lifetime. Lyubimov adds that Charcot's true personality could not be known before the publication of these materials. However, none of these writings has ever been printed. Charcot's son Jean-Baptiste (1867–1936), who had studied medicine to please his father, gave up this profession a few years later and made himself famous as a seafarer and explorer of the South Pole.[36] In 1907, Charcot's son donated his father's precious library to the Salpêtrière; but the resource gradually fell into the most pitiful state of neglect, as did the Musée Charcot.[37]

> The evil that men do lives after them;
> The good is oft interred with their bones.

And so it was with Charcot. It did not take long before his glory was transformed into the stereotype of the despotic scientist whose belief in his own superiority blinded him into unleashing a psychic epidemic. One year after Charcot's death, Léon Daudet, who had been a medical student on his ward, published a satirical novel, Les Morticoles, which gave fictitious names to prominent physicians and ridiculed the Paris medical world of the fin de siècle.[38] Charcot was depicted by Daudet under the name of "Foutange" while Bernheim was called "Boustibras"; faked hypnotic séances at the "Hôpital-Typhus" with "Rosalie" (portraying Blanche Wittmann) were described in a caricatural manner. Another malevolent account of Charcot's Salpêtrière was later given by Axel Munthe in his widely read autobiographical novel The Story of San Michele (1929).[39]

Jules Bois, who was well acquainted with Charcot, relates that during the last months of Charcot's life, the old man expressed his pessimism in regard to the future of his work, which he felt would not survive him for long.[40] In fact, less than ten years had elapsed after his death before Charcot was largely forgotten and disowned by most of his disciples. His successor at the Salpêtrière, Fulgence Raymond, while giving lip service to Charcot's work on the neuroses, himself belonged to the organicist trend in neurology. One of Charcot's favorite disciples, Joseph Babinski, who had made himself known during Charcot's lifetime by his experiments in transferring hysterical symptoms with a magnet from one patient to another,

---

[36] Anonymous, Jean-Baptiste Charcot (Paris, Yacht-Club de France, 1937). See also A. Dupouy, Charcot (Paris, Plon, 1938).

[37] J.-B. Charcot, "Discours prononcé à l'inauguration de la bibliothèque de son père," Bulletin médical, 21 (November 23, 1907).

[38] Léon Daudet, Les Morticoles (Paris, Charpentier, 1894).

[39] Axel Munthe, The Story of San Michele (New York, Duffin, 1929), chap. 17.

[40] Jules Bois, Le monde invisible (Paris, Flammarion, n.d.), 185–92.

now became the main protagonist of a radical reaction against Charcot's concept of hysteria.[41] Hysteria, Babinski claimed, was nothing but the result of suggestion, and it could be cured by "persuasion." The name *hysteria* itself was replaced by the new term *pithiatism*, coined by Babinski. Guillain reports that when he was a young resident at the Salpêtrière in 1899, that is, six years after Charcot's death, there still existed a few of Charcot's hysterical patients who for a small remuneration would act out for students the full-fledged attack of *grande hystérie*.[42] But even these patients eventually disappeared from the Salpêtrière.

As the years went by, Charcot's neurological discoveries were taken for granted and his name became associated with a regrettable and embarrassing episode in the long history of the Salpêtrière. In 1925, his centennial was celebrated at the Salpêtrière with a strong emphasis on his purely neurological achievements and a few rapid apologies about the "slight lapse—*légère défaillance*" that his work on hysteria and hypnotism had been. Psychoanalysts, however, praised Charcot for his work in this regard as a "precursor of Freud." In 1928, a group of Paris Surrealist poets, in their endeavor to counteract all accepted ideas of their time, decided to celebrate the discovery of Charcot's hysteria, which they christened "the greatest poetical discovery of the end of the nineteenth century."[43]

Several years after that, the author of the present essay, then a medical student at the Salpêtrière, met a very old woman patient who had spent almost her entire life there and had known Charcot and his school. She kept talking to herself and had hallucinations in which she was hearing all those men speaking in turn. These voices from the past, which had never been recorded but still resounded in the disturbed mind of that wretched old woman, were all that survived of the glory that had been Charcot's Salpêtrière.

[41] Joseph Babinski, *Recherches servant à établir que certaines manifestations hystériques peuvent être transférées d'un sujet à l'autre sous l'influence de l'aimant* (Paris, Delahaye & Lecrosnier, 1886); idem, "Définition de l'hystérie," *Revue neurologique*, 9 (1901), 1074–80.

[42] Guillain, *Charcot: Sa vie, son oeuvre*, chaps. 13, 14.

[43] Louis Aragon and André Breton, "Le cinquantenaire de l'hystérie (1878–1928)," *La révolution surréaliste*, 4 (1928), 20–22.

5

Pierre Janet, Philosopher

[1973]

PIERRE JANET (1859–1947) offers a remarkable example of the discrepancy that often exists in the history of psychiatry and psychology between the actual importance of the work of a thinker and the significance that is granted to that figure based on his fame and success. In 1889, when Janet published his philosophy dissertation, *L'automatisme psychologique*, and when his first publications appeared on "subconscious fixed ideas" and the psychopathology of the neuroses, contemporaries had the impression that a star of the first magnitude had risen in the firmament of psychology. However, a stereotype formed soon after this, that Janet had repudiated his early work on unconscious mental life, that his ideas were purely descriptive, and that Janetian psychology was static while that of Freud was dynamic. Few people, especially among the new generation of psychiatrists, knew that Janet was in the process of erecting a psychological synthesis that was extraordinary in its scope and audacity. Even fewer people followed his later writings and the orientation of his thought in the direction of philosophy from which it had originated.

Nevertheless, there are signs in the last few years of a renewed interest in Janet. We might recall the scholarly works that have already been dedicated to him by Björn Sjövall (1947), Elton Mayo (1948), Leonhard Schwartz (1951), and John Elmgren (1967). In France, there has even appeared a comparative study of Freud and Janet by Henri-Jean Barraud (1971). Moreover, three collections of appreciative essays about Janet have appeared: a book of *Mélanges* offered by his family and friends in 1939, a special issue of *L'évolution psychiatrique* in 1950, and a special issue of the *Bulletin de psychologie* in 1960.* These diverse writings highlight nu-

"Pierre Janet, philosophe," *Dialogue: Canadian Philosophical Journal/Revue philosophique canadienne*, 12, no. 2 (June 1973), 254–87.

*[Editor's note: The references are: Björn Sjövall, *Psychology of Tension: An Analysis of Pierre Janet's Concept of 'Tension Psychology' Together with an Historical Aspect* [1947], translated by Alan Dixon (Stockholm, Svenska Bokförlaget, Scandinavian University Books, 1967); Elton Mayo, *Some Notes on the Psychology of Pierre Janet* (Cambridge, Mass., Harvard University Press, 1948); Leonhard Schwartz, *Die Neurosen und die dynamische Psychologie von Pierre Janet* (Basel, Benno Schwabe, 1951); John Elmgren, *Pierre Janets psykologi* (Stockholm, Universitetskanslersämbetet, 1967); Henri-Jean Barraud, *Freud et*

merous aspects of the work of Janet; curiously, however, none of the authors of these writings has considered *Janet as philosopher*. A few scholars have acknowledged simply that Janet began his career as a professor of philosophy, almost as if he had to escape from this background in the process of working toward his psychology, which then became his primary lifework.

In reality, the line of evolution of Janet's thought in this regard is comparable to that of Jean Piaget, who erected an enormous system of developmental psychology from an epistemological starting point. To achieve a scientific epistemology, it was first necessary, Piaget believed, to delimit the relevant scientific problems and to explore them with an appropriate methodology capable of guaranteeing a genuine body of knowledge. In this way, Piaget formulated his monumental genetic psychological system, and once this enormous preliminary task was completed, he returned to philosophical matters directly. It is clear, then, that his so-called return to epistemology was only an illusion, since he never really left it in the first place. Exactly the same situation pertains for Janet. Beginning from the field of philosophy, Janet too erected a new psychological synthesis and then returned much later to the philosophical preoccupations from which he had begun.

Janet received a philosophical education as sound as it was possible to get in France at the time. Following his year of philosophical studies at the Lycée Louis-le-Grand in Paris, he spent three years at the École Normale Supérieure in the philosophy section, passed brilliantly the examination for the doctorate, and served as professor of philosophy for twelve years at *lycées* in Châteauroux, Le Havre, and Paris. He compiled no fewer than six philosophy textbooks for college instruction. Janet was exposed to several formative philosophical influences. The first of these was that of his uncle, Paul Janet, the well-known representative of spiritualist philosophy. Next came the influence of classic French philosophy: Descartes, Malebranche, and the Ideologues, especially Maine de Biran, and, among more recent figures, Boutroux, Fouillée, and Jean-Marie Guyau. At the École Normale Supérieure, Janet had been a close friend of Henri Bergson, and there remained during their entire lives a close and reciprocal intellectual relationship between the two philosophers. Janet was little interested in German philosophy, which he was unable to read in the original language; he was much more concerned with the work of the Americans, notably Josiah Royce and William James. Far from abandoning philosophy, Janet

---

Janet: *Étude comparée* (Toulouse, Privat, 1971); *Mélanges offerts à Monsieur Pierre Janet par sa famille, ses amis et ses disciples à l'occasion de ses quatre-vingts ans* (Paris, d'Artrey, 1939); "Hommage à Pierre Janet," special issue of *L'évolution psychiatrique*, fascimile 3 (1950), 343–501; and *Bulletin de psychologie*, special issue in commemoration of Pierre Janet, 14 (November 1960).]

built his entire work on an adjacent philosophical system which always remained the solid intellectual base on which his psychology rested. [. . .]

During the 1960s, in the process of preparing my book *The Discovery of the Unconscious*, which contains an important chapter on Janet, I noticed that Janet's bibliography had never been adequately established. The only known bibliographical listing is located in the special issue of *L'évolution psychiatrique* in Janet's honor (1950, no. 3, 497–501). This record, compiled by R. Diatkine, has been highly useful to scholars; however, it remains very incomplete and contains quite a few errors. The bibliography below is the result of much research, even though it too cannot claim to be exhaustive. Almost all of the references below have been verified against the actual original publications. It might be noted that some of the publications cited are nearly impossible to locate and do not even exist at the Bibliothèque Nationale in Paris. It is my hope that this catalogue will contribute to bringing the work of Pierre Janet out of the historical shadows in which it has been hidden for so long.

BIBLIOGRAPHY OF THE WRITINGS OF PIERRE JANET

COMPILED BY HENRI F. ELLENBERGER

MANUALS OF PHILOSOPHY

1. *Manuel du baccalauréat de l'enseignement secondaire classique* (2e partie, 2e et 3e séries), moderne (2e partie, 2e et 3e séries), PHILOSOPHIE (Paris, Nony, 1894), In–16.
2. *Manuel du baccalauréat de l'enseignement secondaire classique* (2e partie, 1e série), moderne (2e partie, 1e série), Classes de philosophie et de première-lettres. PHILOSOPHIE (Paris, Nony, 1896), In–16.
3. *Manuel du baccalauréat de l'enseignement secondaire* (Classes de philosophie A et B), PHILOSOPHIE, 3e édition (Paris, Vuibert and Nony, 1905), In–. 5e édition (1909) (unchanged).
4. *Manuel du baccalauréat de l'enseignement secondaire* (2e partie), PHILOSOPHIE (Classes de mathématiques A et B). 4e édition (Paris, Vuibert and Nony, 1905), In–16.
5. *Manuel du baccalauréat seconde partie* (Série philosophie), PHILOSOPHIE, *Questions complémentaires* (programme du 3 décembre 1923), avec la collaboration de H. Piéron et C. Lalo (Paris, Vuibert, 1925). (Janet, pp. 109–60).
6. *Manuel du baccalauréat* (2e partie) (Série philosophie), PHILOSOPHIE, 14e édition entièrement refondue (Paris, Vuibert, 1930).

BOOKS

1. *L'Automatisme psychologique* (Paris, Alcan, 1889).
2. *Baco Verulamius alchemicis philosophis quid debuerit* (Angers, Imprimerie Burdin, 1889).

3. *L'Anesthésie hystérique. L'Amnésie hystérique. La Suggestion chez les hystériques* (Evreux, Imprimerie Hérissey, s.d., 1892). (Reproduction of three lectures given at the Salpêtrière in March and April of 1892).

4. *Contribution à l'étude des accidents mentaux chez les hystériques*, Thèse médicale. Paris, 1892–1893, no. 432 (soutenue le 29 juillet 1893) (Paris, Rueff and Cie, 1893).

5. *État mental des hystériques*, Bibliothèque médicale Charcot-Debove, 2 volumes (Paris, Rueff and Cie). I. *Les stigmates mentaux* (Préface de Charcot) (1893). II. *Les accidents mentaux* (1894) (modified reproduction of no. 4).

   5a. German translation: *Der Geisteszustand der Hysterischen: die psychischen Stigmata.* Uebers. von Max Kahan (Leipzig, Deuticke, 1894) (translation of vol. I).

   5b. English translation of vols. I and II by C. Corson, *The Mental State of Hystericals* (New York and London, Putnam's Sons, 1901).

6. *Névroses et idées fixes*, 2 volumes (Paris, Alcan, 1898). Vol. I by Pierre Janet. Vol. II by F. Raymond and P. Janet.

   6a. Russian translation by M. P. Litvinov, *Nevrozy i fiksirovannyja idei, Piera Jane* (St. Petersburg, O. N. Popova, 1903).

7. *Les Obsessions et la psychasténie*, 2 volumes (Paris, Alcan, 1903). Vol. I by Pierre Janet. Vol. II by F. Raymond and P. Janet.

8. *The Major Symptoms of Hysteria* (London and New York, Macmillan, 1907).

   8a. 2nd edition with new material (1920).

   8b. Facsimile of 1920 edition (New York, Hafner, 1965).

9. *Les Névroses* (Paris, Flammarion, 1909).

   9a. Portuguese translation by Dr. Pedro Janet, *Nevroses* (Paris and Rio de Janeiro, Livraria Garnier, 1924).

10. *L'État mental des hystériques. Les stigmates mentaux des hystériques. Les accidents mentaux des hystériques. Études sur divers symptômes hystériques. Le traitement psychologique de l'hystérie*, 2e édition (Paris, Alcan, 1911).

11. *Les Médications psychologiques*, 3 volumes (Paris, Alcan, 1919).

   11a. English translation by Eden and Cedar Paul, *Psychological Healing: A Historical and Clinical Study*, 2 volumes (London, G. Allen & Unwin; New York, Macmillan, 1925).

12. *La Médecine psychologique* (Paris, Flammarion, 1923).

   12a. English translation by H. M. and E. R. Guthrie, *Principles of Psychotherapy* (New York, Macmillan, 1924).

   12b. Reedition of the English translation (Freeport, N.Y., Books for Libraries Press, 1971).

13. *De l'angoisse à l'extase. Études sur les croyances et les sentiments* (Paris, Alcan). Vol. I: *Un délire religieux. La croyance* (1926). Vol. II: *Les Sentiments fondamentaux* (1928).

14. *Psychologie expérimentale*, Comptes rendus du cours de M. Janet (Collège de France) (Paris, Chanine, 1926).

15. *Les Stades de l'évolution psychologique* (Paris, Maloine, 1926).

16. *Psicología de los sentimientos*, Curso desarrollado en los meses agosto y septiembre de 1925 en la Universidad Nacional de Mexico. Versíon del Dr. En-

rique O. Aragon (Mexico, Sociedad de Edicíon y Librería franco-americana, 1926).

17. *La Pensée intérieure et ses troubles* (Paris, Maloine, 1927).
18. *L'Évolution de la mémoire et de la notion du temps* (Paris, Chahine, 1928).
19. *L'Évolution psychologique de la personnalité* (Paris, Chahine, 1929).
20. *La Force et la faiblesse psychologiques* (Paris, Maloine, 1932).
21. *L'Amour et la haine* (Paris, Maloine, 1932).
22. *Les Débuts de l'intelligence* (Paris, Flammarion, 1935).
    22a. Reedition by Imprensa Nacional (Rio de Janeiro, Americ-edit., Collection Connaissances et Culture, 1935).
23. *L'Intelligence avant le langage* (Paris, Flammarion, 1936).

ARTICLES AND PAMPHLETS

1. *Le fondement du droit de propriété*, Conférence de M. Pierre Janet, professeur de philosophie au Lycée, le samedi 10 février 1883. Ligue française de l'enseignement (Cercle de Châteauroux, Imprimerie Gablin, 1883).
2. *Lycée du Havre. Palmarès de la distribution des prix (1884)*, Discours prononcé par M. Pierre Janet, pp. 9–13.
3. "Note sur quelques phénomènes de somnambulisme," *Bulletins de la Société de Psychologie physiologique*, i (1885), pp. 24–32.
   3a. Reproduced in *Revue Philosophique*, xxi (1886), I, pp. 190–198.
4. "Les phases intermédiaires de l'hypnotisme," *Revue Scientifique* (Revue Rose), 3e série, ii (= vol. 23) (May 8, 1886), pp. 577–587.
5. "Deuxième note sur le sommeil provoqué à distance et la suggestion mentale pendant l'état somnambulique," *Bulletins de la Société de Psychologie physiologique*, ii (1886), pp. 70–80.
   5a. Reproduced in *Revue Philosophique*, xxii (1886), II, pp. 212–223.
6. "Les actes inconscients et le dédoublement de la personnalité pendant le somnambulisme provoqué," *Revue Philosophique*, xxii (1886), II, pp. 577–592.
7. "L'anesthésie systématisée et la dissociation des phénomènes psychologiques," *Revue Philosophique*, xxiii (1887), I, pp. 449–472.
8. "Les actes inconscients et la mémoire pendant le somnambulisme," *Revue Philosophique*, xxv (1888), I, pp. 238–279.
9. "Une altération de la faculté de localiser les sensations," Conférence à la Société de Psychologie physiologique, séance du 31 mars 1890, *Revue Philosophique*, xxix (1890), I, pp. 659–664.
10. "Étude sur un cas d'aboulie et d'idées fixes," *Revue Philosophique*, xxxi (1891), I, pp. 258–287, 382–407.
11. "Kyste parasitaire du cerveau," *Archives générales de médecine* (1891), II, pp. 464–472 (VIIe série, tome 28).
12. *Discours prononcé à la distribution des prix au Collège Rollin*, le 30 juillet 1892 (Paris, Chaix, 1892).
13. "Étude sur quelques cas d'amnésie antérograde dans la maladie de la désagrégation psychologique," *International Congress of Experimental Psychology*, second session, London, 1892. (London, Williams & Norgate, 1892) (Janet, pp. 26–30).

14. "Discussion d'une communication de F. W. H. Myers: Sensory Automatism and Induced Hallucinations," *International Congress of Experimental Psychology*, second session, London, 1892 (London, Williams & Norgate, 1892) (Janet, pp. 162–164, 164–165).

15. "Le Congrès international de Psychologie expérimentale," 1–4 août 1892, *Revue générale des Sciences*, iii (1892), pp. 606–616.

16. "Le spiritisme contemporain," *Revue Philosophique*, xxxiii (1892), I, pp. 413–442.

17. "L'anesthésie hystérique," Conférence faite à la Salpêtrière le 11 mars 1892, *Archives de Neurologie*, xxiii (1892), pp. 323–352.

18. "L'amnésie hystérique," Deuxième conférence faite à la Salpêtrière le 17 mars 1892, *Archives de Neurologie*, xxiv (1892), pp. 29–55.

19. "La suggestion chez les hystériques," Troisième conférence faite à la Salpêtrière, le 1er avril 1892, *Archives de Neurologie*, xxiv (1892), pp. 448–470.

20. (Rectification au compte rendu de 1890, p. 55, du Congrès de Psychologie de 1889, à propos de l'attribution à M. Ballet de la communication sur le rétrécissement du champ visuel provoqué par l'attention.) *Archives de Neurologie*, xxiv (1892), p. 459.

21. "Sur un nouvel appareil destiné à l'étude expérimentale des sensations kinesthésiques," *Revue Philosophique*, xxxiv (1892), II, pp. 506–509.

22. "L'amnésie continue," *Revue générale des Sciences*, iv (1893), pp. 167–179.

23. J. M. Charcot, *Clinique des maladies du système Nerveux*, Georges Guinon, ed., ii (Paris, Progrès Médical and Alcan, 1893). Note on the treatment of "Madame D." added to a case history by Charcot, pp. 266–287 (Janet, pp. 287–288).

24. "Quelques définitions récentes de l'hystérie," *Archives de Neurologie*, xxv (June, 1893), pp. 417–438; xxvi (July, 1893), pp. 1–29.

25. "Histoire d'une idée fixe," *Revue Philosophique*, xxxvii (1894), I, pp. 121–168.

26. "Un cas de possession et l'exorcisme moderne," Conférence faite le 23 décembre 1894, *Bulletin des travaux de l'Université de Lyon*, viii, fascimile 2 (December, 1894–January, 1895), pp. 41–57.

27. "Les idées fixes de forme hystérique," Conférence faite à la Salpêtrière le 3 mai 1895, *Presse médicale*, iii (1895), pp. 201–203.

    27a. Reproduced in *Revue de l'Hypnotisme*, ix, no. 12 (1895), pp. 353–367.

28. "Un cas d'hémianopsie hystérique," Conférence faite à la Salpêtrière le 25 janvier 1895, *Archives de Neurologie*, xxix (May, 1895), pp. 337–358.

29. "J. M. Charcot. Son oeuvre psychologique," *Revue Philosophique*, xxxix (1895), I, pp. 569–604.

30. "Rapport sur 'Le merveilleux scientifique' de M. Durand (de Gros)," *Annales médico-psychologiques*, 8e série, 53e année (1895), I, pp. 447–455.

31. "Les délires ambulatoires ou les fugues," Leçon recueillie par le Dr. Pierre Janet (with F. Raymond), *Gazette des Hôspitaux*, lxviii (1895), pp. 754–762, 787–793.

    31a. Abstract in *Les Névroses* (Paris, Flammarion, 1909), pp. 243–246.

32. "Note sur quelques spasmes des muscles du tronc chez les hystériques," *La France médicale et Paris médical*, xxxxii (1895), pp. 769–776.

33. "Résumé historique des études sur le sentiment de la personnalité," *Revue Scientifique* (Revue Rose), lvii (1896), pp. 97–103.

34. "L'influence somnambulique et le besoin de direction," *Dritter Internationaler Congress für Psychologie*, vom 4. bis 7. August, 1896 (Munich, J. F. Lehmann, 1897), pp. 143–145.

   34a. Enlarged version in *Revue Philosophique*, xxxxiii (1897), I, pp. 113–143.

   34b. Reprinted in *Névroses et idées fixes*, i (Paris, Alcan, 1898), pp. 423–480.

35. "Note sur les temps de réaction simple dans leur rapport avec les maladies de l'attention," *Dritter Internationaler Congress für Psychologie*, vom 4. bis 7. August, 1896 (Munich, J. F. Lehmann, 1897), pp. 292–295.

   35a. Reproduced in *Journal de Neurologie et d'Hypnologie*, i (1897), pp. 409–410.

36. "Sur la divination par les miroirs et les hallucinations subconscientes," *Conférence faite à l'Université de Lyon*, ii (July, 1897), pp. 261–274.

   36a. Reprinted in *Névroses et idées fixes*, i (Paris, Alcan, 1898), pp. 407–422.

37. "L'insomnie par idée fixe subconsciente," *Presse médicale*, v (1897), II, pp. 41–44.

38. "Hysterische, systematisirte Contractur bei einer Ekstatischen," *Münchener medicinische Wochenschrift*, xxxxiv (1897), pp. 856–857.

39. "Le Troisième Congrès international de Psychologie," *Revue générale des Sciences*, viii (1897), pp. 22–27.

40. "Une opération chirurgicale pendant le somnambulisme provoqué," *Journal de Neurologie*, ii (1897), pp. 22–24.

41. "Malformation des mains en 'pinces de homard' et asymétrie du corps chez une épileptique" (with F. Raymond), *Nouvelle Iconographie de la Salpêtrière*, x (1897), pp. 369–373.

42. "Hoquets et rots hystériques" (with F. Raymond), *Journal des Praticiens*, xii (1898), pp. 393–398.

43. "Tic de contraction des mâchoires pendant la parole" (with F. Raymond), *Journal des Praticiens*, xii (1898), pp. 529–530.

44. "Obsession érotique chez une hystérique, avec hallucinations, se manifestant pendant le somnambulisme d'une manière beaucoup plus complète que pendant la veille" (with F. Raymond), *Journal des Praticiens*, xii (1898), pp. 609–611.

45. "Perte du sentiment de la personnalité" (with F. Raymond), *Journal des Praticiens*, xii (1898), pp. 625–630.

46. "L'attention volontaire dans l'éducation physique," *Revue Encyclopédique*, ix (1899), pp. 695–696.

47. "Note sur deux tics du pied" (with F. Raymond), *Nouvelle Iconographie de la Salpêtrière*, xii (1899), pp. 353–357.

48. "Note sur l'hystérie droite et l'hystérie gauche" (with F. Raymond), *Revue Neurologique*, vii (1899), pp. 851–855.

   48a. Reprinted in *L'État mental des hystériques* (Paris, Alcan, 1911), pp. 451–457.

49. "Un cas d'hémianopsie hystérique transitoire," *Presse médicale*, vii (1899), II, pp. 241–243.

   49a. Reprinted in *L'État mental des hystériques* (Paris, Alcan, 1911), pp. 458–469.

50. "Objet de l'Institut Psychologique," *Bulletin de l'Institut Psychique International*, dirigé par le Dr. Pierre Janet, i (1900–1901), pp. 85–96.

51. "Société de Psychologie," Première séance à l'Hôtel des Sociétés Savantes le 29 mars 1901. Allocution de M. Pierre Janet. *Bulletin de l'Institut Psychique International*, i (1900–1901), pp. 133–139.

52. "Discussion sur les hallucinations. A la suite de 'Gilbert Ballet: Psychologie pathologique des hallucinations,' *Bulletin de l'Institut Psychologique International*, i (1900–1901), pp. 186–188 (Janet, pp. 188–192).

53. "Une Extatique," Conférence faite à l'Institut Psychologique International le 25 mai 1901, *Bulletin de l'Institut Psychologique International*, i (1900–1901), pp. 209–240.

54. "Discussion sur la rapidité de la réaction consciente. A la suite de Sollier: Sur la rapidité de la réaction consciente," *Bulletin de l'Institut Psychologique International*, i (1900–1901), pp. 286–290 (Janet, pp. 290–292).

55. "Un cas du phénomène des apports," *Bulletin de l'Institut Psychologique International*, i (1900–1901), pp. 329–335.

   55a. Reprinted in *L'État mental des hystériques* (Paris, Alcan, 1911), pp. 499–505.

56. "La maladie du scrupule ou l'aboulie délirante. Le contenu des obsessions," *Revue Philosophique*, li (1901), I, pp. 337–359, 499–524.

57. "Un cas de rythme de Cheyne-Stokes dans l'hystérie. Influence de l'activité cérébrale sur la respiration" (with F. Raymond), *Quatrième Congrès international de Psychologie*, Paris, 20–26 août 1900 (Paris, Alcan, 1901), pp. 524–537; discussion on pp. 537–540.

   57a. Reprinted in *L'État mental des hystériques* (Paris, Alcan, 1911), pp. 484–498.

58. "L'hypnotisme et la psychologie au Collège de France," *Revue de l'Hypnotisme*, xvi, no. 10 (1902), pp. 289–290.

59. "Le syndrome psychasthénique de l'"akathisie' " (with F. Raymond), *Nouvelle Iconographie de la Salpêtrière*, xv (1902), pp. 241–246.

60. "Spasmes et tremblements chez des psychasthéniques" (with F. Raymond), *Nouvelle Iconographie de la Salpêtrière*, xvi (1903), pp. 209–217.

61. "Un trouble de la vision par exagération de l'association binoculaire," *Annales d'Oculistique*, cxxx (July, 1903), pp. 29–41.

   61a. Reproduced in *Bulletin de l'Institut Général Psychologique*, iii (1903), pp. 631–645; discussion on pp. 645–649.

   61b. Reprinted in *L'État mental des hystériques* (Paris, Alcan, 1911), pp. 470–483.

62. "Les maladies déterminées par l'émotion," Conférence faite à l'Union des Femmes de France le 24 février 1904, *L'Union des Femmes de France. Bulletin officiel* (. . .), 7e série, no. 1 (Paris, Masson, 1904), pp. 8–10.

63. "Dépersonnalisation et possession chez un psychasthénique" (with F. Raymond), *Journal de Psychologie*, i (1904), pp. 28–37.

64. "L'amnésie et la dissociation des souvenirs par l'émotion," Communication à la Société médico-psychologique, *Journal de Psychologie*, i (1904), pp. 417–453.

   64a. Abstract in *Les Névroses* (Paris, Flammarion, 1909), pp. 6–8, 40–41, 60, 62.

64b. Reprinted in *L'État mental des hystériques* (Paris, Alcan, 911), pp. 506–544.

65. "La durée des sensations visuelles élémentaires," *Bulletin de l'Institut Général Psychologique*, iv (1904), p. 540.

66. "The Psycholeptic Crises," Paper read by invitation before the Boston Society of Psychiatry and Neurology, October 20, 1904, *Boston Medical and Surgical Journal*, clii (1905), pp. 93–100.

67. "Mental Pathology," *Psychological Review*, xii (1905), pp. 98–117. Modified reprint of a lecture delivered at the Congress of Arts and Science in St. Louis, 24 September 1904. (See also entry no. 71.)

68. *Atti del V Congresso Internazionale di Psicologia tenuto in Roma dal 26 al 30 aprile 1905.* Dr. Sante de Sanctis (Roma, Forzani, 1906). Discours des délégués (Janet, p. 51).

69. "Les oscillations du niveau mental," Conférence faite au Cinquième Congrès de Psychologie, Rome, le 29 avril 1905, *Atti del V Congresso Internazionale di Psicologia tenuto in Roma dal 26 al 30 aprile 1905.* (Dr. Sante de Sanctis (Roma, Forzani, 1906), pp. 110–126.

69a. Reproduced in *Revue des Idées*, ii (1905), pp. 729–755.

70. "A propos du 'déjà vu,'" *Journal de Psychologie*, ii (1905), pp. 289–307.

71. "The Relations of Abnormal Psychology," *International Congress of Arts and Science. Universal Exposition*, St. Louis, 1904, edited by Howard J. Rogers, v (Boston, 1906), pp. 737–753.

72. "Un cas de délire systématisé dans la paralysie générale," *Journal de Psychologie*, iii (1906), pp. 329–331.

73. "On the Pathogenesis of Some Impulsions," *The Journal of Abnormal Psychology*, i (1906–1907), pp. 1–17.

74. "Un trouble de la vision par exagération de l'association binoculaire," *Journal de Psychologie*, iv (1907), pp. 245–246.

74a. English translation as "A Disturbance of Vision due to Exaggeration of Binocular Association," Paper read to the New York Neurological Society on November 28, 1906, *Medical Record*, lxxi (1907), pp. 757–759.

75. "Le besoin d'excitation dans les impulsions psychasthéniques," *Journal de Psychologie*, iv (1907), pp. 346–351.

76. "Letter of Dr. Pierre Janet," *Journal of the American Society for Psychical Research*, i, no. 2 (1907), pp. 73–93.

77. "Théories modernes sur la genèse de l'hystérie," *Compte rendu des Travaux du Premier Congrès International de Psychiatrie, de Neurologie, de Psychologie et de l'Assistance aux Aliénés*, tenu à Amsterdam du 2 au 7 septembre 1907 (Amsterdam, J. H. de Bussy, 1908), pp. 264–270.

78. "Le renversement de l'orientation ou l'allochirie des représentations," *Journal de Psychologie*, v (1908), II, pp. 89–97. Discussion, pp. 147–149.

79. "Délire systématique à la suite des sentiments d'incomplétude chez une psychasthénique," *Journal de Psychologie*, v (1908), pp. 157–160.

79a. "Délire systématique à la suite de pratiques du spiritisme," *Revue Neurologique*, xvii (1909), pp. 432–435.

79b. Reproduced in *L'Encéphale*, iv (1909), I, pp. 363–368.

80. "Un cas de délire somnambulique avec retour à l'enfance," *Journal de Psychologie*, v (1908), pp. 336–.

80a. Reproduced in *L'Encéphale*, iii (1908), II, pp. 104–108.

80b. Abstract in *Revue Neurologique*, xvi (1908), I, pp. 1172–1173. Discussion, pp. 1173–1174.

81. "La perte des sentiments de valeur dans la dépression mentale," *Journal de Psychologie*, v (1908), pp. 481–487.

82. "Le sentiment de la dépersonnalisation," *Journal de Psychologie*, v (1908), pp. 514–516.

83. "Discussion sur la communication de Delmas et Dupouy 'Un cas d'inversion sexuelle masculine,'" *Journal de Psychologie*, v (1908), pp. 516–525 (Janet, pp. 525–526).

84. "Qu'est-ce qu'une névrose?" *Revue Scientifique* (Revue Rose), lxxxiii (1909), pp. 129–138.

84a. Reprinted in *Les Névroses* (Paris, Flammarion, 1909), Conclusion.

85. "Problèmes psychologiques (de l'émotion)," in *Du rôle de l'émotion dans la genèse des accidents névropathiques et psychopathiques*, Compte rendu officiel des séances, *Revue Neurologique*, xvii (1909), II, pp. 1551–1562; participation in general discussion, pp. 1578–1687.

86. "Une Félida artificielle," *Revue Philosophique*, lxix (1910), I, pp. 329–357, 483–529.

86a. Reprinted in *L'État mental des hystériques* (Paris, Alcan, 1911), pp. 545–618.

87. "Les problèmes du subconscient," *Sixième Congrès international de Psychologie*, Genève, 2–7 août 1909, *Rapports et comptes rendus*, ed. Édouard Claparède (Geneva, Kündig, 1910), pp. 57–70.

87a. Reproduced in "Le Subconscient," *Scientia*, vii, année 4, no. 13 (1910), pp. 64–79.

88. "Les problèmes de la suggestion," Jahresversammlung der internationalen Gesellschaft für medizinische Psychologie und Psychotherapie, Brussels, 7–8 August 1910, *Journal für Psychologie und Neurologie*, xvii, Ergänzungsheft (1910–1911), pp. 323–343.

89. "La Kleptomanie et la dépression mentale," *Journal de Psychologie*, viii (1911), pp. 97–103.

90. "Les névroses hystériques," *Le Journal* (Paris) (Thursday, August 8, 1912), no. 7256, p. 6.

91. "La psycho-analyse," *XVIIth International Congress of Medicine*, London, 1913, Section XII. Psychiatry I, pp. 13–64. Discussion, Section XII (II, pp. 51–55).

91a. Reproduced without the discussion in *Journal de Psychologie*, ii (1914), pp. 1–130.

91b. German translation: "Janet über die Psychoanalyse," *Zentralblatt für Psychoanalyse und Psychotherapie*, iv (1914), pp. 309–316.

91c. English translation: "Psychoanalysis," *The Journal of Abnormal Psychology*, ix (1914–1915), pp. 1–35, 153–187.

92. "Valeur de la psycho-analyse de Freud" (Société de psychothérapie, d'hypnologie et de psychologie, séance annuelle du 16 juin 1914), *Revue de Psychothérapie et de Psychologie appliquée*, 29e année, nos. 3, 4 (March–April, 1915), pp. 82–83.

93. "L'alcoolisme et la dépression mentale," *Académie des Sciences Morales et Politiques, Séances et Travaux,* Compte rendu, séance du 7 août 1915, nouvelle série, tome 84 (184e de la collection) (1915), II, pp. 299–311.

   93a. Reproduced in *Revue internationale de Sociologie,* xxiii (1915), pp. 476–485.

   93b. English translation: "Alcoholism in Relation to Mental Depression," *Journal of the American Medical Association,* lxxvii (1921), pp. 1462–1467.

94. "Notice sur la vie et les oeuvres de M. Alfred Fouillée," *Académie des Sciences Morales et Politiques, Séances et Travaux,* Compte rendu (. . .), séance du 8 avril 1916, 76e année, nouvelle série, tome 86 (185e de la collection) (1916), II, pp. 225–253, 392–416.

   94a. Reproduced in the form of a brochure with a photograph of Fouillée (Paris, Firmin-Didot, 1916).

95. "Rapport sur la Fondation Carnot et sur les Fondations Gasne, Augustine Bon, Davillier et Schumacher de Guerry pour 1916," *Académie des Sciences Morales et Politiques, Séances et Travaux,* Compte rendu, séance du 17 juin 1916, 76e année, nouvelle série, tome 86 (185e de la collection) (1916), II, pp. 497–508.

96. "Théodule Ribot" (with Georges Dumas), *Le Temps* (Paris) (December 11, 1916), p. 3.

97. "La tension psychologique et ses oscillations," *Journal de Psychologie,* xii (1915–1917), pp. 165–193.

   97a. Included in Georges Dumas, ed., *Traité de Psychologie* (1923), pp. 919–952.

98. "L'oeuvre psychologique de Th. Ribot," Leçon faite au Collège de France le 11 décembre 1916, *Journal de Psychologie,* xii (1915–1917), pp. 268–282.

99. "Les fatigues sociales et l'antipathie," *Revue Philosophique,* lxxxvii (1919), pp. 1–71.

100. "Les oscillations de l'activité mentale. Les degrés de l'activation des tendances," Cours du Collège de France (1916–1917), *Journal de Psychologie,* xvii (1920), pp. 31–38.

101. "Les oscillations de l'activité mentale. Les degrés de l'activité mentale," Cours du Collège de France (1917–1918), *Journal de Psychologie,* xvii (1920), pp. 38–44.

102. "Un cas de sommeil prolongé avec perte du sentiment du réel," *Journal de Psychologie,* xvii (1920), pp. 665–672.

   102a. "A Case of Sleep Lasting Five Years, with Loss of Sense of Reality," Paper read at the 47th Annual Meeting of the American Neurological Association, Atlantic City, New Jersey, June, 1921, *Archives of Neurology and Psychiatry,* vi (1921), II, pp. 467–474.

103. "Les oscillations de l'activité mentale," *Journal de Psychologie,* xviii (1921), pp. 140–145.

104. "Le centenaire de l'Hôpital Bloomingdale," *Annales médico-psychologiques,* 11e série, 79e année (1921), II, pp. 344–346.

105. "La tension psychologique, ses degrés, ses oscillations," *British Journal of Psychology. Medical Section,* i (1920–1921), pp. 1–15, 144–164, 209–224.

106. "Les deux formes de la volonté et de la croyance dans un cas de délire psych-

asthénique," in *Congrès des Sociétés américaine, anglaise, belge, italienne, et de la Société française de Philosophie*, session extraordinaire tenue à la Sorbonne du 27 au 31 décembre 1921 (Paris, Librairie Armand Collin, 1925) (Janet, pp. 139–169).

107. "La peur de l'action," *Journal de Psychologie*, xix (1922), pp. 459–460.

107a. English translation: "The Fear of Action," *Journal of Abnormal and Social Psychology*, xvi (1921–1922), pp. 150–160.

108. "Discussion d'une communication d'Henri Wallon: Un cas de brusque variation dans la forme de crise d'origine émotive," *Journal de Psychologie*, xix (1922), pp. 551–556 (Janet, pp. 556–557).

109. "Discussion d'une communication de F. L. Arnaud: Sur la sincérité de certains délirants," *Journal de Psychologie*, xix (1922), pp. 557–562 (Janet, pp. 563–566).

110. "A Case of Psychasthenic Delirium," translation of a manuscript of Janet by Francis Devlin, *American Journal of Psychiatry*, i, no. 3 (1922), pp. 319–334.

111. "Psychic Asthenia and Atony" (in French with English title), *VIIth International Congress of Psychology, Oxford, July 26 August 2, 1923*, Proceedings and Papers (Cambridge, Cambridge University Press, 1924), pp. 201–211.

111a. "L'atonie et l'asthénie psychologiques," *British Journal of Medical Psychology*, iv, part I (1924), pp. 1–11.

112. "A propos de la métapsychique," *Revue Philosophique*, xcvi (1923), pp. 5–32.

113. Discours à l'occasion de sa présidence pour 1925 (10 janvier 1925), *Académie des Sciences Morales et Politiques, Séances et Travaux*, Compte rendu, 85e année (1925), I, pp. 164–168.

114. "Les souvenirs irréels," *Archives de Psychologie*, xix (1924), pp. 1–44.

115. "Les états de consolation et les extases. Les sentiments de joie dans l'extase," *Journal de Psychologie*, xxii (1925), pp. 370–420, 465–499.

116. "Discours à l'Institut de France," *Académie des Sciences Morales et Politiques, Séances et Travaux*, Séance publique annuelle du 19 décembre 1925 (Paris, Firmin-Didot, 1925), pp. 3–71.

117. "Psychoneuroses," translation by Elton Mayo of a lecture given by Janet at the Philadelphia General Hospital on October 14, 1925, *The American Journal of Medical Sciences*, clxxi (1926), pp. 781–786.

118. "Le 8e Congrès international de Psychologie, réuni à Groningue du 6 au 11 septembre 1926," *Journal de Psychologie*, xxiv (1927), pp. 348–354.

119. "Social Excitation in Religion," Paper read at the Eighth International Congress of Psychology at Groningen, September 8, 1926, *Psyche* (London), vii, no. 26 (October, 1926–1927), pp. 6–14.

120. "Rapport sur la Suggestion," présenté le 27 novembre 1926 au Congrès de Psychiatrie de Zürich, *Archives suisses de Neurologie et de Psychiatrie*, xx (1927), I, pp. 5–22.

121. "La Peur de l'action," *Revue Philosophique*, ciii (1927), I, pp. 321–336); civ (1927), II, pp. 5–21.

122. "Discussion du rapport de J. Lévy-Valensi: L'automatisme mental . . . ," *Congrès des Médecins Aliénistes et Neurologistes de France et de langue fran-*

çaise, 31e session, Blois, 25–30 juillet 1927 (Paris, Masson, 1927), pp. 168–171.

123. "A propos de la schizophrénie," *Journal de Psychologie*, xxiv (1927), pp. 477–492.

124. "Le sentiment du vide," *Journal de Psychologie*, xxiv (1927), pp. 861–887.
   124a. Abstract in *Annales médico-psychologiques*, 12e série, 85e année (1927), II, pp. 275–277.

125. "Les béatitudes," *Revue Philosophique*, cv (1928), I, pp. 321–366; cvi (1928), II, pp. 106–148.

126. "Discussion d'une communication de Piaget: Les trois systèmes de la pensée de l'enfant," *Bulletin de la Société française de Philosophie*, xxviii, no. 4 (July–September, 1928), pp. 97–141 (Janet, pp. 138–140).

127. "La catatonie et les sentiments," *Congrès des Médecins Aliénistes et Neurologistes de France de langue française*, 32e session, Anvers, 23–28 juillet 1928 (Paris, Masson, 1928), pp. 247–253.

128. "Un cas du vol de la pensée," *Annales médico-psychologiques*, 12e série, 86e année (1928), II, pp. 146–164.

129. "Les sentiments régulateurs de l'action," *Bulletin de la Société française de Philosophie*, xxix (1929), pp. 73–103.

130. "Psychologie et graphologie," *L'Hygiène mentale*, xxv (1930), pp. 191–194.

131. "La force et la faiblesse psychologiques," *Acta. IIIe cours international de perfectionnement pour médecins*, Locarno, 11–26 octobre 1931, Tomarkin-Foundation New York (Siège Européan Locarno, Switzerland, 1931). I. "Les dépenses de l'action," Conférence du 12 octobre 1931, pp. 20–22. II. "Les maladies par faiblesse psychologique et la démence asthénique," Conférence du 13 octobre 1931, pp. 28–30. III. "Les hypothèses sur les lois et la nature de la force psychologique," Conférence du 14 octobre 1931, pp. 35–37.

132. "L'intelligence élémentaire (I): La ressemblance et le portrait," *Revue des Cours et Conférences*, xxxiii (April 30, 1932), pp. 97–110.

133. "L'intelligence élémentaire (II): La psychologie de la forme," *Revue des Cours et Conférences*, xxxiii (May 15, 1932), pp. 211–228.

134. "L'hallucination dans le délire de persécution," *Revue Philosophique*, cxiii (1932), I, pp. 61–98.

135. "Les croyances et les hallucinations," *Revue Philosophique*, cxiii (1932), I, pp. 278–331.

136. "La relativité de la subconscience," *Psychologie et vie*, vi (1932), pp. 3–4.

137. "Les sentiments dans le délire de persécution," *Journal de Psychologie*, xxix (1932), pp. 161–240, 401–460.

138. "Pedro Janet. Nuevo socio correspondiente de la Sociedad Científica Argentina," Discours du président, le Dr. Nicolás Lozano, et de Pierre Janet, le 13 septembre 1932, résumés en traduction espagnole, *Anales de la Sociedad Científica Argentina*, cxiv (1932), II, pp. 308–310.

139. "Les progrès de la science en Argentine," *Journal des Nations américaines. L'Argentine*, nouvelle série, no. 7, 1e année (June 18, 1933) (Janet, pp. 1–2).

140. "Les débuts de l'intelligence," *Revue Bleue, politique et littéraire*, lxxiii (1935), pp. 1–7.
   140a. Reprinted in *Les Débuts de l'intelligence* (Paris, Flammarion, 1935).

141. "Réalisation et interprétation," *Annales médico-psychologiques*, XVe série, 93e année (1935), II, pp. 329–366.

142. "Aux frontières du langage. Le symbole et le signe," *Revue Bleue, politique et littéraire*, lxxiv (1936), pp. 253–259.

142a. Reprinted in *L'Intelligence avant le langage* (Paris, Flammarion, 1936).

143. "Le langage intérieur dans l'hallucination psychique," *Annales médico-psychologiques*, XVe série, 94e année (1936), II, pp. 377–386.

143a. Abstract in *Congrès des Médecins Aliénistes et Neurologistes de France et de langue française*, 40e session, Bâle-Zürich-Berne-Neuchatel, 20–25 juillet 1936 (Paris, Masson, s.d.), pp. 367–369.

144. "Discussion de la communication de L. Schwartz: la psychologie dynamique de Janet à nos consultations," *Congrès des Médecins Aliénistes et Neurologistes de France et de langue française*, 40e session, Bâle-Zürich-Berne-Neuchâtel, 20–25 juillet 1936 (Paris, Masson, s.d.), pp. 370–373 (Janet, p. 374).

145. "Discussion d'une communication de Marcel Monnier: Le traitement des psychoses par la narcose prolongée; sa technique actuelle; ses résultats," *Congrès des Médecins Aliénistes et Neurologistes de France et de langue française*, 40e session, Bâle-Zürich-Berne-Neuchâtel, 20–25 juillet 1936 (Paris, Masson, s.d.), pp. 518–523 (Janet, pp. 523–524).

146. "La psychologie de la croyance et le mysticisme," *Revue de Métaphysique et de Morale*, xliii (1936), pp. 327–358, 507–532; xliv (1937), pp. 369–410.

147. "Le langage inconsistant," *Theoria*, iii (1937), pp. 57–71.

148. "Les troubles de personnalité sociale," *Annales médico-psychologiques*, XVe série, 95e année (1937), II, pp. 149–200, 421–468.

149. "Les signes de l'asthénie psychologique," *La Graphologie scientifique* (1937), pp. 3–12.

150. Discours au IIIe Congrès international de Graphologie, 19–22 septembre 1937, à Paris, *La Graphologie scientifique* (1937), no. 92 (July-December, 1937), pp. 39–40.

151. "L'examen de conscience et les voix," *Annales médico-psychologiques*, 1938, I, pp. 93–99. Discussion on pp. 99–101.

151a. Reproduced in *Scientia* (Milan), lxiii (May-June, 1938), pp. 263–278, 329–344.

152. "Les conduites sociales," *Onzième Congrès international de Psychologie*, Paris, 25–31 juillet 1937, rapports publiés par H. Piéron et I. Meyerson (Paris, Alcan, 1938), pp. 138–149.

153. "Pour le centenaire de Théodule Ribot," Discours prononcé à la Sorbonne le 22 juin 1939, *Revue de Métaphysique et de Morale*, xlvi (1939), pp. 647–657.

154. "Discussion de la communication de J. Devallet et P. Scherrer: Un cas de psychose de dégoût conjugal avec réaction infanticide," *Annales médico-psychologiques*, xcvii (1939), II, pp. 80–86 (Janet, pp. 87–88).

155. "L'acte de la destruction," *Revue générale des Sciences*, li (1940–1941), pp. 145–148.

155a. Reproduced with additions in *Livro de homenagem*, d'Alvaro et Miguel Ozorio de Almeida (Rio de Janeiro, 1939), pp. 354–358.

156. "Perspectives d'application de la psychologie à l'industrie," *Premier cycle d'étude de psychologie industrielle* (6–9 décembre 1943), *Fascicule no. I. Psychologie et Travail* (CEGOS, 1943), pp. 3–8.

157. "La croyance délirante," *Schweizerische Zeitschrift für Psychologie*, iv (1945), pp. 173–187.

158. "Autobiographie psychologique," *Les Études philosophiques*, nouvelle série, no. 2 (April-June, 1946), pp. 81–87.

159. "Le sentiment de l'inspiration et la théorie des sentiments," *Psyché* (Paris), i, no. 2 (December, 1946), pp. 146–149.

N.B. Articles nos. 9, 10, 22, 25, 26, 27, 28, 29, 32, 35, 37, and 40 are also included in *Névroses et idées fixes*, i.

CONTRIBUTIONS TO COLLECTIONS

1. Charles Richet, ed., *Dictionnaire de Physiologie* (Paris, Alcan, 1895), tome I. Articles by Janet on "Aboulie," pp. 9–13; "Amnésie," pp. 431–436; "Anesthésie," pp. 506–513; and "Attention," pp. 831–839.

2. "Traitement psychologique de l'hystérie," in *Traité de thérapeutique appliquée*, directed by Albert Robin, fascimile XV, 2e partie (Paris, Rueff, 1898), pp. 140–216.

   2a. Reprinted in *L'État mental des hystériques* (Paris, Alcan, 1911), pp. 621–688.

3. *Subconscious Phenomena*, by Hugo Münsterberg, Th. Ribot, Pierre Janet, Joseph Jastrow, Bernard Hart, and Morton Prince (Boston, Richard G. Badger, 1910), pp. 53–70.

4. "The Relation of the Neuroses to the Psychoses," *A Psychiatric Milestone. Bloomingdale Hospital Centenary 1821–1921* (New York, Society of the New York Hospital, 1921), pp. 115–146.

5. "La tension psychologique et ses oscillations," in Georges Dumas, ed., *Traité de Psychologie*, 2 volumes (Paris, Alcan, 1923), i, pp. 919–952.

6. "Memories Which are Too Real" (English translation), in Campbell MacFie et al., eds., *Problems of Personality. Studies Presented to Dr. Morton Prince* (New York, Harcourt, Brace & Co., 1925), pp. 141–150.

7. "Fear of Action as an Essential Element in the Sentiment of Melancholia" in Martin L. Reymont, ed., *The Wittenberg Symposium "Feelings and Emotions"* (Worcester, Mass., Clark University Press, 1928), chapter 25, pp. 297–309.

8. "L'analyse psychologique" (English translation), in Carl Murchison, ed., *Psychologies of 1930* (Worcester, Mass., Clark University Press, 1930), pp. 369–373.

9. "Autobiographie," in Carl Murchison, ed., *A History of Psychology in Autobiography* (Worcester, Mass., Clark University Press, 1930), pp. 123–133.

10. "La Psychologie expérimentale et comparée," in *Le Collège de France, 1530–1930. Livre jubilaire composé à l'occasion de son quatrième centenaire*, par MM. A. Lefranc, P. Langevin, etc. . . . (Paris, Presses Universitaires de France, 1932), pp. 221–234.

11. "L'individualité en psychologie," in *L'Individualité*, exposés par M. Caullery, C. Bouglé, Pierre Janet, J. Piaget, and Lucien Febvre. Discussions. Centre International de Synthèse (Paris, Alcan, 1933), pp. 39–50.

12. "La tension psychologique et ses oscillations," in Georges Dumas, ed., *Nouveau Traité de Psychologie*, nouvelle édition, texte de l'édition de 1923 révisé, iv (Paris, Alcan, 1934), pp. 386–411.

13. "Psychological Strength and Weakness in Mental Diseases," in *Harvard Tercentenary Publications. Factors Determining Behavior* (Cambridge, Mass., Harvard University Press, 1937), pp. 64–106.

14. "La psychologie de la conduite," in *Encyclopédie Française*, tome VIII, *La Vie Mentale*, dirigé par Henri Wallon (1938), pp. 08–11 to 08–16.

15. "Les stades de l'évolution psychologique," in *La notion de Progrès devant la science actuelle*, Centre International de Synthèse, 6e semaine (Paris, Alcan, 1938), pp. 49–71.

16. "L'acte de la destruction," in "*Livro de homenagem*," aos Professores Alvaro e Miguel Ozorio de Almeida (Rio de Janeiro, 1939), pp. 354–358.

17. "Le centenaire de Th. Ribot," in *Jubilé de la Psychologie scientifique française* (Agen, Imprimerie moderne, 1939).

18. "Caractères de l'hallucination du persécuté," in Albert Michotte, *Miscellanea Psychologica* (Louvain, Institut Supérieur Philosophique; Paris, Vrin, 1947), pp. 237–253.

19. Contributions au *Vocabulaire technique et critique de la philosophie* (. . .), Société française de philosophie, 5e édition, André Lalande, ed., (Paris, P.U.F., 1947). Observations or comments by Janet in the articles on "Aboulie," p. 3; "Angoisse," p. 57; "Béatitude," p. 106; "Catalepsie," p. 121; "Champ de la conscience," p. 133; "Comportement," p. 151; "Daltonisme," p. 193; "Dégénérescence," p. 203; "Dépersonnalisation," pp. 207–208; "Folie du doute," p. 240; "Subconscient," p. 1014; and "Suggestion," p. 1039.

PREFACES AND INTRODUCTIONS

1. N. Malebranche, *De la Recherche de la vérité*. Livre II. Édité par Pierre Janet (Paris, Alcan, 1886), Introduction, pp. 1–30.

2. Harald Höffding, *Esquisse d'une psychologie fondée sur l'expérience*, édition française, rédigée conformément à la 4e édition danoise (Paris, Alcan, 1900), Preface.

   2a. 2e édition française . . . d'après la 3e édition allemande (Paris, Alcan, 1903), Preface, pp. i–iv.

3. J. Grasset, *Le Spiritisme devant la science* (Montpellier and Paris, Coulet et fils, 1904), nouvelle édition, Preface, pp. vii–xxix.

4. S. Santerre, *Psychologie du nombre et des opérations élémentaires de l'arithmétique* (Paris, Doin, 1907), Preface, pp. i–xiv.

5. Joseph Jastrow, *La Subconscience* (translated from the English) (Paris, Alcan, 1908), Preface, pp. i–x.

6. P. Saintyves, *La Simulation du merveilleux* (Paris, Flammarion, 1912), Introduction.

7. G. Lamarque, *Th. Ribot. Choix de Textes et Étude de l'Oeuvre* (Paris, Rasmussen, s.d., 1925), Preface.

8. A. Gaucher, *L'Obsédé. Drame de la libido* (Paris, Delpeuch, 1925), letter by Janet included in the book, p. xv.

9. W. Drabovitch, *Fragilité de la liberté et séduction des dictatures* (Paris, Mercure de France, 1934), Preface, pp. 8–18.

10. C. Konczewski, *La Pensée préconsciente. Essai d'une psychologie dynamiste* (Paris, Alcan, 1939), Introduction, pp. ix–xiv.

11. Leonhard Schwartz, *Neurasthenie* (Bâle, Benno Schwabe, 1939), Foreword, pp. 7–12.

    11a. Reproduced as the preface to Leonhard Schwartz, *Die Neurosen und die dynamische Psychologie von Pierre Janet* (Basel, Benno Schwabe, 1951), Preface, pp. 19–25.

12. Léon Dupuis, *Les Aboulies sociales. Le scrupule. La timidité. La susceptibilité. L'autoritarisme* (Paris, Alcan, 1940), Introduction, pp. 1–13.

13. Jean Delay, *La Dissolution de la mémoire* (Paris, Presses Universitaires de France, 1942), Preface, pp. xi–xx.

14. R. von Krafft-Ebing, *Psychopathia Sexualis*, 16e et 17e éditions allemandes refondues par Albert Moll (French translation) (Paris, Payot, 1950), Preface, pp. 4–8.

MAJOR BOOK REVIEWS

Revue Philosophique

1. Vol. 21, 1886, I, pp. 97–100; review of Dr. Paul Radestock, *Genie und Wahnsinn, eine psychologische Untersuchung* (Breslau, Eduard Trewendt, 1884).

2. Vol. 22, 1886, II, pp. 188–193; review of Alfred Binet, *La Psychologie du raisonnement, recherches expérimentales par l'hypnotisme* (Paris, Alcan, 1886).

3. Vol. 25, 1888, I, pp. 91–95; review of Dr. A. Baréty, *Le Magnétisme animal étudié sous le nom de force neurique rayonnante et circulaire dans ses propriétés physiques, physiologiques et thérapeutiques* (Paris, O. Doin et J. Lechevalier, 1887).

4. Vol. 27, 1889, I, pp. 511–513; review of Dr. Coste, *L'Inconscient. Étude sur l'Hypnotisme* (Paris, J. B. Baillière, 1889).

5. Vol. 33, 1892, I, pp. 549–554; review of A. Pitres, *Leçons cliniques sur l'hystérie et l'hypnotisme*, 2 volumes (Paris, Doin, 1891).

6. Vol. 34, 1892, II, pp. 516–521; review of Dr. J. Seglas, *Des Troubles du langage chez les aliénés* (Paris, J. Rueff & Co., 1892).

Brain

1. Vol. 16, 1893, pp. 286–302; review of Hack Tuke, ed., *A Dictionary of Psychological Medicine*, 2 volumes (London, Churchill, 1892).

Revue générale des Sciences

1. Vol. 4, 1893, p. 23l; review of Cesare Lombroso, *Les Applications de l'anthropologie criminelle* (Paris, Alcan, 1892).

2. Vol. 4, 1893, p. 397; review of Cesare Lombroso, *The Man of Genius* (London, Walter Scott, 1893).

3. Vol. 4, 1893, p. 512; review of Dr. Paul Richer, *Paralysies et contractures hystériques* (Paris, Doin, 1893).

4. Vol. 5, 1894, p. 89; review of Dr. E. C. Seguin, *Leçons sur le traitement des névroses* (Paris, Doin, 1894).

5. Vol. 5, 1894, pp. 173–174; review of E. Brissaud, *Anatomie du cerveau de l'homme. Morphologie des hémisphères cérébraux ou cerveau proprement dit* (Paris, Masson, 1893).

6. Vol. 5, 1894, pp. 254–256; review of *Brain. A Journal of Neurology* (London), A. de Watterville, ed. (Autumn, 1892–Autumn, 1893).

7. Vol. 5, 1894, p. 941; review of Dr. E. Laurent, *L'Anthropologie criminelle et les nouvelles théories du crime*, 2e éd. (Paris, Soc. Édit. Scientifiques, 1894).

8. Vol. 5, 1894, p. 1002; review of Toussaint Barthélémy, *Étude sur le dermographisme ou dermoneurose vasomotrice* (Paris, Soc. Édit. Scientifiques, 1894).

9. Vol. 7, 1896, p. 493; review of J. Dallemagne, *Les Stigmates anatomiques de la criminalité* (Paris, Masson et Gauthier-Villars, 1896), and J. Dallemagne, *Les Stigmates biologiques et sociologiques de la criminalité* (Paris, Masson et Gauthier-Villars, 1896).

10. Vol. 8, 1897, p. 517; review of J. Dallemagne, *Les Théories de la criminalité* (Paris, Masson et Gauthier-Villars, 1897).

11. Vol. 9, 1898, p. 255; review of A. Proust et G. Ballet, *L'Hygiène du neurasthénique* (Paris, Masson, 1898).

12. Vol. 10, 1899, p. 288; review of Mlle. Georgette Déga, *Essai sur la cure préventive de l'hystérie féminine par l'éducation*, Thèse médicale (Bordeaux and Paris, Alcan, 1899).

13. Vol. 10, 1899, p. 31; review of D. Mercier, *Les Origines de la psychologie contemporaine* (Paris, Alcan, 1899).

14. Vol. 10, 1899, pp. 199–200; review of J. Dallemagne, *Pathologie de la volonté* (Paris, Masson et Gauthier-Villars, 1899).

15. Vol. 11, 1900, pp. 1243–1244; review of Georges Dumas, *La Tristesse et la joie* (Paris, Alcan, 1900).

COURSES TAUGHT AT THE COLLÈGE DE FRANCE*

1900–1901: Th. Ribot, professeur. Premier semestre, Janet: *Du Sommeil et des états hypnoïdes* (Oscillations du niveau mental). Sommeil, rêve, insomnie et hypersomnie, somnambulisme. (Vol. 1, 1901, pp. 26–27).

1901–1902: *Fatigue physique, intellectuelle et en pathologie mentale*. Élévations et abaissements de la tension psychologique. (Vol. 2, 1902, pp. 27–28).

1902–1903: *Émotion chez l'homme sain et le malade*. Émotion—réaction d'un être mis rapidement dans une situation nouvelle à laquelle manque le temps et le pouvoir de s'adapter. (Vol. 3, 1903, pp. 74–77).

1903–1904: *Les Conditions de la conscience*. 1. Relations de dépendance avec le

---

*[*Editor's note*: Information presented in parentheses after each entry indicates the location of Janet's course syllabi in the *Annuaire du Collège de France*.]

cerveau et les fonctions physiologiques. 2. Caractères essentiels de la conscience: durée, variations quantitative et qualitative, étendue, niveau de tension psychologique, tendance à l'unité. (Vol. 4, 1904, pp. 54–56).

1904–1905: *Conditions psychologiques des mouvements des membres*. Sensations kinesthésiques, images de mouvements, localisation latérale et temporelle du mouvement, régulation de la force du mouvement, tendances, actions volontaires. (Vol. 5, 1905, pp. 67–70).

1905–1906: *Modifications de la conscience dans les névroses hystériques*. (Vol. 6, 1906, pp. 65–67).

1906–1907: *Modifications de la conscience dans les névroses psychasthéniques*. Sentiments d'incomplétude, oscillations de la tension psychologique. (Vol. 7, 1907, pp. 57–58).

1907–1908: *Analyse et critique des méthodes de psychothérapie*. Méthodes générales (religieuse, moralisation . . .) et méthodes à base scientifique: hypnose, suggestion, éducation, etc. (Vol. 8, 1908, pp. 70–71).

1908–1909: *Les Emotions, notamment l'émotion dépressive*. (Vol. 9, 1909, pp. 53–54).

1909–1910: *Analyse des tendances et lois de leur réalisation*. Classification en 4 groupes. Réalisation des tendances, degrés de tension et de force, de réalisation. (Vol. 10, 1910, pp. 37–38).

1910–1911: *La Perception*. Relations avec réflexes, tendances régulatrices, tendances lointaines, tendances objectives. L'image du corps propre. Perceptions de situations et d'attitudes. La conscience. (Vol. 11, 1911, pp. 88–91).

1911–1912: *Les Tendances sociales et le langage*. Les tendances grégaires, l'imitation. Les tendances sociales, tendance à la subordination, à la hiérarchie, la suggestion. (Vol. 12, 1912, pp. 38–41).

1912–1913: *Les Tendances intellectuelles élémentaires*. Intellectualisation des objets, des événements, des personnes. Le héros, la mort du héros (application à notre personnalité). (Vol. 13, 1913, pp. 36–39).

1913–1914: *Les Tendances intellectuelles relatives à la recherche de vérité*. Croyance, assentiment, affirmation, etc. (Vol. 14–15, 1914–1915, pp. 80–85).

1914–1915: *Les Tendances rationnelles qui imposent des lois à la conduite et à la croyance*. La conduite réfléchie, la conduite religieuse. Délibération, raisonnement, la décision, le savoir. (Vols. 14–15, 1914–1915, pp. 85–91).

1915–1916: *Les Tendances industrielles et la recherche de l'explication*. L'acte de production. La conduite intentionnelle. La prévision. L'explication. Les recettes techniques. Idée de cause et principe de causalité. Les systèmes, conduite de l'enseignement. *Conduite expérimentale*. La science. Évolution. (Vol. 16, 1916, pp. 55–60).

1916–1917: *Les Degrés de l'activation des tendances*. État de latence, érection. Effort. Pseudo-action, jeu. Consommation de l'action, mécanismes de terminaison. (Vol. 17, 1917, pp. 64–70).

1917–1918: *Les Degrés de l'activité psychologique*. Force, tension. Les formes de paresse intellectuelle (mensonge, timidité, esprit faux, etc.). (Vol. 18, 1918, pp. 50–56).

1918–1919: *Les Oscillations de l'activité psychologique*. Phénomènes de transition (crises, attaques). Circonstances déterminant ces changements. Interprétation des émotions. (Vol. 19, 1919, pp. 52–54).

1919–1920: *Les Oscillations de l'activité psychologique* (leur évolution dans le temps). L'accès épileptique. Le chagrin, les névroses, délires, mélancolies, confusions. Succession et répétition des oscillations psychologiques. Dépressions progressives. (Vol. 20, 1920, pp. 72–74).

1920–1921: *Les Stades de l'évolution psychologique.* Le corps, l'homme, l'individu, le personnage, le moi, la personne, le sujet, l'individualité. (Vol. 21, 1921, pp. 64–65).

1921–1922: *L'Évolution des conduites morales et religieuses.* (Vol. 22, 1922, pp. 83–85).

1922–1923: *L'Évolution de la mémoire et la notion du temps.* L'attente, la mémoire, le présent. L'espace et le temps rationnels. (Vol. 23, 1923, pp. 74–76).

1923–1924: *Étude des sentiments et leur interprétation par l'analyse des mouvements et des conduites secondaires.* Le sentiment du vide. Effort, fatigue, angoisse, joie. (Vol. 24, 1924, pp. 58–59).

1924–1925: *Étude des sentiments sociaux affectifs.* Sympathies et intérêts. Les formes de l'antipathie, les haines, les amours. (Vol. 25, 1925, pp. 99–100).

1925–1926: *Notions sur la psychologie de la conduite, sur les degrés de perfection et force des tendances.* La faiblesse psychologique, les asthénies moyennes, les états démentiels. (Vol. 26, 1926, pp. 44–45).

1926–1927: *La Pensée intérieure et ses troubles.* (Vol. 27, 1927, pp. 76–77).

1927–1928: *Étude de la mémoire et de la notion du temps considérées dans leur évolution psychologique.* La durée. L'Acte du récit. Passé, présent, futur. (Vol. 28, 1928, pp. 33–34).

1929–1930: *La Faiblesse et la force psychologiques.* Actions coûteuses, actions économiques. Divers équilibres entre dépenses et recettes. (Vol. 30, 1930, pp. 67–68).

1930–1931: *Les Délires d'influence et les sentiments sociaux.* Délires de persécution et de grandeur. Hallucinations. Sentiments d'emprise. Faiblesses sociales, timidités, obsessions, phobies sociales. (Vol. 31, 1931, pp. 81–83).

1931–1932: *L'Intelligence élémentaire.* Direction, position, l'outil, rapports de ressemblance, de qualité, de quantité. Le symbole et le signe. (Vol. 32, 1932, pp. 92–93).

1932–1933: *Étude psychologique de la croyance* (quant à son mécanisme). Les notions de rapport. Troubles de la croyance. Croyances réfléchies. Variétés et degrés du réel. Croyances réelles et expérimentales. (Vol. 33, 1933, pp. 101–103).

1933–1934: *Activité de l'esprit et ses oscillations.* Force psychologique et sa tension. Régulation de l'équilibre entre les dépenses de l'action et les forces disponibles. Sommeil, démences. Excitations: jeu, pratiques religieuses. (Vol. 34, 1934, pp. 93–95).

EDITED JOURNALS AND CONGRESS PROCEEDINGS

1. *Quatrième Congrès international de Psychologie,* tenu à Paris du 20 au 26 août, 1900. Compte rendu des séances et texte des mémoires. Publié par Pierre Janet (Paris, Alcan, 1901).

2. *Bulletin de l'Institut Psychique International*, dirigé par Pierre Janet, 1e année, no. 1 (July, 1900), beginning with no. 2 of the first year, retitled *Bulletin de l'Institut Psychologique International*, and beginning with no. 2 of the second year retitled *Bulletin de l'Institut Général Psychologique*.

3. *Journal de Psychologie normale et pathologique*, publié par Pierre Janet et Georges Dumas, 1e année (1904).

6

The Scope of Swiss Psychology

[1957]

THE SUDDEN, rapid, and extensive development of psychological theory and practice in Switzerland represents a unique phenomenon of scientific evolution and cultural mutation. Within a few decades during the late nineteenth and early twentieth centuries, psychology invaded the ideas and institutions of the fields of education, religion, industry, law, social customs, and medicine in Switzerland, resulting in an ever growing awareness of the implications of varied facets of human behavior. This deep penetration of psychology into life and culture has not only increased our knowledge of the human mind but also transformed human personality itself to a hitherto unknown extent.

While this cultural revolution was not limited to Switzerland, it was more remarkable in that country because it started relatively late and was largely unforeseen. Once begun, however, it was more rapid and more complete in that country, which makes its study particularly rewarding. This essay will attempt to sketch cultural and historical backgrounds, to describe the impact of psychology and psychiatry upon Swiss life and institutions, and to consider the rise and present status of psychoanalysis, Jungian psychology, and new trends in phenomenology and existential analysis. I shall conclude with a discussion of the role and development of the psychology of expression and projection and the rise of vocational psychology. Throughout the essay, an effort will be made to consider differences in Swiss and American approaches to the manifold study of personality.

Swiss Cultural Backgrounds

Until the end of the nineteenth century, Swiss culture largely evolved around three independent urban centers of theoretical activity. The oldest

"The Scope of Swiss Psychology," in Henry P. David and Helmut von Bracken, eds., *Perspectives in Personality Theory* (New York, Basic Books, 1957), 44–64; "Der Gesichtskreis der Schweizer Psychologie," in Henry P. David and Helmut von Bracken, eds., *Perspektiven der Persönlichkeitstheorie* (Bern, Hans Huber, 1959), 81–93.

of these centers was Basel, a city renowned for its Renaissance humanism. There Erasmus had made his home, and Felix Platter (1536–1614) pioneered in psychiatry. Basel also produced the philologist Johann Jacob Bachofen (1815–1887), who promoted the hypothesis of matriarchy; Jacob Burckhardt (1818–1897), the great cultural historian; and, most recently, Heinrich Wölfflin (1864–1945), reviver of the history and psychology of art. Basel had a tradition of excellent scholarship allied with highly original thought.

At the opposite end of Switzerland lay Geneva, locus and bulwark of the Calvinist Reformation, the birthplace of Jean-Jacques Rousseau as well as a number of naturalists, linguists, and economists. The Genevan cultural tradition placed special emphasis on pedagogical theory.

Somewhat later than Basel and Geneva, Zurich was recognized as a center of the movement for the Enlightenment. One of its representatives, J. C. Lavater (1741–1801), invented a method of physiognomy and became the ancestor of *Ausdruckspsychologie* (psychology of expression). Another of its citizens was Heinrich Pestalozzi (1746–1827), famous philanthropist and reformer of education. Zurich's cultural tradition was primarily moral and humanitarian. These three local traditions furnished the characteristics that were strongly stamped into Swiss psychology from its very beginnings: a rational approach, respect for the learned professions, humanitarian trends, an interest in education, and a practical orientation to the study of man.[1]

Institutional Psychiatry in Switzerland

Although two outstanding sixteenth-century psychiatric pioneers, Paracelsus and Platter, were Swiss, systematic interest in psychiatry arose in Switzerland only very much later. The first Swiss asylums were founded in the middle of the nineteenth century. However, for two full generations after this, psychiatry was taught only by German professors while many Swiss asylums were operated by German psychiatrists.

An independent Swiss psychiatric school with high standards was founded at the end of the nineteenth century by Auguste Forel (1848–1931). A lifelong student of ants and an extremely versatile mind, Forel distinguished himself in the fields of brain anatomy, hypnotism, forensic psychiatry, psychiatric education, and the public teaching of mental hygiene. In 1879, he was appointed professor of psychiatry at the University of Zurich and director of the Burghölzli, the Zurich psychiatric university clinic.

---

[1] Ellenberger, "La psychiatrie suisse," *L'évolution psychiatrique* (1951), 321–54, 619–44; (1952), 139–58, 369–79, 593–606; (1953), 298–318, 719–51.

Forel transformed this then backward institution into a scientific center of world renown. Through his personal example, his writings, and his teaching, he reemphasized the principle of the psychiatrist's social functions and duties.[2]

It was the good fortune of Swiss psychiatry that Forel found a successor worthy of himself, perhaps even his superior—Eugen Bleuler (1859–1939). Bleuler continued the work of Forel with the same ethical and social principles, while emphasizing more practical methods. He introduced new techniques for the detailed study of patients, adopted fresh ideas, and elaborated mountains of well-established facts into vast syntheses.[3] This may explain why Bleuler was the first to introduce psychoanalysis into university didactic psychiatry and how he came to construct a new theory of dementia praecox, which he termed *schizophrenia*.[4] One of the founders of dynamic psychiatry, he incorporated into his system the new psychoanalytic dimension of the unconscious. As a result, the meaning of psychotic symptoms could be deciphered for the first time, and the therapeutic nihilism of the past gave way to a reasoned optimism. Bleuler thus imbued Swiss psychiatry with a strong psychological emphasis as opposed to the organic approach that had previously prevailed.

Forel and Bleuler directed the Burghölzli for fifty years and were in a position to endow Swiss psychiatry with a durable body of traditions and teachings. Indeed, they created a new type of Swiss psychiatrist whose main characteristics included enormous industry, a passion for detailed clinical data gained from intensive observation, an eclectic and individualized psychological approach to the patient and to the disease, keen interest in forensic psychiatry and criminology, high professional ethics, and a strong sense of social duty. Through their efforts, psychiatry ceased to be an esoteric science incomprehensible to the layman and instead grew in influence far beyond the limits of medical circles.

After these two great pioneers, Swiss psychiatry continued to grow and expand, particularly in the fields of social and child psychiatry. In 1920, Hans Maier, an associate of Bleuler's, opened at the Burghölzli the first *Kinderbeobachtungsstation* (child observation home) for the study of problem children. These institutions became as typical of Swiss psychiatry as child guidance clinics in the Anglo-American countries. Each home evaluates about eighty to one hundred children yearly; every child is carefully observed and examined for three to four months. As illustrated by the work of Moritz Tramer, Jakob Lutz, and Lucien Bovet, child psychiatry in Switzerland has continued to develop remarkably.[5]

[2] Auguste Forel, *Out of My Life and Work* (New York, Norton, 1937).
[3] Eugen Bleuler, *Textbook of Psychiatry* [1916] (New York, Dover Publications, 1951).
[4] Eugen Bleuler, *Dementia Praecox or the Group of Schizophrenias* [1911] (New York, International Universities Press, 1950).
[5] Moritz Tramer, *Lehrbuch der allgemeinen Kinderpsychiatrie*, 2d ed. (Basel, Benno

There has also been an unparalleled extension of forensic psychiatry and reforms in the penal code as expounded by Forel. Swiss civil law now requires a psychiatric report for such cases as prohibition of marriage due to feeblemindedness or psychosis, divorce because of mental illness, court-ordered appointment of a legal guardian, and so on. Most delinquents must also be given a psychiatric examination. Since Swiss forensic reports are generally quite exhaustive and are prepared with extreme conscientiousness, it is not surprising that some mental hospitals have psychiatrists who devote themselves full-time to this service.

The Swiss Penal Code of 1938 was probably the first to proclaim the principle that the "application of penalty in prison or penitentiary shall have an educative value and prepare the prisoner for his return to civil life." As a result, efforts were made to individualize penalties, separate varied categories of convicts, teach new occupations, supervise and assist prisoners after discharge, and extend psychiatric and social services. Most important, perhaps, was the gradual development of a new kind of judge— a judge–psychologist—well acquainted with pertinent psychoanalytic and psychological literature, who studies forensic psychiatric reports in detail and considers the social-psychological as well as the legal aspects of each case.

A further characteristic of Swiss psychiatry is the intensive interest in follow-up studies, taking into consideration both familial and social aspects of different problems, such as the effects of certain operations (interruption of pregnancy, sterilization, and castration), problems of unwed mothers,[6] children of divorced parents, and so on. (Incidentally, marriage counseling is for the most part a psychiatric specialty in Switzerland.) The Second World War and its aftermath also produced increased participation by psychiatrists in the study and care of prisoners of war, refugees, and orphans. Indeed, there are few countries in the world where psychiatry permeates the entire culture so thoroughly, from educational problems to the administration of justice.

Swiss Psychology

If Swiss psychiatry was born in Zurich in the 1880s, Swiss psychology originated in Geneva approximately ten years later. Its two great pioneers were Théodore Flournoy (1854–1920) and Édouard Claparède (1873– 1940). After studying experimental psychology in Leipzig with Wilhelm

---

Schwabe, 1945); Lucien Bovet, *Psychiatric Aspects of Juvenile Delinquency* (Geneva, World Health Organization, 1951).

 [6] Hans Binder, *Die uneheliche Mutterschaft*, 2d ed. (Basel, Benno Schwabe, 1945).

Wundt, Flournoy introduced psychological science to Switzerland. Appointed a professor of psychophysiology at the University of Geneva in 1891, Flournoy demanded that this new chair be annexed to the Faculty of Sciences instead of the Faculty of Philosophy, thus stressing for the first time the purely scientific character of psychology. Nor did he content himself with applying experimental methods to the usual fields of psychological research; he was also deeply interested in the psychology of religion and in parapsychology. His book *Des Indes à la planète Mars* was one of the finest investigations of the unconscious prior to early psychoanalysis.[7]

Claparède, the cousin, pupil, collaborator, and successor of Flournoy, continued his work with the same methods of scrupulous observation and experimentation. Although Claparède was one of the founders of the experimental psychology of testimony and judicial psychology, his primary interest lay in establishing a scientific pedagogy. His *Psychologie de l'enfant*, published in 1905, was a milestone in the history of child psychology.[8] In 1912, Claparède founded the Institut Jean-Jacques Rousseau, later known as the Institut des Sciences de l'Education and now incorporated into the University of Geneva. The Institute has become a world-famous scientific center for the training of special educators and for research in the fields of child psychology and experimental pedagogy.[9]

Pierre Bovet, the first director of the Institut Jean-Jacques Rousseau, and his successor Jean Piaget have accomplished world-renowned work in this field. Originally a logician, Piaget endeavored to elucidate the nature of logical operations by detailed reconstructions of the development of these cognitive operations in the child using the genetic method. This attempt crystallized into an extraordinarily thorough and systematic study, which has now been in progress for more than thirty years. The results have been expounded by Piaget in a dozen very important books and in many articles.[10] Whereas in the United States Arnold Gesell and his school investigated the motor and behavioral development of the child, Piaget was primarily concerned with reconstructing the child's conception of the world and his intellectual functions.

Swiss pedagogy, inaugurated by Rousseau, Pestalozzi, and their followers and placed on a scientific basis by Claparède and the Geneva school, was further enriched by the contributions of such psychoanalysts as Oskar

[7] Théodore Flournoy, *Des Indes à la planète Mars; étude sur un cas de somnambulisme avec glossolalie* (Paris, F. Alcan, 1900).

[8] Édouard Claparède, *Psychologie de l'enfant et pédagogie expérimentale* (Neuchâtel, Delachaux & Niestle, 1946).

[9] Édouard Claparède, *L'éducation fonctionnelle* (Neuchâtel, Delachaux & Niestle, 1931).

[10] Jean Piaget, *Language and Thought of the Child* (New York, Humanities Press, 1950); idem, *The Construction of Reality in the Child* (New York, Basic Books, 1954); idem, *The Child's Conception of the World* (New York, Humanities Press, 1951); idem, *Origins of Intelligence in Children* (New York, International Universities Press, 1952).

Pfister, Hans Zulliger, and Heinrich Meng.[11] After World War I, when the focus of pedagogical interest shifted to the problems of the emotionally disturbed child, great strides were made through the efforts of Heinrich Hanselmann, who initiated a highly efficient system of *Heilerziehung* (therapeutic education). An eclectic and empiricist, Hanselmann took from Claparède, Freud, Adler, and others what seemed to be of most practical value. He established a training center for special teachers in Zurich, organized a model institution, and wrote a basic textbook on therapeutic education.[12] In this way he greatly influenced the development of public school teachers, creating a new type of educator—a combination of teacher, psychologist, and psychotherapist—prepared to deal with the problems of emotionally disturbed children.

Psychoanalysis: Origins and Development

After the birth of Swiss psychiatry and psychology, the most significant theoretical event involved the adoption of psychoanalysis. This was doubly decisive, both for Swiss psychology and for the fate of the psychoanalytic movement.

By 1906, Sigmund Freud had been publishing material about his psychoanalytic method and findings for ten years. Outside of a small group of friends and former patients, however, his ideas had been largely ignored or rejected. At this point, Freud was not a little surprised to hear that his work had been acknowledged in Zurich by the well-known Professor Bleuler and by Bleuler's associate at the Burghölzli, Carl Gustav Jung. In Geneva, psychoanalysis was also becoming accepted in influential university circles.

The first development in Switzerland was the application of classical psychoanalytic concepts to the field of mental diseases. Whereas Freud had limited his study to the neuroses, Bleuler and Jung applied his ideas to the psychoses, hoping to find a means of comprehending the supposedly "absurd" and "senseless" symptoms of these disorders. In 1907, Jung's small book, *On the Psychology of Dementia Praecox*, brought the first stone to the edifice of a psychoanalytic psychiatry of psychosis, which later culminated in the publication of Bleuler's famous volume on schizophrenia in 1911.[13]

[11] See, for instance, Oskar Pfister, *Psychoanalysis in the Service of Education* (London, Kimpten, 1922); Heinrich Meng, ed., *Praxis der Kinder-und Jugendpsychologie* (Bern, Hans Huber, 1951); and Hans Zulliger, *Schwierige Kinder*, 3d ed. (Bern, Hans Huber, 1954).

[12] Heinrich Hanselmann, *Einführung in die Heilpädagogik* (Erlenbach, Rotapfel, 1930).

[13] Bleuler, *Dementia Praecox or the Group of Schizophrenias*; Carl G. Jung, *On the Psychology of Dementia Praecox* (New York, Association of Nervous and Mental Disease Proceedings, 1936).

Meanwhile, an association of Swiss psychoanalysts had been formed in Zurich, including such men as Bleuler, Jung, Pfister, Alphonse Maeder, and Ludwig Binswanger, who soon began to enlarge considerably the scope of psychoanalysis. The Protestant minister Pfister was the first to apply psychoanalysis directly to the education of normal and abnormal children and to interpret the deep psychological meaning of play.[14] Pfister's work in this field was continued by Hans Zulliger, a schoolteacher, who performed outstanding analytic work with difficult children.[15] Pfister was also the founder of the psychoanalytic "Cure of Souls" technique and the first to study the manifestations of morbid religiosity and mysticism with the use of Freudian principles.[16] Another of the early Swiss analysts, Arthur Kielholz, worked with a variety of delinquents and psychopaths, laying the foundations for an analytic criminology.[17]

Thus, Switzerland played a fundamental part in the history of the psychoanalytic movement. Many basic aspects, such as the obligatory training analysis, were introduced by the early Swiss analysts. Unfortunately, however, this initial impetus was greatly retarded by the defections of Bleuler and Jung from the movement and by the dissolution of the Swiss psychoanalytic group from 1913 to 1919. After its reconstitution, the Swiss group never in certain respects caught up again with the international movement. For example, there is no Swiss psychoanalytic institute. Several of the foremost practitioners are lay analysts, including Pfister, Zulliger, and Madame Sechehaye. Still, it may be said that while there is comparatively less "orthodox" thinking among Swiss analysts than many others, the influence of psychoanalysis seems to have permeated everyday life to a far greater extent than elsewhere.

It may also be appropriate at this point to consider briefly several differences between Swiss and American psychoanalytic views. For example, in Switzerland psychoanalysis is ordinarily called *Tiefenpsychologie* (depth psychology), rather than *dynamic psychology*, a term preferred in the United States. This is probably more than a linguistic peculiarity. "Depth psychology" refers primarily to the unconscious and its expression through dreams, parapraxias, and the like whereas "dynamic psychology" is mostly concerned with ego conflicts and defenses. Another difference between the two perspectives stems from the varied conceptual approaches. The dominant American psychoanalytic view emphasizes the almost unlimited flexibility of the human personality, shaped by the life history and social influences of the individual. There is a great deal of

[14] Pfister, *Psychoanalysis in the Service of Education*.

[15] Zulliger, *Schwierige Kinder*.

[16] Oskar Pfister, *The Psychoanalytic Method* (New York, Moffat, 1917); idem, *Analytische Seelsorge* (Göttingen, Vandenhoeck & Ruprecht, 1927).

[17] Ellenberger, "La psychiatrie suisse," 144–45.

emphasis on "reactions to stress" and "interpersonal relations." In Switzerland, however, more attention is typically paid to the relative constancy of the basic character structure, a sociological perspective is less developed, and rather more importance is ascribed to genetics, characterology, and constitutional psychiatry. There is also much emphasis on pertinent studies in comparative psychopathology, physiology, and biology, such as those by Heini Hediger, W. R. Hess, and Adolf Portmann.[18] As reported elsewhere, many attempts have been made in Switzerland to synthesize psychoanalysis either with biology (Meng, Brun, Bally) or with existential analysis (Boss, Blum) or with Piaget's genetic psychology (De Saussure, Odier).[19] Although the Swiss firmly believe in a nucleus of innate, immutable capacities for each person, whether for good or for bad—as contrasted with the primary American belief in unlimited individual flexibility—the paradox remains that Swiss education is highly successful, not only with normal individuals but also with difficult children and with criminals. All this may well carry some sociological implications for the formulation of personality theories.

Jung's Analytical Psychology

Not only did Switzerland adopt psychoanalysis enthusiastically early in the present century, giving it a very personal stamp, it also produced a "depth psychology" of its own in the form of the work of C. G. Jung. Derived substantially from psychoanalysis, and having some similarities to certain Hindu and Oriental philosophies, Jung's system forms a cohesive unity. Jung is far more than a mere "deviant" of psychoanalysis, but the great number of his publications, containing endless repetitions and not a few contradictions, makes it difficult to acquire a precise idea of his teachings.

Jung was born in 1875 into a family of Protestant ministers and scholars. He spent his childhood and youth in Basel, where he also studied medicine. In fact, he belongs to the spiritual family of that strongly imaginative group of Basel scholars previously mentioned. Jung showed a precocious interest in psychological problems, and as soon as he had obtained his medical license, he entered the Burghölzli as a resident. During his nine years in that famous institution (1900–1909), he became Bleuler's first associate, elabo-

---

[18] Heini Hediger, *Wildtiere in der Gefangenschaft* (Basel, Benno Schwabe, 1942); W. R. Hess, *Die funktionelle Organization des vegetativen Nervensystems* (Basel, Benno Schwabe, 1948); Adolf Portmann, *Biologische Fragmente zu einer Lehre vom Menschen* (Basel, Benno Schwabe, 1952).

[19] For a review of these efforts, see Ellenberger, "A Comparison of European and American Psychiatry," *Bulletin of the Menninger Clinic*, 19 (1955), 43–52.

rated the Word Association Test into a means of detecting unconscious complexes, and, together with Bleuler, applied Freud's psychoanalysis to the study of psychoses.[20] He left the Burghölzli in 1909 to devote himself to the private practice of psychotherapy.

From 1909 to 1913, Jung played a prominent part in the psychoanalytic movement, becoming Freud's most energetic collaborator. Several of his contributions at the time were accepted by Freud and incorporated into the psychoanalytic system. After Jung rejected Freud's sexual theory of libido, however, the two men came into conflict, and Jung left the movement permanently. For several years thereafter, his main interest centered on the study of psychological types, including his well-known distinction between "introvert" and "extrovert" characters. Jung supplemented Freud's concept of an individual unconscious and acquired complexes with his theory of collective unconscious with inborn archetypes common to mankind. His book *Psychological Types*, originally published in 1921, contains the principles of his typology as well as several other ideas that he expounded at length during the following thirty years in a long succession of books and articles.[21]

Jung's most important innovation, however, probably concerns the stages and periods of human life. The popular concept of mental growth, peak, and decline had been modified by Freud only in regard to childhood. Freud assumed an initial period of five years marked by an early rise of sexuality, followed by a stage of sexual latency until puberty, with no further structural change after the instinctual emergence during that time. According to Jung, the picture is quite different: life is marked rather by a succession of psychological metamorphoses, one of them being the "turning of life" at the age of 35 to 38, with the two halves of life complementary to each other. Neuroses may be produced as the result of an impediment in the normal development of "individuation," the psychological process by which an individual attains the unity of his total personality, conscious and unconscious. Through this final integration, the "Self," rather than the conscious ego, becomes the center of personality. The fully integrated individual has thus attained that which for centuries was called "wisdom," and in modern language "maturity," and is now a socially more valuable person. Jung's psychotherapy, originally identical to Freud's psychoanalytic method, adopted as its principal aim a way of helping the patient to attain his individuation.

Jung is a fascinating man who leaves an unforgettable impression on many of his visitors. A skillful and experienced psychotherapist, he is also a

[20] Carl G. Jung, *Diagnostische Assoziationsstudien* (Leipzig, Barth, 1906); idem, *On the Psychology of Dementia Praecox*.

[21] Carl G. Jung, *Psychological Types* (New York, Harcourt Brace, 1923).

great scholar, much of whose knowledge has been acquired by personal anthropological study. (He has sojourned among the natives of Uganda and the Pueblos of New Mexico and has twice visited India.) His ideas have provoked great interest among theologians and anthropologists, perhaps more so than among psychiatrists. His opponents assert that his system is nothing but the resurrection of old Gnostic speculations under a modern psychological cloak while his proponents claim that he has annexed to psychology a new field hitherto intermediate between psychology and religion. It is difficult to study his work objectively without feeling the strange seduction of his ideas, and one would wish that they were true! Unfortunately, his work contains more assertions than demonstrations, and it is regrettable that he did not publish at least a few complete case histories of patients treated by his methods.

Phenomenology and Existential Analysis

After World War I, a need to find new theoretical and therapeutic paths arose in Swiss psychological and psychiatric circles. The refined clinical investigations of schizophrenia inaugurated by Bleuler had convinced several psychiatrists that the usual conceptual framework utilized for the description of mental conditions did not provide a real understanding of the states of consciousness experienced by patients. Textbook descriptions of delusions and hallucinations were considered purely verbal formulations, and ordinary concepts proved particularly inept for the expression of the more subtle emotional disturbances and feelings of depersonalization preceding the onset of schizophrenia.

A new conceptual frame of reference, inspired by Edmund Husserl's phenomenology, began to appeal to several Swiss psychiatrists as a more meaningful approach to the analysis of a patient's subjective experiences. Psychiatric phenomenology, initiated by the contributions of Binswanger and Eugene Minkowski, should not be confused with the philosophical system of the same name. It is essentially a method that attempts to study states of consciousness by means of the coordinates of time, space, continuity, and causality, with the aim of achieving a deeper understanding of the patient's inner universe.[22]

In 1931, in a series of studies on mania, Binswanger extended his conceptual framework toward existential analysis. Shortly before this time, the German philosopher Martin Heidegger, a former pupil of Husserl, had published a new existential system, elaborating a phenomenology of human existence as a whole. Binswanger adopted Heidegger's concept of

[22] Ellenberger, "La psychiatrie suisse," 374–79.

"being-in-the-world" and used it, in modified form, as the basis for his revised phenomenological frame of reference. In 1942, Binswanger expounded his new system in a difficult book, followed by the publication of a series of research studies with schizophrenic patients.[23] In the wake of World War II, interest in this line of psychological theorizing continued to grow; Roland Kuhn published several excellent clinical contributions, and Medard Boss and E. Blum attempted a synthesis of psychoanalysis and existential analysis.[24]

Independent of Binswanger, but almost concurrently, Alfred Storch and Hans Kunz also applied existentialist concepts to psychiatric problems. A psychiatrist in the best Basel tradition of scholarship, Kunz pursued his work in the direction of "anthropology," the philosophical study of human nature. His remarkable book, published in 1946, expounds a general theory of human nature and a fresh interpretation of the meaning of imagination. He hypothesized that the fundamental characteristic of man is awareness and anticipation of his own death; many psychological problems are discussed in the light of this theory.[25]

Phenomenology and existential analysis are difficult methods, requiring considerable effort to understand. Nevertheless, increasing interest indicates that they meet a demand. Classical psychological concepts, elaborated by the philosophers of the eighteenth century, are felt to be insufficient, and there is a pressing need for finer methods of psychopathological analysis.

Psychologies of Expression and Projection

Much of the difference between the American and Swiss approaches to psychology is explained by the importance in Switzerland of the concept of *Ausdruckspsychologie* or psychology of expression. This includes a good deal of what is generally considered "projection" in the United States.

Aristotle's theory of the body-mind unit had as a logical consequence the assumption that the body gives expression to the functions of the mind; among other things, this provided a basis for the study of physiognomy. From the time of Aristotle to the present, there has been a little-known but continuous flow of physiognomic literature, from the Greek and Arab periods to the Renaissance and on to Lavater, who is considered the founder of modern *Ausdruckspsychologie*. Although his ideas are now

---

[23] Ludwig Binswanger, *Grundformen und Erkenntnis menschlichen Daseins* (Zurich, Niehans, 1942).

[24] Ellenberger, "La psychiatrie suisse," 377–79.

[25] Hans Kunz, *Die anthropologische Bedeutung der Phantasie* (Basel, Verlag für Recht und Gesellschaft, 1946).

obsolete, Lavater, a pastor from Zurich, was the originator of the great interest in the psychological interpretation of physiognomy, mimicry, gestures, and movements. Historically, graphology is also a branch of the psychology of expression, that is, the interpretation of one particular kind of human movement, handwriting.

The early French graphologists (Michon, Crépieux-Jamin) attempted to collect a variety of isolated graphic signs, endowing each with a specific psychological meaning. In this way, they produced a kind of graphological dictionary, with which they translated handwriting analyses into a system of rudimentary conventional types. This graphological school was subsequently superseded by the work of Ludwig Klages, the true father of modern graphology.[26] Klages was also one of the founders of characterology, the science of the description, analysis, and classification of the various types of personality.[27] His elaborate characterological system provided a refined frame of reference with which to report the findings of graphological analyses. In sharp contrast to the earlier "atomistic" approach, Klages based his analyses on the evaluation of what he called *Formniveau*, that is, an existential quality of handwriting bound to the level of the subject's vitality. This meant that the specific meaning of a particular graphic sign could vary considerably. Graphological analyses made in this fashion adhered to a far higher standard than those prepared according to previous systems.[28]

Although a German citizen, Klages lived in Switzerland for nearly his entire life. There, his graphological method achieved its greatest success and attracted countless students. However, Klages's system was later rivaled by that of the Swiss psychologist Max Pulver, whose more intuitive approach integrated into graphology new concepts derived from psychoanalysis and phenomenology, particularly the phenomenology of space. Pulver's major contributions were his textbook of basic graphology and his studies on the graphological diagnosis of intelligence and the handwriting of criminals.[29]

In Switzerland, graphology is considered today a highly scientific and reliable method. Thousands of graphological analyses are constantly required by industrial and commercial firms as well as by public administrators. These are performed either in the institutes of applied psychology or by private graphologists, some of whom specialize in the study of educa-

[26] Ludwig Klages, *Handschrift und Charakter* (Leipzig, Barth, 1917).

[27] Ludwig Klages, *The Science of Character* (Cambridge, Sci-Art Publishers, 1932).

[28] Ludwig Klages, *Graphologisches Lesebuch* (Leipzig, Barth, 1930); idem, *Was die Graphologie nicht kann* (Zurich, Speer, 1949).

[29] Max Pulver, *Intelligenz im Schriftausdruck* (Zurich, Orell-Fussli, 1949); idem, *Symbolik der Handschrift*, 5th ed. (Zurich, Orell-Fussli, 1948); idem, *Trieb und Verbrechen in der Handschrift*, 7th ed. (Zurich, Orell-Fussli, 1948).

tional or marital problems. The claim is often made that modern graphology is apt to furnish more extensive personality analyses than mere dynamic psychology, and it is always a surprise for Swiss psychologists to
learn that their colleagues in other countries consider graphology unscien-
tific. The reason for this discrepancy may be that *Ausdruckspsychologie*
and characterology are basic disciplines in Switzerland, whereas American
psychiatrists seem largely unaware of these approaches. ("Personology" is
something quite different from characterology.) Conversely, American attempts to use criteria of experimental test psychology to evaluate graphology seem, from the Swiss point of view, questionable procedures.

Although in Switzerland graphology is a basic psychological method,
projective techniques are also used frequently. The first such test was developed in Zurich in the years 1904 to 1906. At that time, psychiatrists were
trying to supplement the methods of clinical examination with the new
procedures of experimental psychology. Bleuler, who believed that the
fundamental problem in schizophrenia was a waning of the strength of
associations, tried to check his hypothesis with the Word Association Test,
an old experimental method devised by Francis Galton and widely used by
Wundt and his pupils. In 1904, intensive research along these lines was
initiated at the Burghölzli under Jung's direction. However, Jung used the
test as a detector of unconscious representations, exploring the dynamisms
of psychosis. Historically speaking, this was the first use of an experimental
psychological method in "depth psychology," but to Jung it was more than
that. He elaborated a classification of associations, dividing them roughly
into verbal and semantic responses, which, he believed, were characteristic,
respectively, of extraverts and of introverts, thus revealing a structural
aspect of personality. It is regrettable that the word *projective* was later
used to designate both the "depth psychological" and the "character structural" aspects of the test, a semantic confusion that may be partially responsible for the many sterile discussions about "projective methods."

It fell to another Swiss psychologist to create a new projective technique
marking enormous progress over its predecessors. Hermann Rorschach
(1884–1922), a man endowed with considerable artistic gifts, a rich cultural background, great versatility of interests, and a profound capacity for
synthesis, died prematurely at the age of 37, shortly after the publication of
his fundamental work, *Psychodiagnostics*.[30] This book gives an outline
of Rorschach's psychological theories, in combination with a synthesis of
Bleuler's associationism, Freud's psychoanalysis, Mourly Vold's research
on kinesthetic representations, Jung's psychological typology, and an ad-

[30] Hermann Rorschach, *Psychodiagnostics* [1921] (New York, Grune and Stratton,
1949). See also Ellenberger, "The Life and Work of Hermann Rorschach (1884–1922),"
Bulletin of the Menninger Clinic, 18, no. 5 (September 1954), 172–219.

ded touch of phenomenology. The test itself, inspired by "klecksography" (a children's game with inkblots popular in Switzerland at that time), contained several elements of Jung's earlier Word Association Method. In the beginning, Rorschach used both techniques, comparing the responses to the words and to the inkblots and similarly measuring the reaction time. As in Jung's test, the inkblots had both a "depth psychological" aspect, that is, the detection of complexes, and a character structural one. Kinesthetic responses were considered characteristic of introversion and color responses of extraversion. However, Rorschach went further than Jung. He developed a new typology, adding to the introversion-extraversion concept the aspects of "dilation" and "coartation," which together form the *Erlebnistypus*. In Rorschach's method, the *Erlebnistypus* played the same role as the *Formniveau* in Klages's graphological system, that is, it was the key to which all other data had to be referred in order to ascertain their exact value. It is perhaps significant that the *Erlebnistypus*, which was for Rorschach and the Swiss tradition the central element of his test, plays a rather negligible role in the American method of interpreting Rorschach's tests.

The success of the Rorschach Test gave the decisive impetus to the elaboration of a whole set of projective techniques in Switzerland as well as in the United States and elsewhere.[31] It would be tempting to study the ways in which the rationales for such projective tests express the different ways of viewing human personality in each country. Murray's Thematic Apperception Test and the Frustration Test of Rosenzweig, for instance, both centering on the investigation of the individual's dynamisms, conflicts, and defenses, are typical for America. Pfister's Color Pyramid Test and Lüscher's Color Choice Test, both oriented toward analysis of a subject's basic character structure, are more representative for Switzerland. Such methods are often inseparably connected with their original system of typology, as has already been noted in the case of Jung and Rorschach. This is particularly true for Leopold Szondi, and it is not surprising that after leaving Hungary, Szondi found an adopted home in Zurich, where his test has been most thoroughly studied and applied.[32]

Consideration of the psychology of expression and projection affords another comment on differences in American and Swiss practices. In Switzerland, projective techniques are used primarily for purposes of "depth psychology" and as tests of character structure. The skill of the interpreter is highly valued and there have been few efforts to utilize mathematical-statistical computations as a means of casting light on a

[31] Richard Meili, *Lehrbuch der psychologischen Diagnostik*, third edition (Bern, Hans Huber, 1955).
[32] Ellenberger, "La psychiatrie suisse," 369–74.

subject's "dynamisms." The profession of clinical psychology, in the American sense, is unfortunately unknown in Switzerland, although its introduction would be well advised.

Vocational Psychology

Yet another important development in Switzerland in the interim between World Wars I and II was the growing interest in aptitude testing and vocational counseling.[33] In 1918, Claparède opened in Geneva the first Swiss laboratory specifically designed to serve that need. However, since in several universities the chair of psychology was occupied by professors more interested in philosophy than in applied psychology, the service demands of interested industrialists went largely unmet until a group of engineers, led by Alfred Carrard, sponsored the establishment of the Psychotechnic Institute in Zurich in 1923. Under the direction of Biaesch, the Psychotechnic Institute developed swiftly, and similar autonomous institutes were soon founded in Basel, Bern, Lucerne, and Geneva.

Although the psychotechnic institutes were established by engineers, it was astonishing how successfully they combined a cautious empiricism in daily practical work with growing alertness to new trends. The Zurich institute soon changed its name to Institut für angewandte Psychologie (Institute for Applied Psychology) and extended its research beyond the testing of specific aptitudes to studies of an examinee's total character. The ensuing publications, such as those of Jean Ungricht and Ulrich Moser, are of high caliber, broad in psychological knowledge and original in thought.[34]

The extensive development of vocational counseling in Switzerland is partly due perhaps to the distinct national psychology and social structures. Whatever the deeper explanation, it seems that correct occupational choice is more vital in Switzerland than in many other countries. Many Swiss towns have public agencies where psychologists provide low-cost or free vocational counseling for young men and women. The time may come soon when every adolescent will receive an extensive examination.

The rise of applied psychology in Switzerland has also produced a new kind of professional man, the "practical psychologist," whose education allies classical psychology, depth psychology, and characterology with intensive training in graphology and a thorough knowledge of the requirements of various trades and occupations. Since one of the main activities of

[33] Franziska Baumgarten, ed., *La psychotechnique dans le monde moderne* (Paris, Presses Universitaires de France, 1952).

[34] Jean Ungricht, *Berufswahl-Lebenswahl* (Zurich, Juris, 1947); Ulrich Moser, *Psychologie der Arbeitswahl und der Arbeitsstörungen* (Bern, Hans Huber, 1953).

practical psychologists is vocational counseling, they have become even better known by people in everyday life than the psychoanalysts are currently in the United States. These social aspects of "practical psychology" are obviously connected with the Swiss approach to problems of personality. If "anybody can do anything," to quote the title of a recent American novel, then vocational counseling becomes superfluous.[35] If, however, aptitudes are bound to a permanent individual character structure, then such counseling based on characterology becomes a vital necessity both for the individual and for society.

Conclusion

Until the end of the nineteenth century, there was no Swiss psychology to speak of. Its rapid and extensive development since that time bears the characteristics of a major cultural mutation. Not only has psychological and psychiatric knowledge increased, but this knowledge has pervaded society and all aspects of life. It has been the purpose of this essay to sketch briefly the origins and current trends in Swiss psychology. Cultural backgrounds, the growth of psychiatry, the beginnings of psychoanalysis, Jungian Analytical Psychology, phenomenology and existential analysis, the psychology of expression and projection, and the ramifications of applied psychology throughout Swiss life and customs have been considered. Where pertinent, similarities and differences between American and Swiss approaches to the manifold study of personality were noted. The extremely broad and deep penetration of psychological ideas and practices today, and man's subsequent increased awareness of himself, suggest that we may be at the beginning of a cultural revolution of incalculable importance.

[35] Betty McDonald, *Anybody Can Do Anything* (New York, Lippincott, 1950).

7

The Life and Work of Hermann Rorschach (1884–1922)

[1954]

THE BIOGRAPHY of a man of genius is more than a contribution to the history of science or art and more than a narrative of success or failure in an individual's vocation. For parallel to an individual's personal struggle for subsistence runs his incessant fight for the achievement of his chosen work. If these two main efforts cannot be reconciled and coordinated, conflicts arise that often end in tragedy. In that respect, few destinies are more poignant than that of Hermann Rorschach, who died prematurely, nine months after the publication of his first book, the *Psychodiagnostics*, just at the time when he had started to develop his thought in a new way and just as he gave hope of other exceptionally promising scientific achievements.

Owing to the circumstances under which it was written, the *Psychodiagnostics* is a very difficult book that gives an extremely incomplete representation of the fundamental conceptions underlying Rorschach's well-known inkblot test. The diagnostic method outlined in the book took an independent course of evolution after its originator's death. During that long and necessary evolution, the connection between the test itself and the original conceptions of the author has become increasingly remote. It has been largely forgotten that Rorschach was not only the inventor of a practical testing method but also a profound thinker and investigator of human nature.

We have no means of knowing how Rorschach would have developed his test if he had survived. However, I am convinced that a deeper insight into the original meaning of the *Psychodiagnostics* could inspire a new develop-

"The Life and Work of Hermann Rorschach (1884–1922)," *Bulletin of the Menninger Clinic*, 18, no. 5 (September 1954), 172–219. Also available as "La vida y la obra de Hermann Rorschach," *Revista de psicología general y aplicada*, 13 (July–September 1958), 561–613; "Leben und Werk Hermann Rorschachs," in K. W. Bash, ed., *Hermann Rorschach: Gesammelte Aufsätze* (Bern, Hans Huber, 1965), 19–69; "La vie et l'oeuvre de Hermann Rorschach," in Ellenberger, *Les mouvements de libération mythique et autres essais sur l'histoire de la psychiatrie* (Montreal, Éditions Quinze, 1978), 229–89; and "La vita e le opere di Hermann Rorschach," in Ellenberger, *I movimenti di liberazione mitica*, 195–248.

ment of the test and also be fruitful for several fields of contemporary psychology. Rorschach's original conceptions, however, have never been fully expounded. This has led me to a difficult attempt to clarify the real meaning of Rorschach's thought by means of a threefold investigation of his life, his personality, and the development of his ideas.

Events of Hermann Rorschach's Life

Hermann Rorschach was born in Zurich on November 8, 1884.* His childhood and youth were spent in the town of Schaffhausen, Switzerland. He studied medicine mostly in Zurich and worked as a resident physician in the asylums of Münsterlingen, Münsingen, and Waldau. He was *Oberarzt* (associate director) of the mental hospital in Herisau when he died on April 2, 1922, at the age of 37, nine months after the publication of his *Psychodiagnostics*. These few facts, and perhaps his stay in Russia, are about all that is generally known of Rorschach. Such details do not give the faintest idea of the fascinating personality described by all Rorschach's friends, and we are, unfortunately, far from the complete and thorough knowledge that would be desirable. Therefore, I shall limit myself to statements of well-established facts, trying to interpret them in their true light so that they may reveal more fully the personality of the man.

Family Background and Parents

Let us recall at first that Switzerland is a federal state whose constitution grants great autonomy not only to the individual "cantons" but also to the communities within each of these cantons. Every Swiss is a citizen not only of Switzerland but also of one particular canton as well as of one particular community. Citizenship of a canton or community does not necessarily imply that the citizen was born there. A Swiss remains a citizen of his home community all his life, whether he lives there or not and even if his parents or ancestors have not lived there for generations, although he may, through complicated formalities, acquire the citizenship of another community and canton.

The Rorschachs were citizens of the canton of Thurgovia in northeastern Switzerland, and their home community was the little town of Arbon on the southern shore of Lake Constance. Hermann Rorschach once made inquiries about his ancestors and ascertained that for several hundred years

*[*Editor's note*: The documentation for this essay takes the form of an extensive bibliography at the end of the article.]

they had not left their "home community." They had been mostly craftsmen and peasants, some of them had been councilmen of the community,
but apparently none had made themselves conspicuous outside of it. Ulrich
Rorschach, the father of the psychiatrist, was born in Arbon and was the
first in his family to break a century-old tradition of settlement there. In
1884 he left Arbon for Zurich, where he stayed for two years and then
established himself definitively in Schaffhausen in 1886. On September 19,
1882, he married Philippine Wiedenkeller, who belonged to a very old
family of Arbon. In the official registers of Arbon and Zurich, Ulrich
Rorschach is entered under the designation of painter. I have not been able
to locate any of his paintings, nor to meet anybody who has seen them, and
there is no evidence that he was remarkable as an artist. In 1886 he was
appointed drawing teacher in the elementary boys' and the secondary
school of Schaffhausen. Ulrich Rorschach is said to have been a good, kind,
and easygoing but rather sickly man and his wife a kindhearted and sociable woman.

Childhood and Youth (1884–1904)

During the Rorschachs' stay in Zurich, Hermann was born in a suburb
called Wiedikon, in a house that at that time was No. 278 on the Halden-
strasse. He was not quite 2 years old when his parents established themselves in Schaffhausen. The canton of Schaffhausen had about 50,000
inhabitants, with approximately 20,000 in the town of Schaffhausen itself.
The town is an international communications center as well as an important industrial, tourist, and cultural center. Few cities along the Rhine rival
Schaffhausen in picturesqueness. The center of town is dominated by several hills, one of them crowned by a big, round fifteenth-century fortress
called the Munot, which is used for special feasts and dances during the
summer. The 700-year-old cloister contains one of the most wonderful
museums of Europe, while the municipal library is rich in bibliographical
treasures. Schaffhausen is at the same time famous for the high quality of its
metallurgy, watches, and textiles. Young Hermann, from early infancy to
late adolescence, lived there in an atmosphere of intellectual, artistic, and
cultural concentration.

The Rorschach family lived at first in an old house, the "Haus zum
Tabor," on the Geissberg hill, a structure with a large, beautiful garden of
which Hermann always kept a wonderful memory. Later they moved to the
Emmersberg hill, and finally they acquired a house that is still in the
family's possession. Leading from the "Munot" to the center of the town is
a long and steep stairway, crossed halfway by a small street, the Sän-
tisstrasse. The Rorschach house was No. 5 on this street.

Hermann was 3 years old when his sister Anna was born (August 10, 1888), and he was 7 when his brother Paul was born (December 19, 1891). His beloved mother died on July 11, 1897, when Hermann was only 12. It seems that the following two years were particularly unhappy for Rorschach. A succession of housekeepers took care of this motherless household with three children until the father married his wife's younger sister, Regina Wiedenkeller, on April 17, 1899. One year later (March 7, 1900), there was born into the family a stepsister named Regina. The stepmother is said to have been a capable and energetic person, but whatever the reasons may have been, an estrangement occurred between her and young Hermann. Soon afterward, Ulrich Rorschach began to suffer from an incurable disease, which finally forced him to give up his activity and to retire in 1902. He died on June 8, 1903, when Hermann was 18 years old.

After completing his studies at the elementary school, Hermann was admitted to the Kantonsschule. He attended this school, renowned for its efficient and capable teaching staff and its high scholastic standing, for six years, from 1898 to 1904. In those days good behavior was considered a matter of course that did not deserve special mention, while only bad behavior was registered in the school's archives. Rector Lüthi, the present director of the Kantonsschule, whom I consulted in this matter, found no mention of Hermann Rorschach, so we can therefore probably draw the conclusion that he was a good boy. We also know that he passed his final examinations with high honors.

In the spring of 1904, eleven pupils of the Kantonsschule Schaffhausen obtained their diplomas. In this class, Oskar Farner, later a well-known theologian and professor at the University of Zurich, ranked first and Hermann Rorschach fourth, with an average of 5.0, with the highest grade being 6. More remarkable than his academic average was the fact that he received equally good marks in each of his subjects.

During the last two years in the Kantonsschule pupils are allowed to join one of the semiofficial, noncompulsory student associations. The initiation ceremony is generally accompanied by some kind of humorous task to be performed by the applicant, a custom similar to the one existing today in American college fraternities. At the same time, the student receives a "cerevis," that is, a nickname by which he is henceforth known to his companions. Thus, in 1903, Hermann Rorschach was admitted into the Scaphusia association, whose members wore a smart cap with the blue and white colors of the fraternity. The archives of the Scaphusia contain several illustrated albums in which the students recorded their activities. Among these illustrations we find several excellent ones signed by Rorschach. A number of photographs show him among his fellow students, a big, healthy, cheerful, and good-looking young man.

It is surely highly significant that in 1903 Rorschach received from his comrades of the Scaphusia the nickname "Klex," a word meaning "ink-blot"! That the future originator of an inkblot test should have been called "Inkblot" by his schoolmates seems too extraordinary to be a mere coincidence. Could it have been that the future psychologist was already fond of playing *Klecksographie*, a game then very popular among Swiss children and consisting of making inkblots on a piece of paper, folding it, and arranging the inkblot in order to give it, for instance, the form of a butterfly? Or did the nickname itself compel him in some way to occupy himself with inkblots until he had elaborated the test? (If this were true, it would be an instance of what Wilhelm Stekel and Karl Abraham call *Verpflichtung des Namens*, that is, "obligation through the name.") Alternatively, it might be that Hermann was named in honor of Maler Klecksel, the hero of a humorous, illustrated story by Wilhelm Busch, one of his favorite authors. (In the colloquial German, *klecksen* means daubing, and mediocre paintings are called *Kleckserei* or *Kleckse*.) In that case, the nickname Klex would only signify that Hermann's schoolmates expected him to become a painter as his father had been.

Be that as it may, at the time when Klex Rorschach was finishing his studies in Schaffhausen, he was far from decided on his future career. He seems to have hesitated a long time between art and the natural sciences. It is reported that in his dilemma young Rorschach wrote to the famous German naturalist Ernst Haeckel in Jena, asking him whether he should choose art or natural science. Haeckel advised him (as might have been expected in view of his own profession) to study natural science. We may presume at this point that young Hermann was unconsciously seeking the confirmation of his own secret wish. He finally decided on medicine but was wise enough not to give up art and to reserve it for his favorite pastime. With his studies in Schaffhausen terminated, Hermann Rorschach decided to move to Zurich to study medicine. He was 19 years old.

Medical Studies (1904–1909)

In Europe at that time, Switzerland possessed the highest standard of medical learning. It was customary for most students to study for a few semesters at various universities, including those in French-speaking Switzerland or abroad, returning for their final studies to their home university. Consequently, young Hermann spent his first semester in Neuchâtel and the following four semesters in Zurich, that is, from the winter of 1904 to October 1906. He then continued for two semesters, respectively, in Berlin and in Bern. His final four semesters, which involved hard and continuous work for the attainment of his medical degree, were again passed in Zurich.

Dr. Walter von Wyss, who was an intimate friend of Rorschach during his studies in Zurich and in Berlin, has told me of Rorschach that "he was an absolutely reliable friend, a thoroughly neat and decent man. Endowed with an astonishing vitality, he mastered his medical studies with little difficulty, was indefatigable, diligent, read much, visited art exhibitions, displayed a deep interest in all human problems and liked to discuss them."

During the earlier part of his studies there occurred two events that, insignificant as they might appear, proved to be of exceptional importance to the young man. The first was an acquaintance, and the second was a dream. While in Neuchâtel, Rorschach took a holiday trip to France and there met an old Russian, an admirer of Tolstoy. It was a crucial event for Rorschach, who was struck as if a whole new world had suddenly opened before him. He now began to feel a passionate interest in Russian culture and the Russian people. Soon afterward, in Zurich, Rorschach became acquainted with the Russian colony there, which included the famous neurologist Constantin von Monakow, a number of emigrants, and Russian students, not to speak of aspiring revolutionaries. He soon began to learn Russian. His friendly relations with the Russians went so far that in 1906, during his semester in Berlin, he was invited to spend a short vacation in Russia, where he was deeply impressed by the country and the people.

The other important occurrence, a dream, also left a powerful impression on Rorschach. About eight years later, he related it in his thesis in the following words:

> In my first clinical semester, I was for the first time present at an autopsy and looked at it with the well-known, respectful eagerness of a young student. The dissecting of the brain interested me particularly, and I joined to it all kinds of reflections about the localization and the cutting up of the soul. The deceased had been an apoplectic; the brain was cut in transverse slices. The following night I had a dream in which I felt my own brain was being cut in transverse slices. One slice after another was cut off from the mass of the hemispheres and fell forward, exactly as it had happened at the autopsy. These bodily sensations (I lack a more precise designation) were extraordinarily clear, and the memory of that dream is even now fairly vivid.

In this dream, to which we will return, we find nothing less than the germinal cell of the whole psychological concept underlying the *Psychodiagnostics* and the Rorschach Test.

Since the beginning of his medical studies, Rorschach had thought of becoming a psychiatrist. If he had hesitated, nothing could have strengthened him in this course as much as choosing Zurich for his last semesters of study. In Switzerland every medical student had to take at least two semesters of a course of clinical and theoretical psychiatry and was examined in both fields at the final examination. The university's psychiatric clinic, the Burghölzli, already a scientific institute of world renown under Auguste Forel, was gaining in reputation from year to year through the work of Forel's successor Eugen Bleuler. Just at the time when Rorschach arrived in Zurich, the city was undergoing what can only be called a psychiatric revolution. A little-known neurologist in Vienna, Sigmund Freud, had advanced a complex of new ideas that were ignored or rejected for ten years, but now were being accepted for the first time in a major university center. The unconscious, which had been timidly explored by Pierre Janet in Paris, Théodore Flournoy in Geneva, and a few others, was with Freud suddenly put in the foreground of psychiatric interest. The unconscious was no longer a philosophical abstraction but a turbulent source of energies, manifesting itself under the mask of dreams, parapraxes, and wit as well as hysterical fits, compulsions, and anxiety. Such conditions could now be cured by bringing into consciousness hidden unconscious representations and conflicts. C. G. Jung, a young alienist at the Burghölzli and an early Freud enthusiast, had just worked out an experimental method, the Word Association Test, as a detector of these unconscious representations. In addition, another striking innovation had just been undertaken: Bleuler and Jung were applying the concepts of psychoanalysis and the Word Association Test not only to the neuroses, as Freud had done, but to the exploration of the psychoses themselves. The apparently "absurd," "incomprehensible," and "senseless" ideas of psychotic patients were being deciphered and interpreted with the help of these methods based on an assumption that seemed incredible at that period of materialistic and organic psychiatry. Students and doctors from all over Europe came to Zurich to investigate these revolutionary ideas. We can easily imagine that this collective enthusiasm extended also to the students who attended twice a week the clinical demonstrations of the famous Bleuler, and among them, young Rorschach must have been not the least interested auditor.

The same period was also a time of strenuous work for Rorschach, for he succeeded in the very difficult feat of completing his medical studies in the minimal time, which was then five years. He passed his final examinations and acquired his federal medical license on February 25, 1909.

At that time Rorschach became engaged to a Russian colleague, Olga Stempelin. After his examinations he took a well-deserved vacation of about two months to visit his new wife's family in Kazan. It was his second journey to Russia. Since Rorschach already knew something of that country and had begun to master the language, his stay there was of great benefit to him. Russia was then a most fascinating country—boundless landscapes, old picturesque towns, and a colorful contrast of peoples, nations, and religions, not to mention an intensely poetic folklore, the people's creative genius, and the sense of beauty—in short, the country was a never-ending source of wonder and delight for the visitor. And yet, Russia was then modernizing with increasing speed, under the influence of powerful personalities. If the asylums there were not worse than in the rest of Europe, the family care of mentally sick patients was the best in the world, and there were quite a number of psychiatrists and psychologists who were receptive to the most modern ideas. (Let it be recalled that the first translation of Freud's *Interpretation of Dreams* was into Russian.) After his intensive and exhausting medical training, Rorschach enjoyed greatly the many varied impressions flowing from the rich Russian world. Every day he was overwhelmed by new perceptions, images, and human contacts. Among the crowd of his new acquaintances there was a young Polish student, Eugène Minkowski, the future phenomenologist. Rorschach readily agreed with his fiancée's suggestion eventually to establish himself in Russia permanently, provided that he should obtain first his doctor's degree (which, in Switzerland, is independent of the federal medical license) and a few years of Swiss psychiatric training.

The Münsterlingen Period (1909–1913)

The young physician now had the choice of beginning in a psychiatric university clinic with a meager salary for an indefinite period or in a cantonal asylum with a modest salary but no university career. As he and his fiancée were both lacking in funds, and with a future position in Russia in view, he chose the second course. Rorschach applied for a residency in the cantonal asylum of Münsterlingen, in Thurgovia, to begin on August 1, 1909. There he could learn practical asylum psychiatry and work on his dissertation.

The asylum of Münsterlingen was in a beautiful site on the shore of Lake Constance. The four hundred patients were housed partly in old cloister buildings, partly in more recent constructions. The medical staff consisted of a director, Doctor Brauchli, and two residents. There were no secretaries and no social workers, and the tasks of the young physicians were manifold, ranging from morning staff meetings and rounds on the wards to organizing entertainments for the patients. But the residents, after the fulfillment of their various duties, had some time left for rowing and swimming in the lake and other amusements. The four years Rorschach spent in Münsterlingen seem indeed to have been happy. On April 21, 1910, he was married to Olga Stempelin by a magistrate in Zurich, and the religious ceremony was performed at the first opportunity in the Russian Orthodox Church of Geneva in the magnificent old Byzantine ritual. In one of the asylum's old buildings the young married couple had a pretty apartment of two rooms with a beautiful view of Lake Constance. Rorschach's brother

Paul came often from Schaffhausen to visit him, and Hermann went often for a trip to Arbon, the home of his parents and ancestors, about fifteen miles east on the shore of the lake. He rapidly made himself popular among the patients, partly by organizing all kinds of feasts, theatrical events, and entertainments.

Concerning his psychiatric work, Dr. Roland Kuhn, the present associate director of the Münsterlingen Mental Hospital, wrote to me: "He photographed the patients, and the old case records still contain many yellowed photos taken by him. . . . His entries in the case records were beautifully written; they are extremely good and far above average of the other case records. In one case, for instance, he discusses the problem of how a picture from a newspaper could be the starting point of hallucinations—which is already the central problem of the form interpretation test." Doctor Kuhn adds that an accurate study of these case histories written by Rorschach would no doubt contribute greatly to a better understanding of some obscure points of the *Psychodiagnostics*.

In fact, Rorschach had begun in Münsterlingen with the firm intention of doing serious research work. The most urgent task was his dissertation for a doctor's degree. Professor Eugen Bleuler agreed on the subject proposed by Rorschach, "On Reflex Hallucinations and Kindred Manifestations." For a Swiss candidate it was proof of independence of mind to propose a subject; most of the Swiss students received from the professor not only supervision but the subject itself. Rorschach accomplished his task slowly and carefully in more than three years. He received the degree of Doctor of Medicine from the University of Zurich on November 12, 1912.

The starting point of Rorschach's thesis is evidently the dream that we have reported above. After having witnessed an autopsy of the central nervous system, Rorschach had dreamt that he felt his own brain being cut in slices. This suggested to him the questions: How can a man experience such delusional perceptions which are physiologically impossible? How are perceptions of one kind transmuted into perceptions of another kind? Rorschach reviews one instance after another of hallucinations occurring as reflex responses to certain perceptions and of the transmutability of perceptions of one sort into perceptions in another sensorial sphere: optic into kinesthetic, kinesthetic into optic, acoustic into kinesthetic, kinesthetic into acoustic, optic into acoustic, acoustic into optic. Rorschach's thesis is not always easy to read. Rorschach obviously did not attempt to give it stylistic qualities, and he had to condense abundant material into fifty-four pages. Furthermore, it is written in the psychological language of the associationist theories taught by Bleuler, which Rorschach apparently did not find completely adequate for his own original thinking. A careful study of the dissertation, however, shows how skillfully he reconciled his clinical observations on his Münsterlingen patients with his studies in the literature on hallucinations as well as his own speculations. The autobiographical component in a work of such a formal nature is striking. Rorschach records not only his initial dream, but a number of observations on himself. He relates, for instance, how as a child he was able to "translate" a toothache into a musical melody; and how he managed to recall in his memory the mental reproduction of certain famous paintings by means of certain movements. He speaks of his bad musical memory and defines himself as a kinesthetic type (a man with predominant kinesthetic images). At the end of 1912, almost simultaneously with his dissertation, Rorschach published a creative paper in the *Zentralblatt für Psychoanalyse* entitled "Reflex Hallucinations and Symbolism." It is a synthesis of the conclusions of his dissertation and the new data of psychoanalysis and at the same time a step further toward his *Psychodiagnostics*.

Meanwhile, the preparation of his dissertation failed to absorb all of his energies, and Rorschach tried other spheres of research. One of his patients in Münsterlingen, who had been committed several times with hebephrenic disorders, had died, and the autopsy had shown a tumor of the pineal gland. The brain was sent to the institute of Monakow, the Russian neurologist in Zurich, and Rorschach performed a microscopical study under Monakow's direction. Rorschach concluded that hebephrenia and brain tumor had nothing to do with each other and published the case in a medical journal. It was a conscientious piece of work but uninspired. Rorschach probably soon understood that brain pathology was not to be his specialty.

Strangely enough, at the same time Rorschach had already found a way leading to his future discoveries, but had not realized it. One of his schoolmates from the Kantonsschule of Schaffhausen, Konrad Gehring, had become a teacher in a school in Altnau, a small town in Thurgovia not far from Münsterlingen, and the two friends still delighted in visiting each other. Gehring came often to Münsterlingen, where he showed picture projections or with his pupils sang popular songs to the patients. Rorschach showed Gehring artistic productions of his patients and how he tested them with Jung's new Word Association Test. He had conceived the idea of testing patients with inkblots and comparing the results with those of the Word Association Test. Gehring proposed to test his school pupils in the same way. I cannot do better than translate here a fragment of Gehring's letter in answer to my inquiry about these experiments: "I gave each of my pupils a piece of paper with the instruction to place an inkblot on it and fold it. Every pupil made his own inkblot, wrote his name and his associations *without* the reaction time. Then the process was repeated on a second piece of paper with new inkblots, associations *with* the reaction time. I gave these productions to Rorschach, and we discussed them. Then we made a new experiment. I showed to every pupil, individually, a piece of paper with inkblots which had been made by Rorschach, and then wrote down the pupil's associations. A further experiment was performed with red inkblots. Rorschach compared the results of the Word Association Test and the associations to inkblots, with his patients and with normal adults." With these experiments, Rorschach's main purpose was to ascertain whether the more gifted pupils generated more fantasy than the less gifted ones. He did not conduct these experiments systematically, nor did he think of publishing the results. Unfortunately, the numerous cards with inkblots that he prepared at that time have been lost.

These early inkblot experiments were carried out in the year 1911. But Rorschach for the time being ended them, as Konrad Gehring explained, because of his growing preoccupation with psychoanalysis. From 1909 to 1913, there was a psychoanalytic group in Zurich, comprising such participants as Bleuler, Jung, Alphonse Maeder, Ludwig Binswanger, and Oskar Pfister. It is very probable that Rorschach came in direct contact with this group, and thus began to occupy himself more and more with the new conceptions of Freud and even to psychoanalyze some patients in the asylum of Münsterlingen.

The *Zentralblatt für Psychoanalyse* (one of the first psychoanalytic periodicals) published a number of Rorschach's short papers, notes, and book reviews between 1912 and 1914. In a paper dealing with a case of "failed sublimation," Rorschach showed how the repressed material within a patient forced its way back into consciousness. In "Clock and Time," he suggested that the interest of certain neurotics in watches was based on an unconscious longing for the mother's breast, while the ticking watch symbolized the heart beating. "Theft of a Horse during Fugue State" was the case report of an epileptic who had stolen a horse with two carriages; in this absurd scenario, Rorschach found an unconscious meaning, or rather a condensation of several unconscious meanings, such as occurs normally in the dream. He used the Word Association Test of Jung as an auxiliary method. A short study of the "Choice of the Friend by the Neurotic" points to the fact that this kind of choice (as with the love choice) is guided by the parental images. "Analytical Remarks on the Painting of a Schizophrenic" is a short but interesting interpretation of the work of a schizophrenic who, copying a painting of *The Last Supper*, gave Christ and the disciples, with the exception of Judas, long hair like women. (This representation by a former patient still exists and is shown to the visitors at the Münsterlingen Mental Hospital.) Another longer study of a drawing by a schizophrenic patient analyzes subtly its various levels of meaning.

At the beginning of 1913, Hermann Rorschach was 28 years old, had his title of Medical Doctor, with four years of mental hospital practice, and had written a few good articles. He began to be known in psychiatric, and especially psychoanalytic, circles. The time had come, however, for him to consider in a concrete way his Russian plans. It was, of course, more complicated than his former trips as a visitor, and he had requirements to fulfill in order to obtain the Russian medical license. In April 1913, Rorschach received his official leave from Münsterlingen and soon afterward entered the asylum of Münsingen near Bern, where he temporarily performed the work of a resident until the end of November. Then, early in December 1913, he left his native country for Russia, where a brilliant future seemed to await him.

The Russian Episode (1913–1914)

It is sometimes alleged that Rorschach spent a very long time in Russia and worked there for years as a psychiatrist. This, however, is false. Since Rorschach left his post in Münsingen at the beginning of December 1913 but returned to practice at the Waldau asylum in Switzerland in July 1914, he could not have been in Russia more than seven months, which time included a trip to the Volga and another to northern Russia where his wife had relatives. Rorschach had been excused from obtaining his Russian medical license because he had found a well-paid position in the Sanatorium Krukovo, a fashionable sanatorium near Moscow housing some of the most distinguished and aristocratic neurotic patients of Russia.

Rorschach had, it is said, a time-consuming but interesting job and lived outside the sanatorium with his wife. But for some reason he suddenly left this excellent position and returned to Switzerland. What happened? It has been said that he was seized by a nostalgic longing for the blue waters of Lake Constance. Other people maintain that he loved Russia too much, and to such an extent that he feared he would forget his own country, be wholly absorbed by the new one, and lose his identity. Mrs. Olga Rorschach, Rorschach's wife, tells me that her husband was not quite satisfied with the kind of work he did in Russia and had no opportunity for scientific work, which he considered his real vocation.

Whatever the deeper reasons may have been, Rorschach realized that it would not be the worst solution to go back to Switzerland and to defer his definitive immigration for a few years, and so, after less than a year, he left Russia. In the meantime, he had lost his position in Münsterlingen, but he soon found an appointment as a resident, with a meager salary, in the Waldau Mental Hospital near Bern, where he began in July 1914. Soon afterward, however, World War I broke out, and he found himself separated by the belligerent countries from his wife, who had remained temporarily in Russia.

The Waldau Period (1914–1915)

Rorschach worked in the Waldau from July 1913 to the middle of October 1915. This new position was less lucrative and probably less interesting than the previous one at Münsterlingen; its main advantage was that it could serve as a possible start for a scientific career. There were only three mental hospitals in German-speaking Switzerland that were at the same time university psychiatric clinics—the Friedmatt (in Basel), the Waldau (near Bern), and the Burghölzli in Zurich. At that time a saying circulated among the psychiatric residents: "If you want to eat well, go to the Friedmatt; if you want to sleep well, go to the Waldau; if you want to learn well, go to the Burghölzli." But it was extremely difficult to obtain a position in the Waldau. There were two senior psychiatrists at the institution with whom Rorschach came into close contact and friendship, W. Morgenthaler and E. Fankhauser. Morgenthaler was a practical and energetic man who later organized a teaching program for the nurses of the Swiss mental hospitals and wrote an excellent textbook on psychiatric nursing; he also founded the interesting Museum of the History of Psychiatry, which still exists today in the Waldau. At that time Morgenthaler was interested in the artistic productions of the psychotic, and Rorschach helped him very efficiently to gather materials for that study. Years later, Morgenthaler proved himself an excellent friend to Rorschach by helping him publish the *Psychodiagnostics*, and, after Rorschach's death, he contributed actively to the propagation of his work. Fankhauser, on the other hand, was more the scholar and thinker, full of original ideas. At that time, Fankhauser was preoccupied by a theory of affectivity which most likely exerted a strong influence on Rorschach's thinking.

During his stay in Münsingen in 1913, Rorschach had heard of certain strange religious sects, and of the founder of one of these, a certain Johannes Binggeli, who had been committed to the Münsingen asylum from 1896 to 1901. Rorschach had been so interested in this fact that he had visited the old man in his village. Now after his return from Russia, his interest in this subject was revived, and he now devoted most of his free time to the study of Binggeli's and other sects. To his amazement, he found that in his own country, not very far from where he now lived, isolated religious sects still existed that were by no means less extraordinary than the Russian sects about which so much was published. Dr. Paul Haeberlin, who in 1915 had been professor of philosophy at the University of Bern, has told me that Rorschach used to visit him and to report enthusiastically about his research. At one point, Rorschach firmly believed that this study of Swiss sects would be his lifework. He went to the remote district of Schwarzenburg to visit these people and study their folklore. He reconstructed their genealogies and gathered numerous documents in the libraries and archives of Bern.

Near Schwarzenburg, Binggeli had founded a *Waldbruderschaft* (forestbrotherhood) comprising a large circle of adherents and a small group of initiated. To the latter, Binggeli taught that his penis was sacred, and he let them adore it. His urine was called "Heaven's Drops" or "Heaven's Balm," and he gave it to his followers as a medication or in place of wine for the Holy Communion. Sexual relations with him were considered a means of expelling the demons from young girls. Binggeli was finally arrested for incest with his daughter. Rorschach discovered that Binggeli's sect was an offspring of an older group, the sect of Anton Unternährer, who at the end of the eighteenth century had also preached the holiness of incest. An ancestor of Binggeli had been head of a community of Unternährer's disciples near Schwarzenburg. Unternährer himself had had precursors in the Schmidlianers. Going back through the centuries, Rorschach found that besides "normal" sects, such as the Anabaptists, the Waldenses, and the Cathares, there had been parallel sects of the same kind as Binggeli's and Unternährer's, all of them in the same regions. Historical documents on the subject went back to the twelfth century, but the same region had already been a hearth of the Arian heresy centuries before.

On the basis of these investigations, Rorschach was able to sketch a general study of past and present Swiss religious sects—a grandiose synthesis of the psychology of religion, sociology, psychopathology, and psychoanalysis. He showed that these sects always appeared in the same regions, which corresponded to frontiers between races, and in populations whose religious enthusiasm contrasted sharply with their lack of political interest. Furthermore, Rorschach demonstrated on a map of Switzerland that the distribution of the sects corresponded exactly to the localities where the weavers lived. In the midst of these populations existed "nuclei of sects," that is, groups of families who throughout the generations furnished followers. Among the disciples of the sects, Rorschach distinguished two kinds: the active ones, often alcoholics or neurotics compensating for inferiority feelings with the help of a missionary activity; and the passive ones through whom an outbreak of repressed libido effects a sudden conversion or transference to one of the sect leaders. Among the leaders of sects, Rorschach also distinguished two types: passive leaders, instituted by the community and without much personal influence; and active ones, who had proclaimed themselves prophets and were either neurotics, such as Binggeli (whom Rorschach diagnosed as a hysterical personality), or schizophrenics, such as Unternährer. According to Rorschach, the schizophrenic prophet exerted a much deeper influence; his teaching contained not only the "low mythology" of the neurotic prophet, resulting from his personal complexes, but the "high mythology" originating from the archetypes of the deep unconscious, which was apt to impress his disciples much more deeply. It is deplorable that Rorschach's very substantial work on Swiss religious sects remained unachieved; but we have at least two most interesting fragments, accounts of the life and teachings of Binggeli and Unternährer in the light of psychoanalytic theory as it existed in Rorschach's time.

Considering that it was conducted in his spare time, Rorschach's actual research on Swiss sects was performed surprisingly quickly, in less than ten months, but the amount of material gathered was so large that Rorschach needed a long time to work it out. Meanwhile, Rorschach's wife had come back from Russia and the meager salary of the Waldau post was now insufficient. The position of associate director of the asylum in Herisau, Switzerland, was available, and his application was accepted. Thus, on October 20, 1915, Rorschach left the Waldau and yet again began his new professional functions on November 1.

The Herisau Period (1915–1922)

The Krombach Mental Hospital was the cantonal asylum of Appenzell in the eastern part of Switzerland, not far from the Austrian frontier. Since its reconstruction a few years before, Krombach had been considered one of the most modern psychiatric facilities in Switzerland. It was, for instance, one of the very few to have the so-called Pavilion System. Instead of one large building, there were at Krombach about a dozen houses arranged in a circle on the top of a hill outside of the little town of Herisau. In the main house, the offices were on the ground floor, the apartment of Director Koller was on the first floor, and the associate director was lodged on the second floor. The associate director had a wide range of responsibilities. For the three hundred patients of the asylum there were only two psychiatrists (the director and his associate) and no residents, no social worker, and no secretaries. One can easily see that there was a heavy load of medical work. Nevertheless, Rorschach introduced an innovation: during the years 1916 and 1917, he organized a course of lectures for the nursing personnel (nothing of the kind had existed previously in any of the Swiss asylums). After two years, the medical staff in Herisau was increased by one resident. Among the three residents who succeeded one another in 1919 and 1920, two, Georg Roemer and Hans Behn-Eschenburg, became pupils of Rorschach.

The canton of Appenzell was in many respects very different from the other regions where Rorschach had worked. In Thurgovia, the native canton of his parents, he felt completely at home. In Münsingen and Waldau, he had learned to know the Bernese and to appreciate their seriousness and their *Gemütlichkeit* (cordiality). In contrast, it seems that Rorschach never accepted certain traits of the Appenzell mentality, for instance, their predilection for malicious wit. The profound difference between the mentality of the Bernese and the Appenzeller, and of the clinical picture they gave when they became mentally sick, interested him very much, and he later commented on it briefly in his *Psychodiagnostics*.

Although the salary of the associate director there was considered relatively good, Rorschach's family expenses were increased by the birth of two children: a daughter, Elisabeth, born on June 18, 1917, and a son, Wadin, born on May 1, 1919. Measured by the Swiss scale, Herisau was far from being an intellectual center, such as Zurich, and a rather uninspiring place. But from the beginning, Rorschach tried to make the best of it and to accomplish some scientific work.

He began by publishing an extremely interesting case he had studied in the Waldau, somewhat similar to the "Theft of a Horse during Fugue State" written during his Münsterlingen period. At that time, he had tried to cure the amnesia of a patient with the help of Jung's Word Association Test and had regretted the impossibility of using hypnosis and psychoanalysis. Now Rorschach used concurrently the three methods of free association, the Word Association Test, and hypnosis, and then compared the findings. The patient in question was a Swiss soldier who had been arrested for desertion when he failed to come back from a military leave. When arrested, the soldier was mentally confused and remembered vaguely that two days before he had had a bicycle accident, after which he had forgotten everything. Rorschach's three methods gave strikingly different perspectives on the case. The free association brought the patient rapidly to vivid daydreams, akin to fugue states and containing many elements of the former fugue state. Jung's Word Association Test revealed nothing of this, but instead gave hints of more important and permanent complexes of the patient, for instance, a deep aversion to his stepfather. Hypnosis revealed little of the fugue state but, strangely enough, brought to light a transitory epileptic delirium that had suddenly appeared during the confusional period. Thus the three methods complemented each other very well in the task of exploring the unconscious of the patient.

Furthermore, Rorschach was now preoccupied with his major work on Swiss sects. He had begun to prepare his abundant material, and one year after his arrival at Herisau, he presented his first communication on this subject to the Swiss Psychiatric Society in Neuchâtel on November 11–12, 1916. This communication is invaluable because it gives us the chief ideas as well as the general outline of the book Rorschach had conceived on the subject. Rorschach never lost sight of this project; he made a further communication on the topic to the Swiss Psychiatric Society in Zurich (October 12–13, 1918) and later spoke about Binggeli and Unternährer to the Swiss

Psychoanalytic Society. In a letter written to Reverend Oskar Pfister a few weeks before his death, Rorschach returned to this subject and mentioned the four hundred to five hundred pages of the planned book.

In the meantime, Rorschach's attention was drawn to new subjects. Psychoanalysis had for several years been one of his great interests. He had already treated some patients psychoanalytically in Münsterlingen from 1912 to 1913. But the theoretical and professional situation of psychoanalysis had by now changed. The original psychoanalytic group of Zurich of 1909 to 1913 had dissolved. At the same time, Freud had developed his conceptions considerably: instead of the drawing into consciousness of unconscious representations and conflicts, Freud now brought the dynamics of transference into the foreground. He was on the verge of disclosing his new "metapsychology." The analytic movement was spreading internationally, and after the end of World War I some Swiss adherents were considering the creation of a new Swiss association. On February 10, 1919, a circular, written by Oskar Pfister, Emil Oberholzer, and his wife Mira Oberholzer, was sent to about fifty people. On March 21, a constitutive assembly was held in Zurich comprising the three initiators and eight participants, among them Rorschach, who was elected vice-president of the new group (the president being Emil Oberholzer). The first official assembly took place on March 24 in the presence of several foreign guests.

It is noteworthy that the early meetings of this regenerated Swiss psychoanalytic organization were devoted mainly to the psychopathology of religion. In the third meeting, Arthur Kielholz spoke about Jakob Boehme; in the fourth and fifth sessions, Rorschach exposed the cases of Binggeli (July 11) and Unternährer (September 19); and in the sixth one, Morel discussed "mystical introversion." During the last three years of his life, Rorschach played a very important part in the activity of the Swiss Psychoanalytic Society, both as vice-president of the organization and with four scientific communications, the two concerning the Swiss sects and two others drawn from his *Psychodiagnostics*. It is certain that he found in the psychoanalytic group a much more congenial atmosphere than in the Swiss Psychiatric Society. His ideas were received there with interest, and certain of his psychoanalytic colleagues, such as Oberholzer and Zulliger, learned his test from him there. He also practiced psychoanalysis with a limited number of patients in Herisau. Rorschach himself had not been analyzed, as a training analysis was not obligatory at that time. To the proposal of certain of his colleagues to undertake it, he replied only that he did not think it necessary.

In the meantime, a decisive change had occurred in the direction of Rorschach's main interests. We have seen that Rorschach arrived at Herisau with the firm intention of organizing on a large scale the rich material he had gathered about the Swiss sects. This project, however, was eventually abandoned, and Rorschach began instead to work feverishly on a new diagnostic inkblot test. There can be little doubt that the stimulating impulse for this new project came from the research work of Szymon Hens. Hens, a young Polish student from Warsaw, had studied in Zurich from 1912 to 1917 and worked for a time at the medical polyclinic there. He had developed an inkblot test of his own and, with the approval of Professor Bleuler, had published it in his doctoral dissertation at the end of 1917. Of course this publication reminded Rorschach of his old experiments with Gehring years earlier in Münsterlingen and returned him to conceptions that had fascinated him since then.

From this day forth, Rorschach devoted himself more and more to this new course of research. Parallel to his work as associate director in the asylum, to his functions in the Psychoanalytic Society, and to his continuing work on Swiss sects, he researched and wrote in a short time his *Psychodiagnostics*. Rorschach's elaboration of the diagnostic cards, the experimentation with patients and with normal people, and his writing of the book, with its many difficulties of publication, were all performed in three years. The book was published in June 1921. But during its protracted publication and afterward, Rorschach's psychological conceptions had taken a new shape and the test a new direction in his mind. Soon after the appearance of *Psychodiagnostics*, he considered the book already obsolete. His last communication to the Psychoanalytic Society, on February 18, 1922, was irrefutable proof to his colleagues of the progress he had made in the use of the techniques expounded in his book and of his improved method of interpretation. Rorschach had discovered his new path to the promise of achievement and success. His fate, however, decreed otherwise; for six weeks later his friends were astounded to hear of Rorschach's sudden and unexpected death. He was 37 years old.

The Death (April 2, 1922)

There are few points in Rorschach's biography that have been so shrouded in legend as the circumstances that preceded and accompanied his death. The best we can do is summarize here a few indisputable facts in their tragic simplicity. On April 1, 1922, Rorschach was admitted, as an emergency patient, to the general hospital of Herisau. He had suffered for a week with abdominal pains, but for reasons unknown to the physician had not come for treatment sooner. The chief physician at the hospital, Dr. Looser, diagnosed a severe diffuse peritonitis with jaundice. Exploratory laparotomy was performed and revealed the condition to be inoperable. The surgical treatment given Rorschach consisted merely of a soft rubber drain in the main incision, with gauze inserted for counterdrainage in a parallel incision. Intravenous infusions were given postoperatively. The patient died on the following morning, April 2, 1922, at ten o'clock. From the autopsy performed the following day, it was difficult to determine whether the cause of death was an acute inflammation or a perforation of the appendix.

Rorschach was buried on April 5 in the Nordheim Cemetery in Zurich on a day of violent wind and snowstorm. The religious service was conducted by his old friend, the pastor and psychoanalyst Oskar Pfister, who told the mourners of Rorschach's stoic attitude toward life and Christian words before death. Bleuler spoke of Rorschach's death as a tragic and irreparable loss not only to his family, friends, and colleagues, but to science as well, and he deplored the fact that no one among them would be capable of continuing this ingenious researcher's work and carrying it to its fulfillment. The grave shows the following inscription:

HERMANN RORSCHACH

Dr. Med.

1884–1922

PSYCHIATER

The Personality of Hermann Rorschach

Hermann Rorschach was a tall, lean, blond man, swift of motion, gestures, and speech, with an expressive and vivid physiognomy. In his first approach to other men, he often appeared reserved, but he was friendly, cheerful, and humorous, and of an even and well-balanced mood. Behind his inherent modesty and unassuming manner, the great variety of his gifts and talents was not easily discernible. According to his friends, he could be a fascinating conversationalist, provided that the topic was of interest to him. He had a peculiar ability to correlate his knowledge in different fields.

There is no doubt that Rorschach had fundamentally an artistic personality. Through his own efforts, he constantly developed and perfected his skill in drawing. A great number of his drawings, especially his albums, are still extant and enable us to make an accurate evaluation of his artistic talents. Not content with mere impressions, he strove at all times for a closer realism. He was particularly good at representing human movements, attitudes, and faces, and he had a curious capacity for drawing sketches of himself in various attitudes as seen from a distance through the eyes of others. Reproductions of animals and landscapes, however, eluded him, as demonstrated by the lack of depth and shading in his drawing of the Basilica of St. Basil the Blessed in Moscow. He did not paint, but he sometimes colored his drawings. He was better at representing forms than using colors. (Incidentally, I have learned from his wife that Rorschach's favorite color was gentian blue, and he mentions several times in the *Psychodiag-nostics* that blue is the favorite color of people who strive for self-control.)

Apart from being a creative artist in his own right, Rorschach was at the same time an excellent art critic, and some of the remarks scattered through his writings about contemporary artists, such as the Swiss painter F. Hodler, are very interesting. He took a keen interest in the artistic productions of psychotics. Konrad Gehring tells me that Rorschach regularly distributed paper, paints, and clay to his patients in Münsterlingen and then studied their productions. Similarly, Dr. Morgenthaler says that Rorschach had remarkable success in getting the Waldau patients to draw, and many products of schizophrenic art that are to be seen today in the museum of the Waldau were obtained through his persistent efforts. Dr. Walter von Wyss of Zurich, one of his closest friends, also confirms that Rorschach as a student had been very fond of visiting art exhibitions and that one of his favorite pastimes had been to compare the effect of a single painting on different people. [. . .]

Rorschach's linguistic talents equaled his artistic abilities. In addition to German (the official and written language of German Switzerland) and the dialect of Schaffhausen, which he spoke in daily life, Rorschach had learned French at school and spoke it well; he also had a fair knowledge of Italian. During his medical studies, both from textbooks and from his wife, he learned Russian, and after his first sojourn in Russia, he spoke it well, his pronunciation being excellent although a little slow. It was in Russian that he conversed with his wife, and he read with her a great number of Russian authors. He had a deep admiration for the Russian classics, such as those by Pushkin, Tolstoy, and Dostoevsky, and he translated a novel of Leonid Andreiew into German for a newspaper. He took pride in showing to his friends an autograph of Tolstoy, which he had received as a present from a Russian who had been acquainted with the great writer. Rorschach was probably not only a great admirer of Russia, but one of the few western Europeans at this time who had a detailed understanding of Russian culture.

Rorschach's interests in natural history, very keen during his school years, remained in the background later in life, with one chief exception: during his stay in Münsterlingen, he managed to acquire a monkey that stayed in the asylum for several months and delighted him with its gestures and grimaces. Minkowski states that Rorschach often showed this monkey to the schizophrenics and used their reactions as a basis for his studies.

Rorschach's preoccupations with the various sciences of man seem to have increased steadily during his life. Some quotations and allusions in his early writings point to his interest in folklore, and later he collected data about popular traditions and superstitions. His interest in folklore concentrated more and more on the world of the religious sects, and he came to have a deep interest in the various manifestations of religion throughout the centuries, with special emphasis on the gnosis. With his extraordinary ability to connect and correlate his knowledge, he envisioned a grandiose synthesis of the history of religion, sociology, and psychopathology. [. . .]

As for his work habits, Rorschach's main characteristic was perhaps the speed with which he worked, while never giving the appearance of undue haste. After a short period of intense application, he would change to another occupation. This highly individual trait differs widely from the customary Swiss working techniques, which are characterized by slow, intensive, and prolonged concentration. Another striking difference lies in Rorschach's use of his free time. The tendencies of the average German-Swiss do not run to hobbies (which they often consider frivolous), but rather to the continuation of their work in their spare time and holidays. Rorschach, however, dismissed his scientific labors at such times and preferred to spend his evenings at home reading and drawing. [. . .] Few people probably understood how much of his creative work was actually the outgrowth of his apparent leisure time. His natural reserve, which was at times mistaken for aloofness, was easily dispelled on closer contact. This fact was regularly borne out by his associates, patients, and asylum personnel alike. Social distinctions were of little importance to him. He had a wide range of acquaintances, but few personal and intimate friends. One of his main virtues seems to have been the *pietas* in the old Latin meaning: a simple, self-evident relationship, without conventionality or exaggerated familiarity, with those to whom one is naturally bound, such as parents, brothers and sisters, spouse, children, and the wider circle of social groups. [. . .] He was not particularly interested in politics, with the exception of the world situation and the Russian revolution. Mrs. Rorschach has told me that he once wrote a number of articles on the communism problem for local Herisau newspapers.

In contrast to his many natural endowments, Rorschach showed a marked inaptitude in all matters of finances and competition, and he was lacking in self-assertion and self-interest. The difficult trick of converting his knowledge into hard cash or into career success was unknown to him, with the result that he was more than once grossly underpaid in his positions and achievements. During his entire lifetime, Mrs. Rorschach told me, he earned only 25 Swiss francs with his test. In spite of these shortcomings, Rorschach seems to have been fully aware of his own value and of the importance of his ideas and concepts. However, he spoke rarely of them, and then only when he was assured of genuine interest and attention. One may assume that at the root of his conceptions he felt a deep awe for the mysteries of the universe, of life, and of humankind. In this sense, he was a religious man, although he does not seem to have paid much attention to conventional organized religion and church life. Like many of the German

Romantic philosophers, he envisioned a stream of the Spirit flowing through the centuries, finding its multiple expressions in the life of peoples and individuals. He suspected that there existed a universal key for deciphering and understanding the world, and the clue to this, he thought, was to be discovered in the realm of creative fantasy. His ultimate answer, and the solution to these problems, he believed he had found at the end of his life. He put forth his ideas in this regard only in an incomplete and veiled form, in his greatest achievement, the *Psychodiagnostics*.

Steps to His Masterpiece

The Mystery of the Psychodiagnostics

The origin of *Psychodiagnostik: Methodik und Ergebnisse eines wahrnehmungsdiagnostischen Experiments* is to us today, and already was for certain contemporaries, a mystery. Nothing would be more erroneous than to consider the book merely the directions for use of a testing method. In truth, as Roland Kuhn has pointed out, the book is nothing less than the grandiose design of a conception of Man, based on totally new psychological conceptions. To quote Kuhn, "like a foundling in an alien world, the *Psychodiagnostics* stands without precedent in the field of general psychiatric literature. Rorschach could not draw on any source which might have yielded previous information on his theme; a fact which stamps him as that rare example of a researcher creating a masterpiece, the *Psychodiagnostics*, almost entirely by his own inventive genius."

Rorschach's book was elaborated far from universities, laboratories, and libraries, in a small mental hospital, by a man who had never studied psychology, attended international congresses, or acquired official titles. His situation reminds us of an earlier case: "How could the little-educated man of Stratford-on-Avon, the actor Shakespeare, possibly create such masterpieces as Macbeth and Hamlet?" Perhaps three centuries from now, someone will try to prove that Rorschach never existed and that the true author of the *Psychodiagnostics*, and of the Rorschach Test, must have been Bleuler or Jung. Fortunately, we are better informed about Rorschach's life than about Shakespeare's, and we believe that our problems can be, for the most part, illuminated.

The isolation and lack of special education of Rorschach has been exaggerated. Although among his colleagues he was one of the very few who had never been a resident in the Burghölzli, he was acquainted with Bleuler, had discussed with him in detail his dissertation, and had remained in touch with him. He had also been a pupil of von Monakow. He was more or less closely acquainted with several of the most original and remarkable psychiatrists of his time, including Jung, Minkowski, and Ludwig Binswanger, as well as with several philosophers and theologians. With his alert and open mind, he drew inspiration from conversations with many men, as well as from less outstanding but learned and original ones, such as Fankhauser. A perusal of his dissertation and early papers shows that he was well acquainted with the psychiatric and psychoanalytic literature of his time. If we add to this that Rorschach had a wide knowledge of certain other fields, such as art, folklore, history of religions, and Russian literature, we are inclined to think he was better prepared than most of his colleagues for a truly original achievement. At the bottom of the alleged "Rorschach riddle" lies perhaps only an old European prejudice that "no scientific work can be performed outside of a university."

Since the *Psychodiagnostics* certainly did not spring from Rorschach's mind as Minerva from the head of Jupiter, it behooves us to consider the way it developed in the author's unconscious and conscious thinking. Nothing is more mysterious to a creative personality than the process of its own creativity. While the conscious mind is occupied with certain problems, the unconscious can travel a separate path marked with flashes of inspiration, dreams, or the stunning effect of the blow of a fortuitous incident on an invisible preoccupation. Thus, while Rorschach eagerly studied the mechanism of reflex-hallucinations, psychoanalysis, and the sociopsychopathology of Swiss religious sects, his mind followed unconsciously other preoccupations, which he constantly picked up and abandoned again, and which finally culminated in his *Psychodiagnostics*.

The Unconscious Way

THE ORIGIN

At the base of Rorschach's thinking were his artistic sensibilities and his attitude of mind. A man can reveal his artistic interests by his creations, by studying the process of artistic creativity, or by appreciating the artistic productions of his fellow men. Rorschach engaged in all three pursuits, but even more, he was interested in *the way other people react in the presence of a work of art*. Rorschach's friend Dr. Walter von Wyss tells me that, when visiting an art exhibition, Rorschach would try to imagine how a certain person would feel viewing a certain painting. In his preoccupation with inkblots, he displayed much the same interest.

Thousands of Swiss children had played klecksography, among them Hermann Rorschach. It is more than probable that he had enjoyed the *Klecksographie* of Justinus Kerner, a strange German physician and Romantic poet well known at that time who arranged inkblots into weird configurations and commented on them with verses reflecting his own depressive mood. But Rorschach did not content himself with making inkblots and looking at inkblots of other people; he manifested his originality with the idea of observing the reactions of children and adults to inkblots and of comparing the reactions of gifted and less gifted children.

THE MÜNSTERLINGEN PREOCCUPATIONS

Kuhn has pointed out the likelihood that Rorschach was familiar with an article by H. Silberer on *Lekanomantie*, which appeared in immediate proximity to one of his own papers in the *Zentralblatt für Psychoanalyse*. The *Lekanomantie* is an old method of divination by looking into a basin full of water, a method similar to crystal gazing. In this essay, Silberer reported on his experiments with this technique to detect unconscious representations, and he compared his findings with those of Jung's Word Association Test. Did this article perhaps inspire Rorschach with the idea of comparing the responses of his patients to Jung's Word Association Test and to inkblots as we know from Konrad Gehring? But Silberer's paper was published serially in 1912 and 1913 while Rorschach's experiments (according to Gehring and to Rorschach himself) were conducted in 1911.

In one of his essays from this period, Rorschach mentions a childhood memory of one of his patients. When 6 or 7 years old, the patient used to look at the humidity spots on the ceiling of his bedroom and to see a form reminding him of a nude woman and of a certain Swiss lake. In an early book review, Rorschach mentions the dream of another patient who dreamt of a painting representing a wonderful landscape and, following the contours with her hand, noticed that they portrayed the figure of her beloved brother. The book under review by Rorschach here seems to have been of special interest to him. It was a study by Pfister titled *Cryptography, Cryptolalia and Unconscious Picture Riddles in the Normal*. Rorschach's studies of morbid mysticism and glossolalia had suggested to Pfister the idea of letting his analysands invent senseless words to which they had to give free associations, or drawing scribbles in which they discovered shapes that proved to have striking connections with the patients' most important complexes. Pfister had also observed that the *Kryptergon* (as he called it) can be a fruitful psychoanalytic tool, provided that it be both produced *and* interpreted by the subject, that is, the associations are poorer if the *Kryptergon* is made by someone else; but, on the other hand, only its author is able to interpret it. A similar preoccupation probably guided Rorschach when he compared the verbal and visual associations of schoolchildren to their own inkblots and to inkblots made by himself. I believe that Pfister's research on *Krypterga* suggested to Rorschach that inkblots contain something intimately personal to the viewer but that these inkblots must be elaborated in such a way that they provide a mirror for the greatest possible number of subjects. The unique value of Rorschach's set of cards is that they are the product of a painstaking elaboration, based on his long familiarity with the world of *pareidolias*. [. . .]

THE ROMANCE OF LEONARDO DA VINCI

Another incident proves how, without being aware of it, Rorschach never lost sight of these sorts of problems. Mrs. Rorschach relates a stirring memory of a day when she and her husband were reading *The Romance of Leonardo da Vinci* by Dmitri Merejkowski. She remembered clearly how deeply impressed her husband had been when she read, in Russian, the following excerpt, a fragment of the alleged diary of Beltraffio, a pupil of Leonardo:

> This evening I saw him, standing under the rain in a narrow, dirty and stinking alley, attentively contemplating a wall of stone, with spots of dampness—apparently one with nothing curious about it. This lasted for a long while. Urchins were pointing their fingers at him and laughing. I asked what he had found in this wall.
>
> "Look, Giovanni, what a splendid monster—a chimera with gaping maw; while here, alongside, is an angel with a gentle face and waving locks, who is fleeing from the monster. The whim of chance has there created images worthy of a great master."
>
> He drew the outlines of the spots with his fingers, and, to my amazement, I did actually perceive in them that of which he spake.
>
> "It may be that many would consider such power of invention absurd," the master went on, "but I, by my own experience, know how useful it is for arousing the mind to discoveries and projects. Not infrequently on walls, in the confusion of different stones, in cracks, in the designs made by scum on stagnant water, in dying embers, covered over with a thin layer of ashes, in the outlines of clouds—it has happened to me to find a likeness of the most beautiful localities, with mountains, crags, rivers, plains and trees; also splendid battles, strange faces, full of inexplicable beauty; curious devils, monsters and many other astounding images. I chose from them what I needed, and supplied the rest. Thus, in listening closely to the distant ringing of bells, thou canst find in their mingled pealing, at thy wish, every name and word that thou mayst be thinking of."

After listening to this passage, Rorschach seemed rapt in thought.

THE HERISAU RESEARCH

For several years, Rorschach put aside his experiments with inkblots, but his mind continued to be preoccupied with similar subjects. While the study of the psychology of Swiss sects had priority with him, he still remained interested in Jung's Word Association Test and in comparing it with other methods for exploring the unconscious. In Herisau, he conceived the idea of devising new tests of his own. He showed to his patients pictures of a green cat, a red frog, and a left-handed woodcutter cutting down a tree with his axe in the left hand. Roemer and Oberholzer reported that for a time he used such picture tests together with his inkblot tests.

We know from the history of science how a scientist, involved in the pursuit of a discovery, often passes by the solution without seeing it, sometimes for several years, until a more or less insignificant incident opens his eyes. In the case of Rorschach, the crucial event was the publication of the Hens Test. Suddenly, at a stroke, Rorschach understood the real nature of the problem he had touched upon and given up in 1911. At the same time, he understood how Hens had missed the opportunity and overlooked the solution. So he tackled the problem himself and soon found the answer. But, of course, he could not have succeeded so quickly if he had not already had in mind a number of original psychological conceptions.

The Conscious Way: Rorschach's Psychological Conceptions

THE STARTING POINT: THE INITIAL DREAM

This leads us to the question of the conscious origin and development of Rorschach's psychological concepts. Here again, however, we must begin with a message from the unconscious, that is, Rorschach's initial dream. We remember how, as a young medical student, Rorschach was deeply impressed by a dream he had had the night after he had been present for the first time at an autopsy. He dreamt that his own brain was being cut into slices exactly as he had seen it done during the autopsy, and he felt these slices falling forward, one after the other, across his forehead. A careful study of Rorschach's dissertation, written some eight years later, shows without doubt that this dream was the nucleus of his work "On Reflex Hallucinations and Kindred Manifestations" and therefore of the *Psychodiagnostics* itself. It must indeed have been a very special dream!

A psychoanalyst would perhaps point out that Rorschach dreamt only of the cutting of his brain, although he had witnessed an autopsy of the entire body. He would think of passive masochistic or even self-destructive tendencies. A pupil of Jung would perhaps go further and speak of *Schicksalstraum* (a destiny dream) being the starting point of a great discovery and connecting it with the tragic death that was to follow it shortly. I will not enter into such considerations but will limit myself to the way Rorschach himself approached his dream.

Here again Rorschach displayed his originality. He did not endeavor to interpret the content of the dream but rather to elucidate its mechanism.

Two questions arose in his mind: How can someone experience in a dream perceptions that are physiologically impossible? And how could a succession of optic images be "translated" into, and reexperienced, as a succession of kinesthetic images? These two questions Rorschach answered years later: we dispose of a much wider range of images than we commonly experience in our daily life, he would conclude. Later on, this was formulated in one of the most important sentences of the *Psychodiagnostics*: "The apparatus with which the individual is endowed for assimilating experiences is a much broader, more extensive instrument than that which he uses in daily life. A person has a number of registers which enable him to experience, but he uses only a few in the ordinary run of living." In addition to the ordinary way of linking perception with perception through the medium of "associations," there is a much more direct way through the kinesthetic system. Through "synkinetic" phenomena, optic perceptions are immediately below the threshold of consciousness, registered in the form of kinesthetic images. These perceptions can be either consciously reexperienced as kinesthetic perceptions or unconsciously retranslated into optic images. The Rorschach Test is therefore nothing else in its first principle than a mirror in which optic stimuli activate kinesthetic images, which are projected in turn into inkblots and are perceived as *pareidolias*. Furthermore, between this dream and the finished *Psychodiagnostics* lie a few basic theoretical conceptions of Rorschach, which we may call "creative introversion," "reproductive extratension," and the *Erlebnistypus*.

CREATIVE INTROVERSION

From his famous dream, Rorschach had drawn the conclusion that certain optic perceptions are unconsciously recorded under the form of latent kinesthetic images. These can be either reactivated and felt by the subject as kinesthetic, conscious perception in his own body or projected, that is, retranslated, into optic images. These peculiar processes are called by Rorschach "synkinetic phenomena." But what else do we know about these kinesthetic phenomena? The textbooks of the day said nothing about them. At this point, it was Rorschach's good luck to discover an author who had treated them extensively.

John Mourly Vold (1850–1907), a Norwegian philosopher, had devoted himself for more than twenty-five years to the study of the psychophysiology of dreams. A small part of Vold's extremely systematic and meticulous research was published posthumously in two volumes in 1910 to 1912. Vold treats the effect of the sexual stimuli on dreams in a half-page in Latin, and the remainder of his 879 pages are devoted almost exclusively to the effect of cutaneous and muscular stimulation on dreams. Vold seems to have totally ignored the research of other authors and to have never heard of psychoanalysis. His book is tedious but contains a number of stimulating facts. Rorschach adopted from him the following important conceptions: (a) Kinesthetic perceptions constitute a fundamental part of our personality, but in the awakened state they are repressed by consciousness, whereas they come back to consciousness during sleep. They furnish the most important material in dreams. (b) Kinesthetic perceptions and movements are antagonistic. When the dreamer awakes, he is able to keep his dreams in mind provided that he remains totally motionless, but as soon as he moves about, they disappear. On the other hand, inhibition of movements stimulates kinesthetic representations. (c) The more inhibited the muscular activity, the more active the kinesthetic imagery becomes. Vold had conducted experiments indefatigably to prove this assertion. To cite only one of them: On the night of February 18, 1901, nineteen of Vold's students went to bed with a woolen tape tied doubly around their left ankle. Their dreams, immediately recorded on the following morning, contained a remarkable number of active movements. One student dreamt he saw horsemen pursuing jumping hares; another that he saw his two brothers running after a herd of cows that flew up a hill; another flew through the streets; and another speedily climbed an incline that in reality was inaccessible. (d) In such experimental dreams, the kinesthetic images can be experienced either as imaginary movements of the dreamer himself, or projected as movements performed by other human beings or by animals having a certain similarity with human beings. Much more infrequently they are projected as movements of objects or of abstract figures. (e) Kinesthetic dreams involve a wide range of kinesthetic representations, from the "wild movements" quoted above to slow movements and static attitudes. Vold considered these static attitudes to be potential, repressed movements. One need only read the chapters on "Movement Responses" in the *Psychodiagnostics* to realize how great the debt of Rorschach is to Vold while at the same time realizing how skillfully Rorschach has incorporated these concepts into a larger framework.

Vold, however, the adept of psychophysiology, had known nothing of the revolution wrought by Freud in the psychology of dreams. The dynamism of wish fulfillment, the censor, the role of childhood remembrances, sexual symbolism—all of these ideas remained unfamiliar to him. One can hardly imagine two dream theories more opposed than those of Freud and Mourly Vold, yet Rorschach audaciously attempted to reconcile and utilize elements from them both. In Rorschach's final model, Vold's kinesthetic factors were the sensorial stuff, the material without which there can be no dream. That material was shaped, however, by Freud's dynamic factors. To quote Rorschach: "Mourly Vold's factors are part of the construction material, the symbols are the workers, the complexes the building craftsmen, the dream psyche the architect of the construction which we call the dream." According to Rorschach, the oneiric symbol appears at the intersection of the kinesthetic material and Freudian dynamism. On the other hand, the more a representation of complex character has stamped itself into the material of the kinesthetic sensations, the more apt it is to be projected, either as a dream symbol or in a psychosis, as a reflex hallucination or—to anticipate the Rorschach Test—as "original movement response."

Furthermore, Rorschach pointed out that not only in sleep and in dreams but in any kind of purely assimilative and creative activity we plunge ourselves into the world of synkinetic phenomena. To this particular kind of interiorization Rorschach later gave the name *introversion*. But we need to understand, as Rorschach himself stressed, that this introversion has nothing in common with the process that Jung designated by the same name. We might call it more precisely "creative introversion" in order to distinguish it from Jung's introversion. Creative introversion is a free, voluntary, transitory turning inward to the realm of kinesthetic phenomena and is the condition for any kind of true fantasy and creativity as well as of an awareness of one's inmost nature. Certain human beings are naturally more adept at the process than others; Rorschach at first called them "kinesthetic individuals," later on "introversives." Because of the antagonism between movement and kinesthetic perceptions, and because inhibition of movement increases the kinesthesias, we are not surprised that the introverts are rather clumsy, awkward individuals. In the *Psychodiagnostics*, Rorschach assigns to the introversives the characteristics of "more individualized intelligence; greater creative ability; more inner life; stable affective reactions; less adaptability to reality; more intensive than extensive rapport; measured, stable motility; awkwardness, clumsiness."

REPRODUCTIVE EXTROVERSION

Such was Rorschach's conception of introversion, a word he borrowed from Jung. But in Jung's teaching, there were two antagonistic forms of personality, the introverted and the extroverted. And what happened to extroversion in Rorschach's system? Here again, his handling of the idea was original. Just as Rorschach had connected kinesthetic perceptions, creativity, and introversion, now he connected color perception, reproductive intelligence, and extraversion.

It is noteworthy that Rorschach's earlier papers contain no references to the factor of color. Only later did he incorporate color into his system. Probably he received suggestions about this point from his learned friend at the Waldau, Dr. Fankhauser. Among other conceptions, Fankhauser imagined a "sphere of emotions" giving a graphic representation of every possible nuance of emotion in a three-dimensional frame; the emotions are considered there as the combination of three pairs of antagonistic emotions. This was an imitation of the "sphere of colors" of Wilhelm Wundt, which gives a graphic representation of the three pairs of complementary colors. Fankhauser was the first to imagine a system of analogies between the colors and the emotional life, as in the systems of Max Lüscher and Hans Werthmüller today. It seems likely that Fankhauser inspired Rorschach's idea of connecting color perception and affectivity, such as red with impulsivity and blue with self-control. As a counterpart to the kinesthetic introversives, Rorschach characterized the color-responding extratensives with "stereotyped intelligence; more reproductive ability; more outward life; labile affective reactions; more adaptable to reality; more extensive than intensive rapport; restlessness, labile motility, skill and adroitness."

THE INTROVERSION-EXTRATENSION SYSTEM

At this point, it should be clear that Rorschach's psychological conceptions have nothing in common with Jung's typology. Rather, they differ from it in several ways: (a) Introversion and extroversion—which Rorschach calls extratension—are not two mutually exclusive constitutional types but two universal psychological functions. They are as little opposed to each other as are, for instance, vision and audition. (b) These two functions are normally mobile and active. At any time, we can turn to the interior world of kinesthetic images and creation that is introversion, or to the world of colors, emotions, and relationships that is extratension. Both functions are necessary for the individual and for mankind. Introversion is the basis of culture and extratension of civilization. (c) In every individual, both functions coexist in a specific proportion that can be measured by the Rorschach Test. The extent of introversion and extratension, and their proportion to each other, is what Rorschach calls the *Erlebnistypus*. Some people are predominantly introversive or extratensive. Others are both simultaneously, even in a large measure; they are the "dilatated." Some others are neither introversive nor extratensive, and they are called "coartated." Between these four types—introversives, extratensives, dilatated, and coartated—all possible forms of transition can exist.

THE *ERLEBNISTYPUS*

This is the core of Rorschach's *Psychodiagnostics*. It is a totally new concept that has no equivalent in prior modern Western psychology. The conception that comes closest to it is the *Karma* of Hindu psychology in its original sense, before it was put in connection with Samsara, that is, with the chain of successive reincarnations. The *Karma* is the continuous elaboration and operation of an invisible nucleus of personality that, although unconscious, is constantly shaped by our conscious acts and thoughts and reciprocally codetermines our conscious acts and thoughts. In other words, it is the inexorable connection between a living being and the totality of his past doings.

Although not identical with this conception, the *Erlebnistypus* shows striking similarities to it. It can be defined as the *inmost, intimate capacity of resonance to life experiences*, and at the same time as a secret elaboration of these new life experiences. It gives the clue to the whole personality. In the mature Rorschach Test, it plays the same role as the *Formniveau* in the graphological system of Ludwig Klages: it is the key to which all other data have to be referred in order to ascertain their exact value. Any psychological manifestation whatever can take infinite meanings according to the formulas of Rorschach's *Erlebnistypus*.

Although the *Erlebnistypus* has a certain stability in each individual, it undergoes fluctuations in daily life: joy dilatates and sorrow coartates. On the other hand, the *Erlebnistypus* undergoes a slow, continuous, autonomous evolution during the span of human life. There are periods of introversion, of extraversion, of dilatation, and of coartation. If we followed these variations from infancy to old age and reported them on a chart, we would obtain a life-curve that is characteristic for each individual. What would happen if we could collect a great number of such life-curves—for instance, those of individuals of the same family or the same occupation—and compare them with those of people of different races and nations? Rorschach was convinced that we would have a most important and efficient tool for anthropological research. He himself began comparative investigations between the people of Bern and Appenzell, and he wished to do research with African Negroes. Mrs. Rorschach has informed me that Rorschach had even asked Dr. Albert Schweitzer, the famous doctor of Lambarene, to perform test investigations along these lines among the natives of the Congo, which unfortunately Dr. Schweitzer did not consider feasible.

The investigation of the *Erlebnistypus* and of the life-curve could be performed, Rorschach believed, either with the help of his test or by other indirect methods. Rorschach believed, for instance, that a systematic study of paintings of past centuries, analyzing the expression of movement and the use of color, would make possible a reconstruction of the mentality of the corresponding epochs. Thus, he considered his *Psychodiagnostics* a universal key for the deciphering and understanding of human culture and civilization throughout all the world and all the centuries.

Such, then, are the basic conceptions on which the inkblot test rests. These have been summarily sketched by Rorschach in the fourth chapter of his book under the title "Results of the Experiment." This fourth chapter of the *Psychodiagnostics* is in my view one of the most powerful fragments on human nature that has been written.

The Birth of the Test

As for Rorschach's test itself, we can now see that it emerged from the confluence of two contemporary currents of psychological thought: the first current concerns Jung's Word Association Test, the first experimental method applied to dynamic psychiatry. Jung used this test as a detector of complexes and isolated a special test syndrome for every mental disease. But perhaps his most original contribution was the formal classification of the answers. Roughly speaking, Jung distinguished internal or semantic associations from external or verbal associations, putting the semantic associations, which he considered characteristic for introverts, on the left side, and verbal associations, characteristic for extroverts, on the right. It is clear that much in the Rorschach Test, details as well as general framework, has been transposed from Jung's Word Association Test.

The second influential current flows from the experimental study of imagination with the help of inkblots. Several attempts in this direction had been made before Rorschach. It is doubtful whether Rorschach knew of the studies of either Whipple in America or Rybakof in Russia; but certainly he knew Hens, for he mentions him in his writings. With eight test cards, Hens had evaluated a thousand children, a hundred normal adults, and a hundred psychotics. In examination, his subjects were allowed to turn their cards as they wished, but Hens did not measure the reaction time. His goal was the study of fantasy, but he had already noticed that other psychological factors intervened. Hens restricted his study to the analysis of the content of the responses, noting that certain responses were predetermined, for instance, by the season, recent political events, or the occupation of the parents. He did not find any noteworthy differences between the content of the responses of the normal and the psychotic adults. Out of his 1,200 subjects, Hens found only two with complexes. At the end of his studies, he offered a few suggestions for future inquiries. Some subjects, he noticed, had the tendency to interpret the whole picture, others only details. Did this pattern have a meaning? His eight cards were all black and white. What could be done with colored cards? Would the comparative testing of members of whole families be interesting? Lastly, might this method be useful some day in the diagnosis of psychoses? "Probably the near future will show it," Hens concluded. Hens's prophecy was soon to be fulfilled by Rorschach.

From the moment when the idea of the test crystallized in Rorschach's mind, it developed very rapidly. He devoted the full year 1918 to the elaboration of inkblot cards and their trials with his Herisau patients. In December 1918, Rorschach presented a preliminary report about the test to the medical association of Herisau, consisting mainly of a few country doctors who showed little understanding. At this point, Rorschach realized the necessity of compiling his findings into book form in order to acquire some kind of academic recognition. His first manuscript for the book with the fifteen original cards was sent to six or seven publishers, all of whom refused it. Julius Springer finally accepted it on the condition that the number of cards be reduced to six. Another report by Rorschach about his work to the Swiss Psychiatric Society meeting on November 1–2, 1919, also stirred little comment. Genuine and intelligent appreciation of his work was expressed by a small group at a meeting of the Swiss Psycho-analytic Association when he addressed it in March 1920. At this time his old friend Morgenthaler, knowing Rorschach's difficulties in locating a suitable publisher, took the matter in hand and was able to arrange for the firm Bircher in Bern to publish the book, but with only ten cards and with certain modifications. Rorschach signed a contract for 1,200 copies of the book with Bircher on May 27, 1920.

The *Psychodiagnostics* was to be ready for publication in October 1920, but owing to recurring difficulties it appeared only at the end of June 1921. If the printing of the book left much to be desired, the printing of the cards was more than unsatisfactory. The cards were reduced in size, the colors changed in print, and the original uniformity of the black areas was repro-duced in a variety of shades, delineating all kinds of vague forms. The printer probably did not expect congratulations for his slovenly work, but as soon as Rorschach saw the proofs he was seized with a renewed enthusi-asm and understood at once the new possibilities that the prints offered. For this reason, no allusion is made to the shades and chiaroscuro in the book itself.

The publication of the book had deprived Rorschach of his cards for long months, and with his pupil Hans Behn-Eschenburg he had created a paral-lel set. In the meantime, Rorschach spoke again to the Swiss Psychiatric Society on November 26–27, 1921, and to the Swiss Psychoanalytic Asso-ciation on February 18, 1922. The test had taken a new and refined devel-opment in his mind, channeling more and more toward a phenomenologi-cal approach. In the end, the publication of the *Psychodiagnostics* was a total failure. The entire stock remained in the basement of Bircher's pub-lishing house, and the few initial reviews were either indifferent or hostile. Rorschach, who had struggled for a long time against a series of obstacles, was exhausted by the terrific output of energy he had sustained in this work and depressed by its failure. It is at this point that he succumbed, taking with him a great part of his secret to the grave.

Evolution and Acceptance of the Rorschach Test

For a number of years, it seemed that the sudden tragedy that had taken Rorschach away might also annihilate his work. His conceptions were in advance of his time so that very few people were able to understand them. The *Psychodiagnostics*, a book written, according to Morgenthaler, "in an incredibly short time," was deficient in organization and clarity. Apart from Bleuler, who had tried the test in the Burghölzli and expressed himself favorably on the result, and a few personal friends, Swiss psychiatrists at first had shown little interest. Psychoanalysts were mainly interested in the test as a possible adjuvant for the analytic technique. During the last year of his life, Rorschach had impressed his contemporaries primarily through his "blind diagnoses" (he is credited with having coined this expression), a procedure that was completely new. But the numerous inkblot tests he had analyzed in writing, and that would have done more than anything else to promote his work, were kept secret by their holders, with the exception of the two published by Ernst Schneider in 1922 and by Emil Oberholzer in 1923.

From the publisher's as well as the author's point of view, the *Psychodiagnostics* had been a failure. The *Schweizer Archiv für Neurologie und Psychiatrie*, the only Swiss psychiatric journal, gave no review of the work. Among the few reviewers, Fankhauser and Flügel did little more than summarize Rorschach's main assertions, without much comment. Kronfeld's review in the *Zeitschrift für experimentelle Psychologie*, although acknowledging Rorschach's originality and the practical value of his test, contained a sharp, inexorable criticism of his methodology and psychological conceptions. This review is said to have depressed him very much. If the *Psychodiagnostics* met with predominating indifference in Switzerland, in Germany the response was overt hostility. On April 20–23, 1921, in Marburg, the German Society of Experimental Psychology held its first congress after a long interruption during World War I. Before a large assembly avid to hear the newest research, Roemer gave a substantial account of the Rorschach Test and advocated its use for vocational counseling. First to speak in the discussion was Professor William Stern, the promoter of "personalism," who broke out in a vehement attack against Rorschach: no test, Stern said, could ever seize and comprehend the human personality; he declared Rorschach's methodology faulty, his evaluations artificial and arbitrary, and his statistics insufficient.

With these words, the destiny of the Rorschach Test was sealed for a long time. Psychologists such as Georg Müller and psychiatrists such as Hoche and Bumke joined Stern in his negative attitude. It was the same stubborn, narrow-minded opposition that had met Freud's psychoanalysis. Since these men controlled the nominations to university positions, a candidate whose list of publications contained a paper on the Rorschach Test would have been automatically excluded. In fact, the problems involved went far beyond the validity of a particular test. Rorschach was in all regards an outsider. An isolated research worker in a small cantonal asylum, his contribution threatened the prejudice, still very strong in the German-speaking countries, that "no scientific work can be performed outside of a university or without the supervision of a university professor." Therefore, the Rorschach Test could not be tolerated. Later, when Rorschach's work achieved world renown, Stern charged one of his pupils, Karl Struve, with the fabrication of a so-called modified Rorschach, the Cloud Test, consisting of three cards showing formless, asymmetrical, gray and black spots, a test intended to investigate the imagination. A humorist declared this test well named since it was "as formless and fleeting as a cloud."

Besides the question of university prestige, a much more acute conflict lay behind the opposition to Rorschach. Following World War I, in Germany and Switzerland, there was a sudden and rapid penetration of psychology into many fields of life, including industry. A number of engineers accused university psychology of being pedantic, formal, and academic. Instead, these critics strove to elaborate economic, practical, and reliable psychotechnical methods for vocational counseling and industrial psychology. This movement, which at the beginning inevitably gave rise to some abuses, was resented by university experimental psychologists as an intolerable usurpation of their own powers. Unfortunately, the Rorschach Test was accused by some people of being one of the new, bogus methods used by the vocational engineers and was discarded as such.

Nevertheless, at the same time the first more constructive attitude toward Rorschach's work began to appear in Switzerland. One year after Rorschach's death, Ludwig Binswanger published a critical study of the *Psychodiagnostics* that was a model of clarity, impartiality, and understanding. Binswanger here deplored the fact that Rorschach had published his book at a time when his knowledge of theoretical psychology was incomplete and he had not yet heard of the Gestalt theory. Although contesting several of Rorschach's ideas, Binswanger stressed the importance of his concepts of color and kinesthetic perceptions, and he highlighted the new problems arising from his work. Rorschach's typology, Binswanger declared, was outstanding, combining an original set of general types with a fine system of individual differentiation. Psychoanalysis, he added, was enriched by this symbolic interpretation of abstract responses and had acquired for the first time a tool for measuring the transformation undergone by the subject in the course of an analysis. Clinical psychiatry gained new methods of investigation. Binswanger concluded by calling the

Rorschach Test a "scientific microcosm" reflecting the larger fields of psychiatry and psychology.

However, in spite of Binswanger's manifesto, the development of the Rorschach Test in Switzerland was slow. From 1922 to 1935, not a single communication about it was given at the meetings of the Swiss Psychiatric Society. During this long period of latency, small groups of Rorschach students were formed throughout Switzerland which met to discuss one or two Rorschach protocols, after which the case history was revealed and compared with the findings of the participants. Among such groups, the "Swiss tradition" of the Rorschach was developed and interesting research was performed. The most important progress in this area was due to Hans Binder, who in 1932 introduced the concept of chiaroscuro in the test technique and analyzed thoroughly the psychological substrata of the experiment.

Finally, the years before the outbreak of World War II saw the triumph of the Rorschach Test throughout the scientific world. In the United States, where the test had been introduced by David Levy and S. J. Beck, outstanding theoretical contributions were made by Bruno Klopfer. In 1936, the *Rorschach Research Exchange* was published, and in 1939 the Rorschach Institute was founded in New York City. Later, the *Psychodiagnostics* was translated into English, French, and Spanish. This success surprised, and sometimes disquieted, even the most enthusiastic Swiss adherents. On June 26 and 27, 1943, the Swiss Psychiatric Society held in Münsterlingen a congress devoted exclusively to the Rorschach Test and its psychiatric applications. And the asylum of Münsterlingen itself, where young Rorschach had performed his first experiments some thirty years earlier, had become, under Director Zolliker and Dr. Kuhn, a center of studies of the Rorschach Test. [. . .]

Hermann Rorschach: A Contribution to the Psychology of Genius

Although our knowledge of the life of Rorschach is far from being sufficient for a full study of his genius, we may ascertain briefly what parts heredity and environment, natural endowment and life events, played in his accomplishments and attempt to evaluate his place in the realm of creative minds.

Rorschach's father and mother belonged to old families that for centuries had been established in the same place and had produced long successions of honest, capable, hardworking people. The stimulating influence of environment is also obvious in the formation of Rorschach's personality. Schaffhausen, a place of high cultural achievement, is a good example of what the historian G. Ferrero called a "qualitative civilization." This is evidenced by the fact that within a few years the Kantonsschule gave rise to several outstanding men, including the theologians Adolf Keller and Oskar Farner, and the psychiatrist Binswanger, who was Rorschach's senior by only four years.

In his constitutional endowment, Rorschach united quickness of mind and versatility with an aptitude for synthesis and contemplation. As a schoolboy he was notable for the equality of his achievement, in contrast with some other famous men. Rorschach learned with incredible speed and ease, almost as if playing. He was perhaps referring to himself in his book when he mentioned "the child for whom learning is too easy, so easy that he does not attain the physiologically—or at least socially—necessary degree of coartation." This might have been the reason for his long hesitation in the choice of his future occupation.

Rorschach's intellectual versatility might have been a danger for him had it not been compensated for by his capacity for synthesis. In his early article "Reflex Hallucinations and Symbolism," one is amazed by the intellectual boldness of the young resident, reconciling associationist psychology, psychoanalysis, Jung, Bleuler, and his own original ideas. Later on, he displayed the same ability on a larger scale in his studies on Swiss religious sects and still more so in his *Psychodiagnostics*.

But versatility and aptitude for synthesis enable truly creative work only if combined with the need for contemplation and vision. Kuhn has pointed out the importance of Rorschach's interest in the mysterious and occult. Another subject of his contemplation was the unwinding of the past: his interest turned from the study of his own genealogy, to the genealogy of Swiss sects' founders, to the rise and fall of the sects themselves, and finally to the vicissitudes of the human spirit as a whole. This explains why, experimenting with a projective test, Rorschach was not content with his present findings, but endeavored to reconstruct the evolution of *Erlebnistypus* from early childhood to old age and thought of similar reconstructions of past centuries.

Currently, we simply know too little of Rorschach's life to attempt a dynamic psychological interpretation. However, the death of his mother when he was 12 years old must have had a profound influence on him. It is also noteworthy that, after he left Schaffhausen as a student, Rorschach never felt bound to the town. Schaffhausen was also too small for him. A Swiss town of 50,000 inhabitants with its own government, cantonal assemblies and council, ministerial departments and administrations, where every man is involved in politics, promotes a spirit of exclusiveness and narrow-mindedness called *Kantönligeist* (little canton spirit) that repelled him, whereas "Mother Russia," for instance, was boundless, hospitable, and fascinating. The disappointment of the Russian episode, in 1914, might have affected Rorschach as a second loss of a mother and led him to an increased introversion and visualization of the past centuries.

But the germinal cell of the *Psychodiagnostics* had already emerged from Rorschach's unconscious under another form, described by the physician V. von Weizsäcker under the name *logophania*. At times, a new idea or theory can be the result of conscious, voluntarily directed thinking, or the result of a life event or situation, or the product of a personal psychological predicament of its author. However, a new idea can also originate directly from a bodily perception, which is what Weizsäcker calls a logophania. Such was the *Psychodiagnostics*, issuing from the kinesthetic perception of a dream.

Wilhelm Ostwald, in his studies on geniuses, distinguishes between "classical" and "romantic" geniuses. The classical genius is slower, the romantic quicker, be it for the apperception of reality, in the creative process, or in the development of the lifework. Ostwald's description of the "romantic" fits Rorschach very well, whereas Freud would be a good example of the "classical." The romantic gives earlier proofs of his superior intellectual capacities; he soon discovers a field which he masters and where he becomes outstanding; he shows an all-absorbing mind and a precocious audacity of thought; he overflows with ideas and projects; he has a greater faculty for enthusiasm and a greater need for communication, and he works and produces quicker and often gives his finest achievement earlier in life. Sometimes he has finished his lifework at an age when the classical genius begins his: Freud published the *Interpretation of Dreams* at 43 years of age, while Rorschach was dead at 37.

The classical genius, in contrast, is more concerned with the systematic elaboration and formal perfection of his works. He finishes a work before starting another one, in contrast to the romantic, who leaves unfinished projects. According to Ostwald, the greatest danger for the romantic is exhaustion through overwork. Ostwald sketched a psychopathology of the creative mind and stressed the role of a very special kind of exhaustion, the exhaustion of creative work, which cannot be compared with any other kind of exhaustion. Unfortunately, what Ostwald describes fits only too well with what we know about Rorschach's last months.

Psychosomatic medicine and the "Analysis of Destiny" of Leopold Szondi have incited modern psychology to search for the meaning of sickness and death in relation to time, circumstances, and personality. Can it be a coincidence that Rorschach died at the age of 37, a time corresponding to what Jung calls the "turning of life," which is frequently accompanied by a life crisis? Rorschach himself in his paper on Swiss sect founders observed that the age of 35 years is marked by an increased introversion. At this crucial point, Rorschach found himself in a critical life situation and was beginning to doubt whether he had not missed his career. As an asylum psychiatrist, he had few prospects for the future except to become an institutional director, a position entailing considerable administrative functions, which he disliked. His fervent wish for doing scientific research could have been satisfied only in a university clinic, but it was too late for him to secure a position there.* The only solution, Rorschach decided the last year of his life, was to leave Herisau and start a private practice as a psychoanalyst in Bern or Zurich. This was a relatively new specialty at the time and one that implied a considerable risk. Rorschach needed his strength to make this final vital transition, but he was exhausted from his work. Although he kept the same cheerful facade, a few friends knew how deeply concerned he was, and how depressed he was by the failure of his book.

It would be tempting to speculate about what would have happened if Rorschach had survived to lead a full life. Certainly he would have had a difficult time at first; but his scientific fame would have spread slowly with the development of his work. His book on Swiss sects would have been epoch-making for the psychology of religion. A few years later, the second edition of the *Psychodiagnostics* would have followed, enriched by the integration of Gestalt psychology, phenomenology, and other newer techniques. The evolution of Rorschach's thought was leading him toward phenomenology. He was personally acquainted with Minkowski and Binswanger, whose first contributions to psychiatric phenomenology appeared just one year after Rorschach's death. With his versatility and power for synthesis, he might well have given us a new anthropology and a new psychiatry, a synthesis of experimental psychology, psychoanalysis, and phenomenology. [. . .]

Unfortunately, the *Psychodiagnostics* is for us today only the outline of an unachieved masterpiece, and from Rorschach's other works we possess but fragments of fragments. They are what Paul Valéry said of Leonardo da Vinci's works, "the debris of nobody knows what grandiose games." Hidden and disguised by later structures, they are like majestic ruins which the archeologist tries to reconstruct in their original pattern in an effort to ascertain their true meaning and sometimes also to erect at their base a place of personal admiration.

---

*[*Editor's note*: At this point, readers may well have perceived the biographical parallels between the author and subject of this essay. Both Rorschach and Ellenberger were Swiss psychiatrists with itinerant careers, who worked as associate directors of cantonal asylums, spent a number of years in Schaffhausen, and were frustrated professionally and intellectually by their administrative duties. Both men were trained medically but maintained extensive interests in the humanities, including the arts, religion, anthropology, and popular folklore. Rorschach and Ellenberger were also intrigued by Russian culture and history, and both married Russian women.]

SOURCES AND BIBLIOGRAPHY

THE LIFE OF HERMANN RORSCHACH

Verbal and Written Statements by Contemporaries

I want first to express here my thanks to Mrs. Olga Rorschach, who gave me a wealth of information about her husband and showed me a great number of his drawings and photographs as well as miscellaneous objects made by him and various documents. Hermann Rorschach's stepsister, Mrs. Regina Möckli-Rorschach, also provided me with a great deal of interesting information.

Among the numerous other people who gave me details about Rorschach, I would like to mention particularly Dr. Walter von Wyss of Zurich, his university comrade and lifelong friend; Alt Reallehrer Konrad Gehring of Rüdlingen, his schoolmate and collaborator in the first experiments in the Münsterlingen period; Professor Carl Haeberlin of Basel, the well-known philosopher; Drs. Eugène Minkowski of Paris and Miecislav Minkowski of Zurich; Dr. Walter Morgenthaler of Bern; Reverend Oskar Pfister, the "grand old man of Swiss psychoanalysis"; and Dr. Emil Oberholzer and Georg Roemer, the first collaborators and students of the Rorschach Test.

Documents Provided by Archives

For this essay, I consulted and received information from the following archives: Archives of Kantonsschule, Schaffhausen; Archives of the Students' Association Scaphusia, Schaffhausen; Eidgenössisches Gesundheitsamt (Federal Office of Public Hygiene), Bern; Town Registry Office of Arbon, Thurgovia; Town Registry Office of Zurich; Town Registry Office of Schaffhausen; Secretariat of the University of Zurich and of the University of Bern. Also, Dr. O. Gsell, director of the Canton Hospital of Herisau, investigated the medical archives of the hospital and supplied me with an account of the fatal disease and the death of Hermann Rorschach. Dr. Roland Kuhn, associate director of the Münsterlingen Mental Hospital, sent interesting details of the case histories written by Rorschach from 1909 to 1913.

Contemporary Printed Documents

Festschrift zum 75. Stiftungsfest der Scaphusia, Schaffhausen (1933), 91.
Internationale Zeitschrift für ärztliche Psychoanalyse, 6 (1920), 101–9; 7 (1921), 516–21; 8 (1922), 242–43, which provides short summaries of the proceedings of the Swiss Psychoanalytic Society.
Jahrbücher Appenzell-Ausserrhodische Heil-und Pflegeanstalt in Herisau (1915–1922).
Jahrbücher Thurgauische Irrenanstalt Münsterlingen (1909–1913).
Jahrbücher bernischen kantonalen Irren-Anstalten Waldau, Münsingen und Bellelay (1913–1915).
Schweizer Volkskunde, 5 (1915), 75.
25 Jahre Appenzell A. Rh. Heil- und Pflegeanstalt in Herisau (Herisau, Buchdruckerei Schlapper, 1933).

Biographical Sketches

Hans W. Maier, "Dr. Hermann Rorschach," *Schweizerische medizinische Wochenschrift*, 52 (1922), 730.

Miecislav Minkowski, "Hermann Rorschach," *Schweizer Archiv für Neurologie und Psychiatrie*, 10 (1922), 318–20.

Isidor Fischer, *Biographisches Lexikon der hervorragenden Aertze der letzten fünfzig Jahre* (Berlin and Vienna, Urban & Schwarzenberg, 1933), 2:1320.

Olga Rorschach, "Über das Leben und die Wesenart von Hermann Rorschach," *Schweizer Archiv für Neurologie und Psychiatrie*, 53 (1944), 1–11.

Georg Roemer, "Hermann Rorschach und die Forschungsergebnisse seiner beiden letzten Jahre," *Psyche*, 1 (1948), 523–42.

Roland I. Kuhn, "Rorschachvorlesung," vol. 2, "Praktische Rorschachkunde" (Undated photocopied manuscript that gives details about Rorschach's Münsterlingen period).

THE PUBLICATIONS OF HERMANN RORSCHACH

A complete bibliography of Rorschach's publications has not yet been compiled. The following list should be considered as provisional.

Articles and Books

1. "Ueber 'Reflexhalluzinationen' und verwandte Erscheinungen" ["On Reflex Hallucination and Kindred Manifestations"]. Medical dissertation also published in *Zeitschrift für die gesamte Neurologie und Psychiatrie*, 13 (1912), 357–400.
2. "Zum Thema 'Sexualsymbolik,'" *Zentralblatt für Psychoanalyse*, 2 (1912), 365.
3. "Ein Beispiel von misslungener Sublimierung und ein Fall von Namenvergessen" ["An Instance of Failure in Sublimation and of Forgetting of a Name"], *Zentralblatt für Psychoanalyse*, 2 (1912), 403–6.
4. "Zum Thema: Uhr und Zeit im Leben der Neurotiker" ["Clock and Time in the Life of the Neurotic"], *Zentralblatt für Psychoanalyse*, 2 (1912), 606–8.
5. "Zur Symbolik der Schlange und der Kravatte" ["On Symbolism of the Serpent and the Tie"], *Zentralblatt für Psychoanalyse*, 2 (1912), 675.
6. "Reflexhalluzinationen und Symbolik" ["Reflex Hallucinations and Symbolism"], *Zentralblatt für Psychoanalyse*, 3 (1912), 121–28.
7. "Pferdediebstahl im Dämmerzustand" ["Theft of a Horse during Fugue State"], *Archiv für Kriminal-Anthropologie und Kriminalistik*, 49 (1912), 175–80.
8. "Zur Pathologie und Operabilität der Tumoren der Zirbeldrüse" ["On the Pathology and Operability of the Tumors of the Pineal Gland"], *Beiträge zur klinischen Chirurgie*, 83 (1913), 451–74.
9. "Analytische Bemerkungen über das Gemälde eines Schizophrenen" ["Analytic Remarks on the Painting of a Schizophrenic"], *Zentralblatt für Psychoanalyse und Psychotherapie* 3 (1913), 270–72.
10. "Ueber die Wahl des Freundes beim Neurotiker" ["On the Neurotic's Choice of a Friend"], *Zentralblatt für Psychoanalyse und Psychotherapie*, 3 (1913), 524–27.

11. "Analyse einer schizophrenen Zeichnung" ["Analysis of a Schizophrenic Drawing"], *Zentralblatt für Psychoanalyse und Psychotherapie*, 4 (1914), 53–58.

12. "Gebet gegen Verzauberung" ["A Prayer against Magic Enchantments"], and "Gebet gegen Bettnässen" ["A Prayer against Enuresis"], *Schweizer Volkskunde*, 7 (1917), 30–31.

13. "Assoziationsexperiment, freies Assoziieren und Hypnose im Dienst der Hebung einer Amnesie" ["Word Association Experiment, Free Associations and Hypnosis Used for the Cure of Amnesia"], *Correspondenz-Blatt für Schweizer Ärzte*, 47 (1917), 898–905.

14. "Einiges über schweizerische Sekten und Sektengründer" ["On Swiss Sects and Founders of Sects"], *Schweizer Archiv für Neurologie und Psychiatrie*, 1 (1917), 254–58.

15. "Weiteres über schweizerische Sektenbildungen" ["Further Studies on the Formation of Swiss Sects"], *Schweizer Archiv für Neurologie und Psychiatrie*, 2 (1919), 385–88.

16. "Sektiererstudien' ["Studies on Founders of Sects"], *Internationale Zeitschrift für ärztliche Psychoanalyse*, 6 (1920), 106–7. (Rorschach's summary of his lectures on Binggeli and Unternährer).

17. "Ein Mord aus Aberglauben" ["A Murder Because of Superstition"], *Schweizer Volkskunde*, 10 (1920), 39–43.

18. "Ueber ein wahrnehmungsdiagnostisches Experiment" ["On an Experiment of Perception Diagnosis"], *Schweizer Archiv für Neurologie und Psychiatrie*, 6 (1920), 360–61.

19. *Psychodiagnostik. Methodik und Ergebnisse eines wahrnehmungsdiagnostischen Experiments (Deutenlassen von Zufallsformen)* [*Psychodiagnostics: A Diagnostic Test Based on Perception*], vol. 2 of the collection *Arbeiten zur angewandten Psychiatrie*, edited by Dr. W. Morgenthaler (Bern, Bircher, 1921).

20. "Experimentelle Diagnostik der Affektivtät" ["Experimental Diagnosis of Affectivity"], *Schweizer Archiv für Neurologie und Psychiatrie*, 11 (1922), 147–48.

21. "Zur Auswertung des Formdeutversuchs für die Psychoanalyse" ["The Evaluation of the Form Interpretation Test for Psychoanalysis"], *Zeitschrift für die gesamte Neurologie und Psychiatrie*, 82 (1923), 240–74.

22. "Zwei schweizerische Sektenstifter (Binggeli und Unternährer)" ["Two Swiss Founders of Sects"], *Imago*, 13 (1927), 395–441.

Major Book Reviews and Article Abstracts by Rorschach

In *Zentralblatt für Psychoanalyse*, 1913–1914:
Wilhelm Steckel, *Der Zweifel*; K. Bonhöffer, *Die Psychosen im Gefolge von akuten Infektionen*; P. Schröder, *Intoxikationspsychosen*; O. Bumke, *Gerichtliche Psychiatrie*; E. Schultze, *Das Irrenrecht*; Emil Redlich, *Die Psychosen bei Gehirnerkrankungen*; Alfred Hoche, *Dementia paralytica*; W. Spielmeier, *Die Psychosen des Rückbildungs-und Greisenalters*; M. Rosenfeld, *Die Physiologie des Grosshirns*; Max Isserlin, *Psychologische Einleitung*; Theodor Kirchhoff, *Geschichte der Psychiatrie*; Alfred Gross, *Allgemeine*

Therapie der Psychosen; J. Wagner von Jauregg, *Myxödem und Kretinismus*; N. E. Ossipow, *Reflections and Hesitations about a Case of Degenerative Psychopathy*; M. M. Assatiani, *The Psychological Mechanism of the Symptoms in a Case of Hysteric Psychosis*; L. J. Bjeloborodow, *Psychoanalysis of a Case of Hysteria*; N. N. Schreider, *Psychotherapeutic Remarks*; W. N. Lichnitzky, *The Fundaments of the Present Rationalistic Psychotherapy*; J. Kannabich, *Hystero-Cyclothymia and a Few Words on Suicide*; N. A. Wyrubow, *Cyclothymia and Its Combinations*; M. M. Assatiani, *The Conception of the 'Conditioned Reflexes' and Its Application to the Symptoms of the Psychoneuroses*; I. A. Birstein, *A Dream of W. M. Garschin (A Psychoanalytic Study on the Question of Suicide)*; N. E. Ossipow, *'The Memoirs of an Insane,' an Uncompleted Work of L. N. Tolstoy*; W. Itten, *Beiträge zur Psychologie der Dementia Praecox*; Oskar Pfister, *Kryptolalie und unbewusstes Vexierbild bei Normalen*.

In *Imago*, 1921–1922:
G. A. Wehrli, *Krankheitsdarstellungen in den Winterzeichnungen der Dakota-Indianer mit einigen Parallelen aus europäischen Kinderzeichnungen*; G. A. Wehrli, *Die inneren Körperorgane in den Kinderzeichnungen mit ethnographischen Parallelen*; A. Knabenhans, *Die Erziehung bei den Naturvölkern*; Raymond de Saussure, *A propos d'un disciple d'Unternährer*.

Publications of Research Made under the Direction of Rorschach

Hans Behn-Eschenburg, *Psychische Schüleruntersuchungen mit dem Fordeutversuch (Psychological Research with Schoolchildren with the Form Interpretation Test)* (St. Gallen, Zollikofer & Cie, 1921). This important study was performed under the direct and constant supervision of Rorschach and contains a summary of the test, which is said to have been written by Rorschach himself.

Test Interpretations by Rorschach

A large number of "protocols" with Rorschach's own interpretations are known to exist. Since many of these protocols were performed after the publication of the *Psychodiagnostics*, their publication is highly important for Rorschach studies. It is hoped that the holders of these documents will come forth and make them available. Only a small number of such tests have been published as yet. Besides the well-known test illustrating Rorschach's last conference, posthumously published by Oberholzer (see No. 22 above under "The Publications of Hermann Rorschach") and incorporated in the second and all subsequent editions of the *Psychodiagnostics*, the following are known to exist:

Ernst Schneider, "Ueber Psychodiagnostik," *Die Schulreform* (Bern), 16 (1922–1923), 37–51, 84–91, 120–24.
Ernst Schneider, "Eine diagnostische Untersuchung Rorschachs auf Grund der Helldunkeldeutungen ergänzt," *Zeitschrift für die gesamte Neurologie und Psychiatrie*, 159 (1937), 159.

Ernst Schneider, "Original-Ausarbeitungen von Hermann Rorschach," *Rorschachiana III, Beiheft No. 19, Schweizerische Zeitschrift für Psychologie und ihre Anwendungen* (Bern, Hans Huber, 1950), 5–24.

RORSCHACH'S SOURCES

Rorschach owed the greatest part of his formal psychiatric knowledge to his teacher, Eugen Bleuler. He had also read much of Freud, Jung, and the central European psychoanalysts up to the date of his death. Furthermore, he is known to have read and been influenced by the following texts:

Justinus Kerner, *Die Klecksographie* (1857).
Dmitry Merejkowski, *Leonardo da Vinci* (1902). (The fragment quoted is an excerpt from the English translation by Bernard Guilbert Guerney, *The Romance of Leonardo da Vinci* [New York, Random House, 1931], 168.)
John Mourly Vold, *Ueber den Traum: Experimental-psychologische Untersuchungen*, edited by O. Klemm, 2 volumes, (Leipzig, Barth, 1910–1912).
Herbert Silberer, "Lekanomantische Versuche," *Zentralblatt für Psychoanalyse*, 2 (1912), 383–401, 438–50, 518–30, 566–87.
Oskar Pfister, "Kryptolalie, Kryptographie und unbewusstes Vexierbild bei Normalen," *Jahrbuch für psychoanalytische und psychopathologische Forschungen*, 5 (1913), 117–56.
William Stern, *Die differentielle Psychologie in ihren methodischen Grundlagen* (Leipzig, Barth, 1911).
Szymon Hens, *Phantasieprüfung mit formlosen Klecksen bei Schulkindern, normalen Erwachsenen und Geisteskranken* (Zurich, Speidel & Worzel, 1917).
E. Fankhauser, *Ueber Wesen und Bedeutung der Affektivität* (Berlin, Springer, 1919).

Inkblot Tests before Rorschach

Simon H. Tulchin, "The Pre-Rorschach Use of Ink Blot Tests," *Rorschach Research Exchange*, 4 (1940), 1–7.
Franziska Baumgarten-Tramer, "Zur Geschichte des Rorschachtests," *Schweizer Archiv für Neurologie und Psychiatrie*, 1 (1943), 1–13.
Saul Rosenzweig, "A Note on Rorschach Pre-history," *Rorschach Research Exchange*, 8 (1944), 41–42.

APPRECIATIONS OF RORSCHACH'S WORK

Early Reviews of the Psychodiagnostics

E. Fankhauser, *Schweizerische medizinische Wochenschrift*, 3 (1922), 1288.
Arthur Kronfeld, *Zeitschrift für angewandte Psychologie*, 20 (1922), 290–93.
J. G. Flügel, *Internationale Zeitschrift für ärztliche Psychoanalyse*, 8 (1922), 362–65.

Later Important Studies

Ludwig Binswanger, "Bemerkungen zu Hermann Rorschach's *Psychodiagnostik*," *Internationale Zeitschrift für ärztliche Psychoanalyse*, 9 (1923), 512–23.

Hans Binder, "Die Helldunkeldeutungen im psychodiagnostischen Experiment von Rorschach," *Schweizer Archiv für Neurologie und Psychiatrie*, 30 (1932), 1–67, 233–86. (An extensive analysis of the psychological factors involved in the test).

Hans Binder, "Die klinische Bedeutung Rorschachschen Versuches," *Schweizer Archiv für Neurologie und Psychiatrie*, 53 (1944), 12–29.

Roland Kuhn, "Ueber Rorschach's Psychologie und die psychologischen Grundlagen des Formdeutversuches," *Schweizer Archiv für Neurologie und Psychiatrie*, 53 (1944), 29–47.

Albert Reibmayr, *Die Entwicklungsgeschichte des Talentes und Genie*, 2 volumes (Munich, J. F. Lehmann, 1908).

Wilhelm Ostwald, *Grosse Männer* (Leipzig, Akademische Verlagsgesellschaft, 1910), 317–407.

Georg A. Roemer, "Ueber die Anwendung des psychodiagnostischen Verfahrens nach Rorschach auf Fragen der Berufsberatung," *Seventh Congress for Experimental Psychology, Marburg, April 1921*, edited by Karl Bühler (Jena, Gustav Fischer, 1922), 165–67.

William Stern, "Ein Test zur Prüfung der kindlichen Phantasietätigkeit (Wolkenbilder Test)," *Zeitschrift für Kinderpsychiatrie*, 5 (1938), 5–11.

Franziska Baumgarten-Tramer, "Der Rorschach Test im Licht der experimentellen Psychologie," *Schweizer Archiv für Neurologie und Psychiatrie*, 54 (1944), 3–41.

Part Three

THE GREAT PATIENTS

8

Psychiatry and Its Unknown History

[1961]

THE HISTORY of science constitutes one of the most important aspects of the collective memory of humanity. Inside this large edifice, the history of psychiatry forms a rather modest part, which is not surprising considering that psychiatry itself, as a science, is of quite recent origin. If I bring to your notice here some thoughts about this limited chapter in the history of science, it is because for several years recently, I was in charge of teaching the history of psychiatry. Now, the more deeply I read the writings of earlier psychiatrists as well as the few biographical accounts that we possess of their lives, the more the specific link between the biography, the theory, and the psychiatrist's historical influence seemed to me to become complex and obscure. It is surely difficult to explain why some pioneers of psychiatry produce a powerful movement of ideas, some others a simple momentary fashion, and still others remain unknown for a long time. It is possible that some of these facts can be explained by social phenomena, such as changes within the social population to which practitioners or patients belong. Furthermore, it would be fine to believe that the advancement of psychiatry always results from the application of a rigorous and objective method, based on the formulation of hypotheses, and supported by accurate measurements and statistics. These methods, of course, retain their validity; but, at the source of many of the most significant psychiatric discoveries, we find with surprising frequency the presence of irrational speculations, personal intuitions, and emotional preoccupations of all sorts. Above all, it seems to me that two typical situations, which I would like to examine in this article, have appeared recurrently in the history of psychiatry. The first one is the situation of a psychiatrist, deeply affected personally by neurotic symptoms, which he succeeds in overcoming eventually in such a way that a permanent insight into psychiatric science results from it. The second one, historically and psychologically more complex, is the situation of a psychiatrist who has made one of his patients—most often a *female* patient and generally a *hysterical* one—a special object of psychological investiga-

"La psychiatrie et son histoire inconnue," *L'union médicale du Canada*, 90, no. 3 (March 1961), 281–89; "La psiquiatría y su historia desconocida," *Revista de neuro-psiquiatría*, 26 (1963), 1–18.

tion. The psychiatrist develops unconsciously with this patient a long, complex, and quite ambiguous relationship the result of which will be very fruitful for medical science.

Let us begin with the first situation, the story of the psychiatrist who has to face his own neurosis or the neurotic elements in his own personality. When a psychiatrist is in such a state, he may take his own illness as an object of description and publish his own critical self-observations, either under his own name or under an assumed name. He may also attempt to fight against this neurosis, which may worsen its nature or may lead to the development of new therapeutic methods.

To my knowledge, the oldest example of this phenomenon involves the English writer Robert Burton, the famous author of *The Anatomy of Melancholy*, the first edition of which was published in 1628.[1] Burton was not a physician, but his book became a classic medical work of the seventeenth century. The word *melancholy* had at that time a very imprecise meaning and included almost every mental illness and neurosis as well as many familiar character types. Therefore, Burtonian melancholy had to be divided and subdivided in order to classify its innumerable forms. Burton declares that this classification is "a labyrinth of uncertainty and errors," and yet he undertakes it nonetheless. Among the kinds of melancholy he describes with the help of many quotations is "melancholy arising from study." Here, Burton mostly describes his own psychological story in the sorrowful portrait he draws of "scholar's melancholy." Let us note incidentally that "scholar's melancholy" was considered for a long time afterward a specific morbid entity; it was again described in detail in the eighteenth century, for instance, by the Swiss physicians Auguste Samuel Tissot and Johann Georg Zimmermann. For generations, being struck down by this illness was considered proof of intellectual distinction.

By the middle of the eighteenth century, "melancholy" was already waning as a fashionable illness; it was being superseded by "hypochondria." It was then claimed that hypochondria was more frequent in England than elsewhere, which explains the name "the English illness" often attributed to it. One of the most famous descriptions of the phenomenon was provided by George Cheyne in his book *The English Malady*, published in 1733.[2] Cheyne supported his account of classic hypochondriacal illness with several clinical observations, and the longest and the most interesting is the observation he made of himself. Subsequent to Cheyne's book, hypochondria fared well; a series of distinguished people were struck by it, including James Boswell, Samuel Johnson's famous

---

[1] Robert Burton, *The Anatomy of Melancholy* (Oxford, John Lichfield, 1621).
[2] George Cheyne, *The English Malady* (London, Strahan, 1733).

biographer who published a series of chronicles in *The London Magazine* from 1777 to 1783 entitled "The Hypochondriack."[3]

In the nineteenth century, two new illnesses emerged again to replace hypochondria, which had gone out of fashion. One of these new disorders, "neurasthenia," was formulated in the United States by George Beard in 1869 as a fundamentally modern and American illness; and the other one, "emotive delirium," was described in France by Bénédict-Augustin Morel in 1868.[4] Beard remained discreet about the origin of his theory as well as about the identity of the patients he took as his clinical prototypes. Morel, however, when depicting "emotive delirium" (later on, labeled "phobia"), made a number of curious observations which he linked with scenes from his own life, including the illness of the uncle of a young man he once tutored. Another case of the disease was Morel himself, who told how, after a bout of typhoid fever, he suffered for a long time from pathological fear of staying alone and of falling over a precipice.

We can see now that descriptions of three major historical neuroses—melancholy, hypochondria, and emotive delirium—were illustrated by authors who included auto-observations as a significant part of their descriptions. Unfortunately, we do not know how many other physicians have suffered from nervous symptoms which they did not think they could reveal to posterity but which they used in order to understand their patients better, to create new methods of psychotherapeutic treatment, and to erect new psychological theories. Among this group also appear perhaps the two greatest pioneers of the modern, scientific study of neurosis: Pierre Janet and Sigmund Freud.

The biography of Pierre Janet (1859–1947) is very underresearched. Yet we do know that Janet suffered in his youth from a religious crisis of sufficient intensity that his educational studies had to be stopped for a few months.[5] Following this crisis, Janet was able to finish his studies, and little by little he lost the shyness that previously used to paralyze him. If we read with close attention Janet's psychological writings, and if we compare some of his passages with what we know about their author's personality, there is little doubt that Janet often talks about himself when describing "the difficulties of action," "the cost of social actions," and diverse other manifestations of the neurosis he designated by the name *psychasthenia*.

Fortunately, we are much better informed about Freud than Janet. Freud took special precautions for disguising many of the personal facts that he

[3] James Boswell, *The Hypochondriack*, reprinted and edited by Margaret Bailey (Stanford, Calif., Stanford University Press, 1928).

[4] B. A. Morel, "Du délire émotif," *Archives générales de médecine*, 6th ser., 7 (1866), 385–402, 530–51, 700–707.

[5] Hélène Pichon-Janet, "Pierre Janet: Quelques notes sur sa vie," *L'évolution psychiatrique*, 3 (1950), 345–55.

evoked in his writings. However, we now possess a selection of Freud's
letters to his friend Wilhelm Fliess as well as many other curious and
moving details in his biography written by Ernest Jones.[6] We know, for
instance, that Freud, from 1890 to 1900, and especially between 1897 and
1900, suffered personally from symptoms that he himself called neuras-
thenic. It is also during those three years that he started his "self-analysis,"
which eventually led him to discover in himself an unconscious hatred for
his father and, from this, to formulate the theory of the Oedipus complex.
These experiences also allowed Freud to improve his method of dream
interpretation. Therefore, it is not an exaggeration to say that without
Freud's own neurosis—and above all without his long and heroic effort to
analyse and overcome this neurosis—psychoanalysis as we know it today
would not have come into being.

Next among the most famous other psychiatrists of our century is Ivan
Petrovitch Pavlov, a figure whom Soviet Russians today officially consider
the founder of their school of psychiatry. Pavlov, as is well known, was first
a professional physiologist, and he came only very late—around 1921,
when he was 72 years old—to the experimental study of the neuroses. At
that time he took a sudden interest in psychiatry. It seems, however, that
this evolution of his interests was precipitated by a little-known episode. In
1927, Pavlov underwent a surgical operation for a biliary lithiasis. In the
course of his convalescence, he developed a cardiac neurosis, which he
described himself in an article published in the Russian newspaper
Klinitcheskaya Meditsina in 1930.[7]

Now, without further discussion, let us proceed to a second series of historical cases. In these instances, a psychiatrist has taken as an object of systematic study a hysterical female patient with whom he becomes involved,
without his knowledge, in a rather ambiguous relationship. Why a hysterical patient in particular? Surely this is not by chance. Hysteria is an extremely curious illness, which has given rise over the years to many theories
and about which there is still no medical agreement, if there ever will be.
One thing, however, is certain: in pronounced cases, this affection reveals a
process that the British psychologist Frederick Myers called the "mythopoetical functions of the unconscious." The unconscious, Myers observed, seems constantly to be busy creating stories and myths. At other

    [6] Sigmund Freud, *Aus den Anfängen der Psychoanalyse* (London, Imago, 1960) (see,
among many others, the letter dated April 19, 1894, pp. 92–94); Ernest Jones, *The Life and
Work of Sigmund Freud*, 3 vols. (New York, Basic Books, 1953–1957), vol. 1, chaps. 13, 14.
    [7] M. K. Petrova, "Posleoperatsionnyi nevroz serdtsa, tchastyu analizirovannyi samin
patsientom-fisiologom," *Klinitcheskaya Meditsina*, 8 (1930), 937–40. A copy of this extremely rare article was obligingly conveyed to me by Professor P. Kupalov of Leningrad.

times, these stories and myths remain unconscious or appear in dreams. Sometimes, they appear as nice tales that the individual tells to himself, which are then waking dreams. Sometimes, these stories are acted out, as in cases of somnambulism, hypnosis, fugues, possession, and psychic trances. And, finally, sometimes the work of the mythopoetical function expresses itself through the language of a bodily organ, as with hysteria. In the past, hysteria was nicknamed "the great malingerer," precisely because it could imitate almost every illness: paralysis, anesthesia, blindness, nervous attack, and so on. Throughout the nineteenth century, hysteria was studied extensively, not only because among neuroses it was the strangest and most multiform, but also because it was closely related to some fundamental mysteries of the human mind. One could say that modern dynamic psychiatry emerged entirely from the study of hysteria.

The first of the major pioneers of dynamic psychiatry was the Austrian physician Franz Anton Mesmer (1734–1815), the founder of the doctrine of animal magnetism. We know that Mesmer first settled in Vienna, where he was leading the ostentatious life of a wealthy, bourgeois patron of the arts. One day, however, he began to treat some townspeople with magnets and was rather successful. Based on these experiences, Mesmer took into his house in 1773 a certain Miss Oesterlin, who was 29 years old.[8] Oesterlin had been afflicted for many years with extraordinary symptoms, including convulsions, which repeated themselves with amazing periodicity. As he was treating her with magnets, Mesmer began to realize that the real curative agent here was not the magnets but the personal influence that he himself exerted on the patient. He made this discovery on the historic date of July 28, 1774. Mesmer then decided that he personally emitted a specific magnetic fluid with therapeutic effects. Miss Oesterlin was soon completely cured and was later able to marry the son of Mrs. Mesmer's first marriage.

Another still more important patient soon succeeded Oesterlin. Maria Theresia Paradis was the daughter of an influential figure in Vienna. She was a talented pianist who had been blind from birth and who was also a godchild of the Empress Maria-Theresa. Maria Paradis had been treated unsuccessfully by the best physicians in Vienna but was reputedly incurable. Mesmer, however, took Maria into his house in 1777 to magnetize her. One day, a miracle occurred, and Maria declared that she had recovered her powers of sight. At first, Maria's family was delighted, but in time they became strangely reserved. The recovery of the blind pianist, to tell the truth, was not in the financial interest of either the family or the patient. In

---

[8] Franz Anton Mesmer, *Mémoire sur la découverte du magnétisme animal* (Geneva and Paris, Didot, 1779).

time, Maria's family came and took their daughter out of Mesmer's home, and the patient now declared that she had again gone blind.[9] At that moment, Mesmer left Vienna. His sudden departure from the city has been diversely interpreted. His experience with the case of Maria Paradis was almost certainly the reason. Significantly, Mesmer's wife remained in Vienna at this time, and Mesmer in fact never saw her again.

Mesmer then came to Paris to pursue his career. In Paris, after many trials and tribulations, he set up his medical practice. He built up a clientele, founded a flourishing school, and provoked a tempest of controversies. Eventually, his doctrine of animal magnetism was condemned by a Royal Commission of inquiry. In 1785, after being discredited, Mesmer suddenly left France and his many recent followers. Historians have been able to reconstitute only a part of his travels during the following twenty years. Like his sudden leaving of Vienna, Mesmer's departure from Paris may be understood in different ways. It is unlikely that the reason was the negative verdict by the Royal Commission, because he still had many disciples in Paris. However, we do know that on April 16, 1784, at the Lent Spiritual Concert at the Tuileries, a young blind pianist gave a harpsichord recital. It was Maria Theresia Paradis. The Baron Melchior Grimm, who attended the concert, wrote a letter recording that "everyone in the hall turned and looked at Mesmer, who unwisely had come to the concert. He noticed this and sustained there one of the biggest humiliations of his life."[10] Maria Paradis remained in Paris six months after this, and her presence must have made Mesmer feel ill at ease. He reacted to the situation as he had the first time, by running away.

As for the heroine of the story, Maria Theresia Paradis, musical dictionaries tell us that she went on to lead a brilliant career, playing at the major European courts, composing songs, sonatas, cantatas, a melodrama, and an opera, and founding a music school where she gave singing and piano lessons. It is impossible retrospectively to determine what the nature of her blindness was, whether a hysterical blindness that was temporarily cured or real blindness with a temporary pseudo-recovery resulting, again hysterically, from self-suggestion.

The doctrine of animal magnetism became widely diffused in France and Germany. In the cultural movements of the early nineteenth century, it played a part comparable to that of psychoanalytic ideas in the twentieth century. Certain German Romantic doctors and philosophers thought for a while that magnetism might provide a way to explore the soul of the universe and could constitute the basis for an experimental metaphysics. A

[9] Franz Anton Mesmer, *Précis des faits relatifs au magnétisme animal jusques en avril 1781* (London, 1781).

[10] Cited in Joseph Wohleb, "Franz Anton Mesmer," *Zeitschrift für die Geschichte des Oberrheins*, n.s., 53 (1940), 33–130.

curious episode in this line of investigation concerned a woman named "the Seeress of Prevorst," who was made famous by the German poet and physician Justinus Kerner.

Kerner is recognized today as one of the minor poets of the Romantic period. Medicine owes to him the discovery of the toxic food infection called botulism. But we often forget that Kerner was also one of the most important figures in the origins of dynamic psychiatry. Kerner was a country physician in the small town of Weinsberg in Würtemberg. In November 1826, he received an extraordinary patient, Friedericke Hauffe, whom he quickly took into his house where he could observe her closely. She ended up staying there almost until the time of her death in 1829, three years later.

Friedericke Hauffe, a poor uneducated country woman, was often in a state of "magnetic sleep" in which she was said to be "more awake than anyone" and during which she revealed considerable clairvoyant gifts. Kerner, along with a small group of philosophers and theologians, began to study her. He made many experiments concerning Friedericke's sensitiveness to certain plants, minerals, and animal products, and he gathered with much care her revelations about the spiritual world. Kerner recorded the result of these studies in a book, *The Seeress of Prevorst* (1829), which achieved a prodigious success in its own time.[11] This work was challenged by some contemporaries, and Kerner was often accused of having been duped by "a hysterical woman." But to that we can only answer that, if so, he was in good company, because the clairvoyant also received the attentions of the philosophers Görres, Baader, Schelling, Schubert, and Eschenmayer as well as the theologians David Strauss and Friedrich Schleiermacher. Kerner made many efforts to study Hauffe objectively. But neither he nor his colleagues seem to have suspected that the mere fact of studying a subject, with the clear expectation in advance of the apparition of some phenomena, could have an iatrogenic influence on the development of those phenomena. Historically, *The Seeress of Prevorst* represents the first monograph devoted to the in-depth study of a single patient. It retains its value today as a study of the "mythopoetical function of the unconscious" and what it can do when given time and auspicious circumstances.

Kerner conducted his work at a period when magnetism prospered in Europe. But soon thereafter, medicine became dominated by a new intellectual tendency, positivism, and magnetism and hypnosis fell into disgrace. However, around 1880, an antipositivist reaction gradually set in. We owe the revival of the study of hypnosis and a deepening of the investigation of hysteria mainly to the famous French neurologist Charcot. Un-

---

[11] Justinus Kerner, *Die Seherin von Prevorst: Eröffnungen über das innere Leben und über das Hineinragen einer Geisterwelt in die unsere*, 2 vols. (Stuttgart and Tübingen, J. G. Cotta, 1829).

fortunately, Charcot's studies were corrupted by certain methodological errors and by the fact that his clinical work on hypnosis was based on a too limited number of subjects (according to Janet, only three hysterical women). Among these patients, however, the *prima donna* Blanche Wittmann deserves special mention. The role patients have played in the edification of modern dynamic psychiatry has been much too neglected; unfortunately, it is difficult to gather reliable documents about this subject. I have been unable to find any information about Wittmann's origins or life before she entered the Salpêtrière Hospital in Paris. According to A. Baudouin, Wittmann was young when admitted to Charcot's service, where she quickly became one of the favored subjects.[12] Wittmann was the chosen patient to use any time that the doctors wanted to demonstrate in front of an important audience Charcot's famous three stages of hypnosis. According to Frederick Myers, she was not only a type, but the prototype, of the phenomenon.[13] She was nicknamed "the Queen of the Hysterics," and she is the figure represented in the famous painting by André Brouillet that shows Charcot and Joseph Babinski on each side of a female patient in the middle of a hysterical attack.

For unknown reasons, Blanche Wittmann at one point left the Salpêtrière and entered the Hôtel-Dieu in central Paris, where she was treated by Jules Janet, the brother of Pierre Janet.[14] Modifying the hypnotic technique used by Charcot and his students, Jules Janet discovered to his surprise a second personality in the patient, Blanche II. Blanche II revealed that she had always been there, conscious and alert, when Blanche I was hypnotized. For years, she had mutely and angrily witnessed the endless experiments that Blanche I was submitted to. As the personality of Blanche II was more stable than that of Blanche I, Jules Janet attempted to maintain her as long as possible in this second state. When she left the Hôtel-Dieu, Wittmann had literally become somebody else.

Wittmann's further story is known to us only through Baudouin's memoir.[15] Returning to the Salpêtrière, Wittmann took a small job at the laboratory of medical photography. Later on, after Charcot's death, when the first radiography laboratory was opened, she was employed there. She was authoritarian and temperamental, and she became angry if people asked her about her earlier dramatic history, which she now denied. As the

[12] A. Baudouin, "Quelques souvenirs de la Salpêtrière," *Paris-médical*, 15, I (May 23, 1925), x–xiii.

[13] Frederick Myers, *Human Personality and Its Survival of Bodily Death*, 2 vols. (London, Longmans, Green and Co., 1903), 1:447.

[14] Jules Janet, "L'hystérie et l'hypnotisme, d'après la théorie de la double personnalité," *Revue scientifique*, 3d ser., 15 (May 19, 1888), 616–23.

[15] Baudouin, "Quelques souvenirs de la Salpêtrière," x–xiii.

dangers of radium were not known at the time, Wittmann was one of its first victims. Several of her limbs were successively amputated, and the last years of her life were a calvary which she stoically endured. She died a martyr of science.

As mentioned above, one of the most important pioneers of twentieth-century dynamic psychiatry was Janet, who first studied in the field of philosophy and only later turned to medicine and psychology. In a short autobiographical notice, Janet related how, when he was 22, he arrived at Le Havre in western France to teach philosophy at the city *lycée*.[16] A physician and friend, Dr. Gibert, brought to his attention a woman, named Léonie B., who exhibited strange clairvoyant talents and who could be hypnotized from a distance. It was a stroke of luck for a young philosopher looking for a dissertation topic! On Janet's request, Gibert brought Léonie to Le Havre, where Janet could study her for several years. Janet noticed that Léonie, too, when hypnotized, revealed a distinct second personality, Léonie II, very different from the first one; by intensifying the hypnotic trance, he could even make appear a third personality, Léonie III. Each of these personalities had a very clear-cut nature and each differed in important ways from the other two. The case of Léonie provided the central subject matter for Janet's philosophy doctorate, his famous book *L'automatisme psychologique* of 1889.[17]

Janet assures us that Léonie's life was an extraordinary novel that he would write someday—which, unfortunately, he never did. Léonie was the daughter of a poor rural family from Normandy. In her youth, she had suffered from somnambulism and various hysterical troubles. She had also revealed great gifts of clairvoyance, and a group of men looking for a treasure in an old castle cellar had supposedly used her talents with success. She had been mesmerized by the best-known French hypnotists of the time. Frederick Myers, who once met Léonie, described her as "a fundamentally simple and honest person, a strong countrywoman with a slow and heavy physiognomy, and limited intelligence and vocabulary."[18] But Léonie proved an ideal subject for a hypnotist. She could even be hypnotized from a distance, merely through the thought commands of the hypnotist, as Janet once demonstrated. These experiments became controversial and attracted a lot of attention to the young Janet. The Society for Psychical Research in London sent a special delegation to Le Havre to observe Léonie. A report about his experiments was published; but Janet noted

[16] "Pierre Janet," in Carl Murchison, ed., *A History of Psychology in Autobiography*, 2 vols. (Worcester, Mass., Clark University Press, 1930), 1:123–33.

[17] Pierre Janet, *L'automatisme psychologique* (Paris, F. Alcan, 1889).

[18] Frederick Myers, "On Telepathic Hypnotism . . . ," *Proceedings of the Society for Psychical Research*, 10 (October 1886), 127–88.

"with surprise and regret" that people, while citing him, forgot to write to obtain accurate information about the case. He also felt that the reports written by many visitors were reckless.[19]

We do not know what happened to Léonie after Janet left Le Havre. For some time, Charles Richet as well as a number of English parapsychologists studied her.[20] As for Janet, he never disavowed his early researches on Léonie; but the direction of his work changed quite notably after this, and later in his career he had many reservations about so-called parapsychological phenomena.

Also among the early leading figures of dynamic psychiatry in our century is the Swiss psychologist Théodore Flournoy (1854–1920). A student of Wilhelm Wundt and professor of experimental psychology at the University of Geneva, Flournoy undertook to study the psychics of Geneva with a strict psychological methodology. He found a very gifted local psychic, Elise Muller (better known under the pseudonym of "Hélène Smith"), and he studied her from 1894 to 1900. During her psychic trances, Hélène Smith related and mimed to Flournoy some scenes from her many former lives. She reported that she had been Queen Simandini of the Indies in the fifteenth century and later Marie Antoinette. She said that she had also traveled, by thought, to the planet Mars, whose inhabitants she described and whose language she spoke fluently. Flournoy described and analyzed Hélène Smith's case in depth in a well-known book, *From India to the Planet Mars* (1900).[21] In his book, which became a best-seller, he was led to the following conclusions: the three great "cycles"—the Hindu, the Versaillian, and the Martian—experienced by Hélène constituted three "novels of the subliminal imagination" which were fed by forgotten childhood memories and readings. (Flournoy was actually able to identify some of the childhood readings.) These subliminal creations expressed a regression of the psychic's personality to different ages—the Martian cycle to age 12, the cycle of Marie Antoinette to age 6, and so forth. The cycles also represented an "embryology" and a "teratology" of the mind. Each of the novels constituted an imaginary realization of unfulfilled dreams as well as an effort for Hélène to compensate for her present boring and depressing daily existence as a lowly saleswoman.

We can see clearly that Flournoy anticipated several notions developed later by Freud. However, he underestimated the role of one of these notions, the transference, because he did not understand the part that he himself was playing in the development of the psychic's subliminal novels. During

[19] "Pierre Janet," in *A History of Psychology in Autobiography*, 123–33.

[20] Charles Richet, "Expériences sur le sommeil à distance," *Revue de l'hypnotisme*, 2 (1888), 225–40; R.A.H. Bickford-Smith, "Experiments with Madame B. in September 1889," *Journal of the Society of Psychical Research*, 4 (1889–1890), 186–88.

[21] Théodore Flournoy, *Des Indes à la planète Mars* (Geneva and Paris, Kundig, 1900).

her "Hindu" trance, for instance, Hélène identified Flournoy as her ancient husband, King Sivrouka. With admirable art, she mimed one day the poignant scene of the *suttee* in which she actually threw herself on the bed of her deceased "husband" to be burnt with him. Flournoy does not seem to have guessed the symbolic meaning of this scene, so evident for psychoanalysis. In his book, Flournoy talked about Hélène with obvious admiration, whereas in later publications he showed a certain disappointment. Furthermore, the publication of the book provoked from Hélène a sharp reaction of hostility to Flournoy.

We mostly know the rest of Hélène's story thanks to a book by Waldemar Deonna, *De la planète Mars en Terre Sainte*, published in 1932.[22] A wealthy and generous American woman, it seems, full of admiration for Hélène, gave her a sufficient fortune to allow her to spend the remainder of her life devoted to her psychic preoccupations. That very day, Hélène left her humble job as a salesclerk, breaking the only link that bound her regularly with reality. She shut herself up at home, concentrating on her dreams and visions, and then began to practice automatic painting in a state of somnambulistic trance. Among other things, she made a number of very curious paintings that were honored after her death in an exhibit held in Geneva and Paris.

We come now to the story of the famous woman who rests at the origins of psychoanalysis and who was known for a long time only by the pseudonym of "Anna O." In 1953, Ernest Jones revealed the patient's name as Bertha Pappenheim. The first account of Anna O.'s illness, written by Josef Breuer, was published by both Breuer and Freud in their *Studies on Hysteria* of 1895.[23] But the facts of the case related by Breuer had occurred much earlier, between 1880 and 1882. Anna O.—or, rather, Bertha Pappenheim—belonged to a distinguished Austrian Jewish family. She was, according to Breuer, very intelligent and physically attractive and had received a quite refined education, speaking German, French, and Italian. However, by age 21, she had been compelled to settle into a monotonous life at home that contrasted with her strong intellectual vitality. She found comfort only by telling herself interminable stories, which she called her "private theater." Breuer adds that "the sexual element in her nature was surprisingly underdeveloped."

When Breuer was first called to see her, in December 1880, Pappenheim presented a small museum of hysterical symptoms. Breuer treated her with hypnosis. By April 1881, a certain amelioration in her condition was quite noticeable. At this point, however, the patient's father died unexpectedly,

---

[22] Waldemar Deonna, *De la planète Mars en Terre Sainte. Art et subconscient. Un médium peintre: Hélène Smith* (Paris, Boccard, 1932).

[23] Josef Breuer and Sigmund Freud, *Studien über Hysterie* (Vienna, Deuticke, 1895).

which the patient received as a psychological shock. She now began to suffer somnambulistic crises, and she entered periods of momentary self-hypnosis that corresponded to the time of Breuer's daily visits to her. In this state, the patient would then relate to Breuer the hallucinations she had experienced during her episode of somnambulism. One day, Pappenheim told Breuer the specific circumstances that had first marked the appearance of a certain symptom. To the physician's surprise, that very symptom disappeared at once. The patient then began to tell Breuer the circumstances that had surrounded the appearance of each of her innumerable symptoms, and every one disappeared progressively. This technique is what the patient herself named the "talking cure," or her therapy by "chimney-sweeping" (*Kaminfegen*). Breuer adopted the idea, substituting for the popular phrase *chimney-sweeping* the more decorative Greek term *katharsis*. However, Pappenheim's treatment was consuming an enormous amount of time. Breuer was now coming to the Pappenheim house twice a day, and at times he spent several hours at a time with the patient. Then one day the patient declared spontaneously to Breuer that she wanted to be cured by the end of June 1882, and for this reason she redoubled her efforts with her "talking cure." On the last day, she had a final hallucinatory crisis, after which her symptoms disappeared, and she went on vacation. But, Breuer adds, she still required much more time before recovering completely.

Such is the account of the case of Anna O. as published by Breuer. But Jones has provided us with a more complete version, relying on original information given primarily by Freud himself, whose wife was a personal friend of the patient.[24] Jones tells us that Mrs. Breuer became very jealous of her husband's young patient (just as Mrs. Mesmer had probably been of Maria Paradis 150 years earlier). This situation in fact motivated Breuer to hasten the end of the treatment. However, the evening after his final session with Pappenheim, he received an urgent call saying that the patient was in labor. It was, of course, a hysterical pseudo-delivery, the culmination of a hysterical pregnancy that had developed during the previous months without Breuer's knowledge. Breuer hypnotized the patient to quiet her down, and the next day he left with his wife for Venice. Jones tells us that the result of this trip was the conception of a girl. As for Pappenheim, she was sent to a sanatorium for nervous disorders, where her state was for a long time considered quite grave. It was said that she nonetheless inflamed the hearts of the physicians there, so that her mother had to come and take her back to their home.*

---

*[*Editor's note*: For additional information about Pappenheim's later medical career, see Chapter 9, "The Story of 'Anna O.': A Critical Review with New Data."]

[24] Jones, *Life and Work of Sigmund Freud*, 1:223–26.

When she was about 30, a remarkable transformation occurred in Pappenheim's life and character. At this point, she not only recovered totally but emerged as a superior personality. Renouncing a private life, she henceforth devoted herself to social good works. With the cooperation of Rabbi Jacob Marcus, director of the American Jewish Archives in Cincinnati, Ohio, I was able to gather the following information: For about twelve years, Pappenheim directed a young girls' orphanage in Frankfurt. She then began to travel to the Balkan countries, the Middle East, and Russia in order to investigate illegal prostitution and the white slave trade. In 1904, she founded the Jüdischer Frauenbund (League of Jewish Women) and, in 1907, a teaching institution affiliated with this organization.[25] Among her numerous remarkable writings from this period are short stories and plays inspired by various current social themes, travel letters, studies of the Jewish woman's condition, and criminality in Jewish circles.[26] Later on, her activity took on an increasingly religious dimension. Pappenheim believed that the best way of raising up the cultural level of the Jewish people of central Europe was to publish again in a modernized form the early works that had nourished Jewish piety in past centuries, such as the *Mass Book* and the *Women's Bible*.[27]

It remains unknown if Bertha Pappenheim ever suspected the eminent part she played in the origins of psychoanalysis. Freud, who knew from Breuer the story of Pappenheim's illness and treatment, was fascinated by the case and was forever asking Breuer for more details about it. Owing to Freud's encouragement, Breuer finally agreed to publish the case; but he never again employed the treatment of the "talking cure." Freud, however, was less inhibited than Breuer and pursued the method with other patients. Over time, he changed the technique little by little until he had formulated the method of psychoanalysis.

Finally, there is Carl Gustav Jung, an early follower of Freud who broke from him later on to establish a psychological school of his own. To tell the truth, however, Jung's psychological research considerably predated his encounter with Freud. Specifically, several of Jung's most important ideas first appeared in his dissertation written for the medical degree. This disser-

---

[25] Salomon Wininger, ed., *Grosse jüdische National-Biographie* (Cernauti, Druck "Orient," 1925), 366.

[26] Bertha Pappenheim, *Kämpfe: Sechs Erzählungen* (Frankfurt am Main, J. Kauffmann, 1916); idem, *Tragische Momente: Drei Lebensbilder* (Frankfurt am Main, J. Kauffmann, 1913); idem, *Sisyphus-Arbeit: Reisebriefe aus den Jahren 1911 und 1912* (Leipzig, P. E. Linder, 1924); idem, "The Jewish Woman in Religious Life," *The Jewish Review* (January 1913).

[27] *Allerlei Geschichten, Maasse-Buch*, translated and edited by Bertha Pappenheim (Frankfurt am Main, J. Kauffmann, 1929); *Zeenah u-Reenah, Frauenbibel*, translated and edited by Bertha Pappenheim (Frankfurt am Main, J. Kauffmann, 1930).

tation, published in 1902, was entitled *On the Psychology and Pathology of So-Called Occult Phenomena*. It contains the detailed case history of a young milliner who, at age 15, revealed psychic gifts.[28] This young woman began to hold sessions in Zurich with a group that included Jung, who was then a 21-year-old medical student and who became the group's secretary. For two years, the woman provided revelations during séances, quite a few of which recalled the visions of Friedericke Hauffe, Kerner's famous patient. Similar to Flournoy's prize psychic, Hélène Muller, Jung's medium evoked her previous existences. She asserted that in her earlier lives she had been the ancestor of most of the people she knew, including Jung himself. Jung noticed that the many spirits that manifested themselves during these parapsychological sessions could be classified into two groups—either dark and taciturn or exuberant and a little crazy. Now, not uncoincidentally, these were the same two aspects of the young person's character, which constantly seemed to shift between two extremes. Moreover, there appeared to this woman the spirit of a superior essence, named Ivènes, who completely differed from the others by her serious, thoughtful, well-balanced personality. Jung proposed that this spirit represented the emergent adult personality of the psychic being elaborated in her unconscious. Coming from an old Basel family now in decline, the young woman was inhibited, because of both her neuropathic constitution and her strict upbringing. Through these dramatic mediumistic performances, Jung believed, her unconscious mind was attempting to overcome these obstacles to her psychological maturation.

Thanks to the assistance of Dr. Carl A. Meier in Zurich and of Jung himself, I obtained some additional information on the destiny of this important young woman.[29] First, it is permitted today to reveal that the woman in question was none other than Jung's own cousin on his mother's side of the family. Further, after a certain stage in the séances, the young woman began to fall in love with Jung. Jung, however, did not realize this; nor did he notice that she was carefully presenting her psychic revelations to please him. However, when he did finally figure out what was going on, he ended the sessions. This sudden termination was fortunate for the patient, because it obliged her in a sense to come back to reality. She left Zurich for Paris, where she worked for a while in a clothing atelier. She then turned to high fashion, set up her own business, and created clothes of rare beauty and originality. Jung once paid her a visit in Paris and discov-

[28] Carl Gustav Jung, *Zur Psychologie und Psychopathologie sogenannter occulter Phänomene* (Leipzig, Mutze, 1902).

[29] C. G. Jung, *Notes on the Seminar in Analytical Psychology, Conducted by Dr. C. G. Jung, Zurich, 23 March to 6 July 1925, Arranged by Members of the Class* (1926). Extracts from this private publication have been provided to me by Dr. Carl A. Meier with the authorization of Dr. Jung.

ered that she had almost completely forgotten her youthful psychic sessions. Shortly after this, however, she suffered from pulmonary tuberculosis and died prematurely.* [. . .]

It remains for us to conclude. As we can see from the material presented above, the history of dynamic psychiatry is inseparable on the one hand from the history of the neuroses of its founders and on the other from the story of a succession of remarkable women. These hysterical women, during a particular period of their lives, were minutely studied and intensely treated by a psychiatric clinician. The physician often allowed himself to be misled for a long time by his patient—or, rather, by the mythopoetical operations of the patient's unconscious—as well as by his own illusions and expectations. As Goethe once observed:

Halb zog sie ihn, halb sank er hin

[Half she pulled, half he let himself fall down]

Once the mistake was recognized, however, it was translated into a gain for both doctor and patient. If we put aside the cases of the Seeress of Prevorst, who died of a serious physical illness, of Hélène Smith, in which a stranger's intervention disturbed the situation to her disadvantage, and of Janet's Léonie, whose later life remains obscure, we can confirm that all of these women, once freed from their youthful hysterias, became outstanding personalities who deserve our recognition and respect.

On the other side, the clinician who studied these patients so intently often underwent a change of orientation in his ideas, if not in his very career, as a result of the encounter. Sometimes it was less the doctor himself who profited from the experience than one of his students or successors. In this way, the lessons offered by Breuer's Anna O. most profited Freud while Hélène Smith's case was better understood by Jung than Flournoy. It has been largely owing to the experience of cases of this sort that dynamic psychiatry today has learned the value of preliminary training and "didactic analyses" for future psychotherapists, which allow them to become conscious of their own potential psychological investments in cases in order to be able to neutralize them. In psychiatry as elsewhere, it is true that our mistakes, once overcome, often become our best guide.

*[Editor's note: The preceding paragraph, written in 1961, should be compared with Chapter 11, "C. G. Jung and the Story of Helene Preiswerk" (1991), in which Ellenberger gives a fuller, and considerably less positive, presentation of the medium's life after ending the séances and leaving Zurich.]

9

The Story of "Anna O.": A Critical Review with New Data

[1972]

FOR SOME YEARS now, psychiatric historiography has been at an important turning point. The belief is beginning to develop that in order to write the history of psychiatry satisfactorily, it is inadequate to be a practicing psychiatrist interested in the history of the profession. It will not do to have two historical methodologies, one for psychiatric history and another for all other forms of historical research. One expression of this change in orientation took place at a symposium held in April 1967 at Yale University devoted to methodological problems in the history of psychiatry.[1] Severe criticisms were lodged at this conference against the traditional methodologies of the field.

Two critical points in particular recurred: first, there has been "the cult of the hero." According to this approach, a single figure is taken as the central point of the history of the discipline. The key figure (whether it be Weyer, Pinel, Freud, or someone else) is established as "a genius" while all those who come before him are designated as "precursors" and those who come after are either "disciples," "rivals," or "apostates." (The resemblance of this hagiographical vision to the Nietzschean conception of history is noteworthy: a small number of supermen dominate history and in the intervals there is only a "race of dwarfs—*ein Gezwerge.*") It should be evident that such a perspective makes impossible any objective evaluation of the facts, personalities, or ideas in psychiatric history and risks any number of errors and distortions of perspective.

A second methodological shortcoming concerns uncritical reliance on source materials of a second, third, and fourth order and neglect of primary sources. The combination of these two deficiencies leads inevitably to the

"The Story of 'Anna O.': A Critical Review with New Data," *Journal of the History of the Behavioral Sciences*, 8, no. 3 (July 1972), 267–79; "L'histoire d'"Anna O.': Étude critique avec documents nouveaux," *L'évolution psychiatrique*, 37, no. 4 (1972), 693–717; and "Il caso di 'Anna O.,'" in Ellenberger, *I movimenti di liberazione mitica*, 153–74.

[1] The results of this symposium were published as George Mora and Jeanne Brand, eds., *Psychiatry and Its History: Methodological Problems in Research* (Springfield, Ill., Charles C. Thomas, 1970).

formation of historical myths, and it is by this means that certain domains of the history of psychiatry have come to be obscured by a thick cloud of legend. This situation is particularly apparent with the history of psychoanalysis, which has just begun to emerge from its initial hagiographical stage.

A small number of genuinely objective historical researches in this area have been made already. Siegfried and Suzanne Bernfeld, the first in this regard, have conducted investigations in the Vienna Archives on the childhood, educational studies, and scientific beginnings of Freud. Josef and Renée Gicklhorn have made important discoveries in the archives of the University of Vienna concerning his university career. Two American psychoanalysts, Ilse Bry and Alfred Rifkin, have probed deeply the question of the critical reception accorded to some of Freud's first publications and have dispelled the former belief according to which these works were received at the time only with criticism or contemptuous silence. But the scholars—psychoanalysts and nonpsychoanalysts alike—who have engaged in these sorts of critical studies have discovered the obstacles in their way and the hostility, at times masked by a superficial politeness, with which their work is received by those who adhere to the official legends.

In my report at the Yale symposium, I reviewed the four basic rules for an objective historical methodology in the history of psychiatry: (1) take no facts for granted; (2) verify everything; (3) place all materials in their historical context; and (4) firmly separate the facts from the interpretation of the facts. These are the simple principles that I attempted to apply in my recent book *The Discovery of the Unconscious*. [. . .] The present article represents a new contribution to the objective study of the history of dynamic psychiatry. It is hoped that it will encourage other scholars to refrain from reproducing indefinitely some of these well-known official legends and instead to explore for themselves the relevant primary sources and to study these sources in their full, original context.*

The Problem of Anna O.

To this day, the most elementary account of psychoanalysis begins with the story of a mysterious young woman, "Anna O.," whose numerous hysterical symptoms disappeared one by one as Josef Breuer was able to make her evoke the specific circumstances that had led to their appearance. The patient herself called this procedure the "talking cure" or "chimney-sweeping," while Breuer called it "catharsis." Anna O.'s treatment took

---

*[*Editor's note*: The preceding five introductory paragraphs appear only in the French edition of this article (pp. 693–96).]

place from 1880 to 1882, but the case history was published only thirteen years later, that is, in 1895, in Breuer's and Freud's *Studies on Hysteria.* From that time on, Anna O.'s story has been cited as the prototype of a cathartic cure and as one of the basic occurrences that led Freud to the creation of psychoanalysis.

Today, the veil of legend surrounding the foundation of psychoanalysis has been only partly lifted by objective research. In the following essay, we will examine Anna O.'s story in the light of the historical-critical method in order to ascertain what can be considered historically certain, possible but doubtful, and definitely legendary. After a brief summary of Breuer's original report of 1895, we will make a survey of all subsequent researches about Anna O., following the chronological sequence of the investigations. We will then bring to light two newly discovered documents, one being a hitherto unknown case history of the patient, written in 1882 by Breuer himself, and the second one a follow-up report written in the Bellevue Sanatorium, in Kreuzlingen, Switzerland, where Anna O. was transferred in July 1882.[2] Furthermore, we will explore what new light these documents throw upon the understanding of Anna O.'s famous story.

Breuer's Original Report of 1895

According to Breuer, Anna O. was 21 years of age at the time she fell ill in 1880. Anna O. belonged to a well-to-do family. She was very intelligent, attractive, kind, and charitable but apparently also moody and stubborn. The family was extremely puritanical, and, Breuer says, "the sexual element was surprisingly undeveloped" in the patient. There was, he added, a marked contrast between the refined education she had received and the monotonous home life she led. This brought Anna O. to escape from her daily domestic situation into long daydreams that she was in the habit of calling her "private theater." However, these daydreams did not interfere with her daily activities, and the other family members were not aware of them.

Anna O.'s illness, as described by Breuer in 1895, went through four chronologically sharply delimited periods:[3]

1. The *period of latent incubation* ran from July 1880 to December 1880. The starting point of Anna O.'s case was a severe physical illness of

---

[2] The author is immensely indebted to Dr. Wolfgang Binswanger, the present director of the Bellevue Sanatorium, in Kreuzlingen, who provided him with photocopies of both documents and gave him permission to utilize them for historical purposes.

[3] Josef Breuer and Sigmund Freud, *Studien über Hysterie* (Leipzig and Vienna, Deuticke, 1895), 15–37.

her beloved father. Anna O. gave her father intensive care, staying up during the nights and resting in the afternoons. But over time she became exhausted and had to be kept away from him. Soon thereafter, Anna O. began to suffer from intense coughing, and she experienced long episodes of sleepiness and agitation in the afternoons. According to Breuer, Anna O. also had at that time all kinds of hidden symptoms that neither her family nor she herself suspected. But Breuer did not see her during that period; it must be remembered that his description of her symptoms—overt or hidden—was a later reconstruction.

2. The *period of manifest psychosis* in Anna O.'s sickness ran from December 1880 to April 1881. During that period Anna O. was under Breuer's care, and she remained in bed from December 11, 1880, to April 1, 1881. A great variety of symptoms appeared within that short time, beginning with ocular disturbances, followed by paralyses, contractions, zones of tactile anesthesia, and linguistic disorganization. She spoke an agrammatical jargon composed of a mixture of four or five languages. Her personality was now split into one sad, "normal," conscious person, and one morbid, uncouth, agitated person who had hallucinations of black snakes. It happened that for two weeks Anna O. remained completely mute, but Breuer knew that this had followed a certain incident that was emotionally painful. After he was able to bring her to talk about this incident, the patient started to speak again. At this point, however, Anna O. talked only in English, although still understanding what people told her in German. In the late afternoons she experienced what she called (in English) her "clouds," that is, a kind of drowsiness. In this state, she could be easily hypnotized. Breuer usually visited Anna O. during these spells; she told him her daydreams, which were mostly stories of an anxious girl around sick persons. During the month of March there came a gradual improvement, and she left her bed for the first time on April 1, 1881.

3. The *period of "continuous somnambulism alternating with more normal conditions"* went, according to Breuer, from April to December 1881. The death of Anna O.'s father, on April 5, 1881, was a severe psychological shock to the patient. After two days of deep stupor, a new set of severe symptoms appeared. Anna O. manifested a "negative instinct" against her close relatives and recognized no one, except Breuer, who for some time even had to feed her. She spoke nothing but English, and now apparently she was unable to understand what was also said or written in German.

About ten days after her father's death, another medical consultant was called. Anna O. manifested "negative hallucinations" toward him, or, in other words, she behaved as if she did not perceive his presence. The consultant tried to force her attention by blowing some smoke at her face. This attempt was followed by a terrific attack of anger and anxiety. On the same evening, Breuer had to leave for a journey. When he came back, he found that Anna O.'s condition had worsened greatly. During his absence she had refused to eat, and she had fits of intense anxiety and ghastly hallucinations. Breuer began to hypnotize her again in the evenings, and she told him about her recent hallucinations, whereupon she was again relieved. The personality contrast was now between the disturbed mind of the daytime and the clear mind of the night hours.

Because Anna O. had begun to manifest suicidal impulses, it was felt that she should no longer be kept at home, and—much against her will—she was transferred to a country house near Vienna on June 7, 1881. After three days of great agitation, she quieted down. Breuer visited Anna O. there every three or four days. Her symptoms now appeared in a regular cycle and were relieved by Breuer's hypnotic sessions. The patient remained quiet after Breuer's visits, but during the intervals had to be given fairly high doses of chloral.

It was found that no one but Breuer could practice what she now called her "talking cure" or "chimney-sweeping." While Breuer was on a vacation trip, one of his colleagues attempted to give her the same treatment but failed. Nevertheless, her condition gradually improved. She played with a Newfoundland dog and visited a few poor people in the neighborhood. In the fall of 1881, she went back to Vienna, where her mother had moved to another house. However, her condition became worse in December 1881, so that she had to be taken back to the country house.

4. The *fourth period* of Anna O.'s illness extended from December 1881 to June 1882. A very remarkable, twofold change occurred in the illness as recorded by Breuer and Freud. First, there developed over this period a difference with regard to the multiple personality. There still were the "normal" and "sick" personalities, but the main feature was that the sick personality lived 365 days earlier than the healthy one. Thanks to the diary her mother kept about her illness, Breuer was able to check that the events Anna O. hallucinated had occurred, to the day, exactly one year earlier. The patient sometimes shifted spontaneously and rather abruptly from one personality to the other, and Breuer could even provoke the shifting by showing her an orange.

The second modification concerned the nature and content of the talking cure. One time, while under hypnosis, the patient told Breuer how her difficulties in swallowing water had started after she had seen a dog drinking from a glass. Having told Breuer this, the symptom disappeared. This initiated a new kind of treatment. Anna O. would relate to Breuer, in reverse chronological order, each appearance of a given symptom with exact dates until she reached the original manifestation and initial event, and then the symptom would disappear. Obviously, this was an extremely time-consuming procedure. Breuer gives as an example of the symptoms the patient's transient states of deafness. He found seven subforms of this symptom, and each of them constituted one of the "series" that Breuer had to treat separately. The first subform, "not hearing when someone came in," had occurred 108 times, and the patient had to tell the detail of each one of these 108 occurrences in reverse chronological order, until Breuer reached the first manifestation, an instance when Anna O. had once not heard her father entering the room. But the six other subforms of the "not hearing" symptom as well as each other symptom had to be treated for themselves with a similar procedure. Breuer eradicated each symptom in this tedious way. Finally, the last symptom was traced back to a specific incident. While nursing her sick father, Anna O. had once experienced a hallucination of a black snake, had been agitated by this, and had muttered a prayer in English, the only one that came to her mind. As soon as Anna recovered this memory, the paralysis in her arm vanished, and she was then also able to speak German. The patient had then decided and announced in advance that she would be cured by June 1882, on the anniversary of her transfer to the country house, and in time for her summer vacation. At that time, Breuer says, "she left Vienna for a trip, but needed much time until she recovered her psychic equilibrium. Since then she enjoys a fully good health."

The current accounts of Anna O.'s illness tend not to emphasize the unusual features of that story, such as the peculiar form of multiple personality during the fourth period (that is, one person living in the present and the other 365 days earlier). Above all, it is absolutely not so that "it sufficed to recall the circumstances under which the symptom had appeared," the point explicitly stated by Breuer. Rather, Anna had to recall each instance when the symptom had occurred, whatever the number, in the exact reverse chronological order. Anna O.'s illness was not a "classical case of hysteria" but a unique case of which, to the author's knowledge, no other instance is known, either before or after her.

From Breuer to Jones

The story of Anna O. remained for a long time an anonymous case history that psychoanalysts and nonpsychoanalysts faithfully copied from book to book and with a certain tendency toward oversimplification. The case was proclaimed as the prototype of a cathartic cure. Pierre Janet's claims of priority to the catharsis concept, based on his cases of Lucie (1886), Marie

(1889), and a few other ones after 1890, were rejected on the grounds that he had been anticipated by Breuer. At times, a few doubts were also expressed passingly about the accuracy of the diagnosis. In 1952, for instance, Charles Goshen contended that Anna O., as well as the other patients described in the *Studies on Hysteria*, had in fact been schizophrenics.[4]

For many years, very few new details emerged about Anna O.'s extraordinary case. In 1924, Freud suggested that in treating his patient Breuer had been the unwitting victim of "transference love."[5] Then, in a seminar given in Zurich in 1925, Carl Gustav Jung stated that Freud had once confided in him that the patient had actually not been cured.[6] Jung stated that this famous first psychoanalytic case "so much spoken about as an example of brilliant therapeutic success was in reality nothing of the kind. . . . There was no cure at all in the sense of which it was originally presented." And yet, Jung added, "the case was so interesting that there was no need to claim for it something that did not happen."

Next, in 1953, Ernest Jones revealed—much to the family's displeasure—the true identity of the patient: Bertha Pappenheim. In his famous biography of Freud, Jones published a new version of the story.[7] Unfortunately, it is not clear to what extent Jones documented himself in Freud's unpublished correspondence or simply reported from memory details he had heard many years earlier. According to Jones's version, Freud had told him that Breuer had developed a strong "counter-transference" toward his patient so that Mrs. Breuer became jealous, and Breuer decided to bring the treatment quickly to an end. However, on that same evening, Breuer had been called to the patient's bedside to find her in the throes of a hysterical childbirth, the logical termination of a phantom pregnancy that had slowly developed without Breuer's awareness. Horrified, Breuer hypnotized Anna O. and then "fled the house in a cold sweat." On the next day, according to Jones, Breuer left with his wife for Venice to spend a second honeymoon, which resulted in the conception of a daughter, Dora. As for the patient, she was removed to an institution in Gross Enzersdorf and remained very sick for several years. In the sanatorium she inflamed the heart of the psychiatrist in charge, so that her mother had to come from Frankfurt, where the Pappenheims were now living, and take her back home there. Later, Anna O. recovered, developed a remarkable social activity, and with great energy devoted her life to the cause of the emancipation

---

[4] Charles E. Goshen, "The Original Case Material of Psychoanalysis," *American Journal of Psychiatry*, 108 (1951–1952), 830–34.

[5] Sigmund Freud, *Medizin in Selbstdarstellung*, 4 (1924), 15.

[6] *Notes on the Seminar in Analytical Psychology Conducted by C. G. Jung*, Zurich, March 23-July 6, 1925, as arranged by members of the class (Zurich, 1926) (unpublished typescript).

[7] Ernest Jones, *The Life and Work of Sigmund Freud*, 3 vols. (New York, Basic Books, 1953–1957), 1:223–26.

of women and the care of orphan children. Jones's version of the story, however, was in many important points incompatible with that of Breuer. Now, owing to the revelation of the patient's true identity, new avenues are open toward objective biographical research of this subject.

Who Was Bertha Pappenheim?

Bertha Pappenheim, it turns out, was by no means an unknown figure in Jewish circles. A short biographical note on her was already to be found in the *Grosse jüdische National-Biographie*, edited by S. Winiger. Pappenheim's death in 1936 was commemorated with a special forty-page issue of a journal she had founded, the *Blätter des jüdischen Frauenbundes*, with introductory notes by Martin Buber and Max Warbi, and with substantial accounts of her life, writings, and social activities.[8] Material toward her biography had been gathered but was unfortunately destroyed during World War II. A number of biographical details have been collected by Mrs. Ellen Jensen in Denmark,[9] and a short monograph was published by Mrs. Dora Edinger in 1963.[10]

Bertha Pappenheim belonged to an old, distinguished Jewish family. Her grandfather, Wolf Pappenheim, a prominent personality of the Pressburg ghetto, had inherited a great fortune. Her father, Siegmund Pappenheim, was a well-to-do merchant in Vienna. The family belonged to the strictly orthodox Jewish community. Little is known of her childhood and youth. Bertha spoke English perfectly and read French and Italian. According to her own account, she led the usual life of a young lady of high Viennese society, with a great deal of needlework and with outdoor activities including horseback riding. It was reported that, after her father's death in 1881, she and her mother left Vienna and settled in Frankfurt am Main. In the later 1880s Bertha devoted herself fully to philanthropic activities. For about twelve years she was the director of an orphanage in Frankfurt. She traveled in the Balkan countries, the Near East, and Russia to inquire into prostitution and white slavery. In 1904 she founded the Jüdischer Frauenbund (League of Jewish Women), and in 1907 she established a teaching institution affiliated with that organization. Among her writings are travel reports, studies on the condition of Jewish women and on criminality

---

[8] *Blätter des jüdischen Frauenbundes für Frauenarbeit und Frauenbewegung*, 12 (July–August 1936).

[9] Ellen Jensen, "Anna O.: Ihr späteres Schicksal," *Acta psychiatrica et neurologica scandinavica*, 36 (1961), 119–31. See also Jensen, "Anna O.—A Study of Her Later Life," *Psychoanalytic Quarterly*, 39 (1970), 269–93.

[10] Dora Edinger, ed., *Bertha Pappenheim: Leben und Schriften* (Frankfurt am Main, Ner-Tamid-Verlag, 1963).

among Jews, and a number of short stories and theatricals (which reveal more concern with social problems than true literary talent). In her late years she reedited ancient Jewish works into modernized form, including a history of a prominent ancestor. Toward the end of her life, she was depicted as a deeply religious, strict, and authoritarian person, utterly selfless and devoted to her work, who had retained from her Viennese education a lively sense of humor, a taste for good food, and the love of beauty, and who possessed an impressive collection of embroideries, china, and glassware. When Hitler seized power and began to persecute the Jews, Pappenheim discouraged their emigration to Palestine or other countries. She died in March 1936, perhaps too early to realize that she had been mistaken in this regard. After World War II she was remembered as an almost legendary figure in the field of social work, to the extent that the government of West Germany honored her memory by issuing a postage stamp with her picture.

In the biographical notices of 1936 about Pappenheim, there was not a single mention of a severe and protracted nervous illness in her youth. She was said to have left Vienna for Frankfurt with her mother after her father's death in 1881. Clearly, there exists an enormous discrepancy between the descriptions of Bertha Pappenheim, the philanthropist and pioneer of social work, and of Breuer's hysterical patient, Anna O. One means of filling this gap would be to place the person into the context of Viennese life of the early 1880s. Obviously, Bertha Pappenheim had nothing in common with the "sweet girl" (*das süsse Mädel*) of Arthur Schnitzler's plays and novels. Many Jews of higher social strata kept the strict puritanical mores that had been those of their parents or grandparents in the ghetto. However, they had access to the privileges and pleasures of the Austrian wealthy bourgeoisie. Bertha had received a fine education, she enjoyed outdoor activities, and she attended the theater; but none of this could lead her to an independent or professional life, because the universities were still closed to women at this time. We thus find in her situation a contrast between the ambitions aroused in her and obstacles set to the realization of these ambitions. The same contrast is found in the story of several prominent hysterical women of that time.[11]

Furthermore, Juan Dalma[12] has shown the connection between Anna O.'s cure and the widespread interest in catharsis that followed the publication in 1880 of a book on the Aristotelian concept of catharsis by Jacob

[11] See, for example, the stories of Catherine Muller and Helene Preiswerk in *The Discovery of the Unconscious* (New York, Basic Books, 1970), 315–17, 689–91.

[12] Juan Dalma, "La catarsis en Aristóteles, Bernays y Freud," *Revista de psiquiatría y psicología médica*, 6 (1963), 253–69; idem, "Reminiscencias culturales clásicas en algunas corrientes de psicología moderna," *Revista de la Facultad de Medicina de Tucumán*, 5 (1964), 301–32.

Bernays, the uncle of Freud's future wife.[13] For a time, Dalma establishes, catharsis was one of the most discussed subjects among Viennese scholars and intellectuals and one of the topics of conversation in sophisticated Viennese salons. A contemporary historian of literature even complained once that, following the treatise of Bernays, there had been such a craze for the topic of catharsis that few people remained interested in the history of drama.[14] In other words, the time was ripe for catharsis to develop as a psychotherapeutic procedure.

The Author's Own Research: Biographical Background

During the preparation of my book *The Discovery of the Unconscious*, I conducted in Vienna a special inquiry into the case of Bertha Pappenheim. The first task was simply to identify exactly the characters of the story. In the *Heimat-Rolle* of the Vienna Community Archives, I found the following information: Bertha's father, Siegmund Pappenheim, merchant, was born in Pressburg on June 19, 1824; he died in Vienna on April 5, 1881. This is exactly the date given by Breuer as that of the death of Anna O.'s father and thus a confirmation of the identity between Anna O. and Bertha Pappenheim. Pappenheim's mother, Recha Goldschmidt, was born in Frankfurt am Main on June 13, 1830. Siegmund and Recha had three children, all of them born in Vienna: Henriette, born on September 2, 1849, Bertha, on February 27, 1859, and Wilhelm, on August 15, 1860. Henriette, who was ten years older than Bertha, died in early youth. The family lived for many years in the Jewish quarter of Leopoldstadt, but moved to Liechtensteinerstrasse in 1880.[15]

A few details about Pappenheim can be found in the *Memoirs* of one Sigmund Mayer.[16] Mayer had been acquainted in the ghetto with old Wolf Pappenheim, a man of a rather humble condition who, following an unexpected inheritance, had been metamorphosed into a wealthy patrician. All the Pappenheims were distinguished people, Mayer says. Mayer was well acquainted with Wilhelm (Bertha's brother), whom he depicts as an accomplished gentleman, strongly identified with the Jewish tradition but open

---

[13] Jacob Bernays, *Zwei Abhandlungen über die Aristotelische Theorie des Drama* (Berlin, Wilhelm Hertz, 1880).

[14] Wilhelm Wetz, *Shakespeare vom Standpunkt der vergleichenden Literaturgeschichte* (Hamburg, Haendeke & Lehmkübe, 1897), 1:30.

[15] Incidentally, this street was quite close to the Berggasse, where Freud was to live from 1891 to 1938.

[16] Sigmund Mayer, *Ein jüdischer Kaufmann, 1831 bis 1911. Lebenserinnerungen* (Leipzig, Duncker & Humblot, 1911): 49–50.

to all modern ideas, and who owned perhaps the most complete library on socialism to be found in Europe.

Further, Bertha Pappenheim was related to prominent Jewish families from her mother's side, too. This is shown in an extremely rare book that Pappenheim and her brother Wilhelm published privately in 1900. It is a German translation of the memoirs of an illustrious ancestor, Glückel von Hameln (1645–1724).[17] The translation is supplemented with a series of genealogical tables. One learns here of the connections of the Gold-schmidts with numerous well-known Jewish names, including the families Gomperz, von Portheim, Homburger, Friedländer, and Oppenheim.

Coming now to Jones's version of Bertha's illness, we find difficulty reconciling it on numerous points with the ascertainable facts. First of all, Breuer's last child, Dora, was born on March 11, 1882, as evidenced by the *Heimat-Rolle* in Vienna. Thus she could not possibly have been conceived after the supposed terminal therapeutic episode of June 1882. The approx-imate date of Dora's conception (June 1881) would rather coincide with the date of Bertha's transfer to the country house, but there is no evidence that Breuer interrupted the treatment at this time. (This was instead the beginning of the period when he went to visit her every few days and when her symptoms developed in the form of a regular cycle.) Second, there never existed a sanatorium in Gross Enzersdorf. Mr. Schramm, who wrote a history of this locality, told the author that Jones must have confused Gross Enzersdorf with Inzersdorf, also a suburb of Vienna, where there was a fashionable sanatorium. Upon inquiry, the author learned that the In-zersdorf sanatorium was now closed and that its medical archives had been transferred to the main Viennese Psychiatric Hospital. However, no case history of Bertha Pappenheim could be located there.[18]

Now, in Dora Edinger's biography of Bertha Pappenheim there was a photograph of Bertha with the date "1882" showing a healthy-looking, sporting woman in riding habit, in sharp contrast to Breuer's portrait of a homebound young lady who had no outlets for her physical and mental energies. Thanks to the help of Edinger, I received the authorization to examine the original of this photograph. As was usual at that time, the picture was stuck on a piece of cardboard, and the date "1882" had been embossed on the picture by the photographer. The name and address of the photographer could no longer be deciphered. However, when the picture was examined under special lights in the laboratory of the Montreal City

[17] *Die Memoiren des Glückel von Hameln . . . Autorisierte Uebertragung nach der Aus-gabe des Prof. Dr. David Kaufman von Bertha Pappenheim* (Vienna, Verlag von Dr. Stefan Meyer und Dr. Wilhelm Pappenheim, 1910).

[18] For assistance in my inquiries on this matter, I am indebted to Mr. Schramm, mayor of Gross Enzersdorf, Mr. Karl Neumayer, mayor of Inzersdorf, and Dr. W. Podhajsky, director of the Viennese Psychiatric Hospital.

THE STORY OF "ANNA O."

Police, the name of the town "Constanz" appeared along with a part of the address.[19] This discovery led to the question: What was Bertha doing in riding habit in Konstanz, Germany, at the time when she was supposed to be severely sick in a sanatorium near Vienna? Mrs. Edinger suggested to me that the patient could have been treated in one of the sanatoria that existed in that part of Europe. In fact, there was one famous such sanatorium, in the little Swiss town of Kreuzlingen, quite close to Konstanz: the Bellevue Sanatorium. I asked the present director of the Bellevue Sanatorium, Dr. Wolfgang Binswanger, if by chance the medical archives contained a case history of Bertha Pappenheim. I learned from him that Bertha Pappenheim had actually sojourned there as a patient from July 12 to October 29, 1882. The patient's file contained two documents: a copy of a case history written by Breuer himself in 1882 and a follow-up medical report written by one of the doctors of the Bellevue Sanatorium.

Breuer's Unknown Report of 1882

The name of Breuer does not appear in the document dated 1882, but this document quite obviously originates from him. It is the story of the same patient told by the same physician; whole sentences are almost identical to those of the *Studies on Hysteria*. It consists of a manuscript of 21½ pages of large size, manifestly a copy written by a layperson because a number of technical words are misunderstood, left blank, or corrected by another hand. The report of 1882 contains numerous details that were left out in the later published version, but it ends rather abruptly at the end of the "third period" of Bertha's illness. The time has not yet come for a publication of this complete document, but we will provide here a cursory view of the early case history, stressing the points where it furnishes new information or differs from the printed 1895 report.*

First, Breuer's 1882 report offers a more complete picture of the family constellation. Bertha, we learn, had difficulties with her "very serious" mother. Her brother (never mentioned in the *Studies on Hysteria*) plays a role; she sometimes had quarrels with him. There are several references to her "passionate love for her father who pampered her."[20] Breuer confirms that the sexual element in Bertha was "astonishingly undeveloped" and

---

*[*Editor's note*: Breuer's report, along with other documents pertaining to Pappenheim's residence at the Bellevue Sanatorium, has now been translated and printed in full in Albrecht Hirschmüller, *The Life and Work of Josef Breuer: Physiology and Psychoanalysis* (New York and London, New York University Press, 1989), 276–307.]

[19] Thanks are due to Dr. Jörg Schuh-Kuhlmann, who performed this investigation, and to the Montreal City Police Laboratory for its valuable contribution to this point of psychiatric history.

[20] ". . . in leidenschaftlicher Liebe zu dem sie verhätschelnden Vater."

says that he had never found it represented in the immense amount of her hallucinations. Bertha had never been in love, "insofar as her relationship to her father did not replace it, or rather was replaced by it."[21] Two other features in Bertha's character are stressed: her stubborn, childish opposition to medical prescriptions; and her opposition to religion—"She is thoroughly unreligious. . . . Religion played a role in her life only as an object of silent struggles and silent opposition"[22]—although, for her father's sake, she outwardly followed all the religious rites of her strictly orthodox Jewish family.

As early as the spring of 1880, we read further, Bertha had begun to suffer from a facial neuralgia and muscular jerks. What Breuer called the "first period of the illness" ran from July 17 to December 10, 1880. Breuer states that he did not see the patient during that time. All of what he related about her symptoms during that period he learned later from the hypnotized patient, and the patient herself, in her conscious state, knew only what Breuer told her about it. To these hypnotic revelations belongs the story of the initial symptom. During the night of July 17–18, while her father was sick and the family waited for the arrival of a surgeon from Vienna, it happened that Bertha experienced a vivid hallucination of a black snake crawling out of the wall to kill her father. She wanted to drive the snake away, but could not move her right arm; she saw her fingers as transformed into many little snakes with tiny skulls, instead of the nails. She was filled with anguish, tried to pray, but could not speak until she found an English sentence. At this point the spell was interrupted by the whistling of an engine. It was the train that brought the surgeon from Vienna. A great number of other symptoms are also described; many of them occurred during a peculiar state of absentmindedness that Bertha termed (in English) "time-missing." Her visual perceptions were strangely distorted. Looking upon her father, she saw him as a skeleton and his head as a skull. After having once been shaken by her brother, she became momentarily deaf, but from that time onward a transient deafness appeared whenever she was shaken. A great number of other symptoms developed, too, but, Breuer says, no one around her even noticed them.

At the beginning of September 1880, the family went back to Vienna (it is not stated where they were before). Bertha devoted herself to nursing her sick father. However, her symptoms became aggravated, and a "nervous cough" appeared. Breuer saw her for the first time at the end of November on account of a "hysterical cough." He recognized at once that she was mentally sick—something that seemed to have escaped her family's notice.

[21] ". . . soweit nicht ihr Verhältnis zum Vater dieses ersetzt hat oder vielmehr damit ersetzt war."

[22] "Sie is durchaus nicht religiös. . . . Eine Rolle in ihrem Leben spielte Religion nur als Gegenstand stiller Kämpfe und stiller Opposition."

The second period (the "manifest illness" of Breuer's case history of 1895) thus began shortly after Breuer's first visit. Bertha remained in bed from December 11, 1880, to April 1, 1881. In his 1882 report, Breuer gives a lengthy description of that period of the disease, which does not add very much to what he recorded in 1895. In 1882, however, he laid more emphasis upon Bertha's "truly passionate love" for her father.[23] The period when she remained mute for two weeks (in 1882 Breuer called it an "aphasia") occurred, Breuer says, after she had once been hurt (*gekränkt*) by her father. After being prevented from seeing her father, she felt a longing (*Sehnsucht*) for him. During that period of Bertha's illness, Breuer was concerned with an organic diagnosis and considered in particular the possibility of a tubercle in the left *fossa Sylvii* with a slowly expanding chronic meningitis. However, the "nervous" character of her cough, and the tranquilizing effect of Breuer's listening to the stories she told him in the evenings, led him to think of a "purely functional ailment."[24]

Breuer's report of 1882 also gives a great number of hitherto unknown data about the mysterious third period of Bertha's illness. First, we learn why her father's death was such a shock to her. During the previous two months Bertha had not been allowed to see him and had continuously been told lies about the state of his health. In spite of her lasting anxiety, there had been some improvement in Bertha's illness, and she had got up for the first time on April 1. On April 5, at the moment when her father was dying, she called her mother and asked for the truth, but was appeased, and the lie went on for some time longer. When Bertha learned that her father had died, she was highly indignant: she had been "robbed" of his last look and last words. From that time onward, a marked transformation appeared in her condition: acute anxiety developed along with a kind of dull insensitivity and distortions in her visual perceptions. Human beings appeared to her as waxen figures. In order to recognize someone, she had to perform what she called (in English) a "recognizing work." The only person she immediately recognized was Breuer. She manifested an extremely negative attitude toward her mother and to a lesser degree toward her brother.

We also learn that the consulting psychiatrist who came to examine her about ten days after her father's death was none other than Richard von Krafft-Ebing. The story of his intervention in the case is related with the same details as in the published version, save that we learn the fact that the smoke he blew into her face was from a burning piece of paper! Unfortunately, nothing is said of Krafft-Ebing's diagnosis and recommendations.

In view of the difficulty of keeping Bertha at home, and because of several suicide attempts, it was decided to transfer her to Inzersdorf. However, it

[23] ". . . ihre wahre leidenschaftliche Liebe."
[24] ". . . dass es sich doch rein funktionelles Leiden handle."

was not in the fashionable sanatorium there of Drs. Fries and Breslauer, but in a kind of cottage close to the sanatorium (Breuer called it in 1882 a *Villa*, in 1895 a *Landhaus*), so that she could be kept under the daily care of the psychiatrists of that institution while still being visited by Breuer every few days. The transfer was performed "without deceit, but by force" on June 7, 1881.[25]

In that month of June, Bertha's illness reached its acme, and from that time on there were periods of slow improvement and relapses. Breuer, as we know, came frequently, and he was able to soothe her by listening to her stories. But his task was not always easy. He had to use much persuasion and to introduce the story with the English sentence: "And there was a boy . . . ," and she had to feel his hands to make sure of his identity. Dr. Breslauer did not enjoy the same success and had to give her chloral.

Breuer tells further of a five-week vacation from whence he came back in the middle of August (whether or not he went to Venice is not mentioned in the report). On his return, he found Bertha again in a pitiful condition, "emotionally very bad, disobedient, moody, nasty, lazy."[26] It also looked as if her fantasy of a pregnancy was exhausted. She gave distorted accounts of what had irritated her during the last days. There was also an unexpected development at this point. Breuer's report of 1882 brings a new, more complete version of the discovery of the "talking cure." He found that certain of the patient's whims or fancies (he called them by the French word *caprices*) could disappear when traced back to the "psychic incitements" (*psychische Reize*) that had been at their origin. (Let us recall that even earlier Bertha's "aphasia" had disappeared when Breuer could get the patient to recall that the symptom had started after having been offended by her father.) But the patient had taken to quite a few other "fancies." Thus, she went to bed with her stockings on, and then sometimes woke up at two or three in the morning and complained that she had been left to go to bed in her stockings. One evening she told Breuer that while her father was sick, and she had been forbidden to see him, she used to get up in the night, put her stockings on, and go listen at his door, until one night she was caught by her brother. After she told Breuer of this incident, the stockings "fancy" disappeared.

The following occurrence (described in the *Studies on Hysteria* as being the first one) concerns the story of a little dog. For six weeks Bertha refused

---

[25] Details about the Inzersdorf sanatorium may be found in Heinrich Schlöss, ed., *Die Irrenpflege in Oesterreich in Wort und Bild* (Halle, Carl Marhold, 1912), 241–53. The institution had been founded in 1872 by Dr. Hermann Breslauer (a former assistant of Professor Leidensdorf) and Dr. Fries. The main building was the former castle of a noble family; there was a large English garden. All kinds of neurotic and psychotic patients were treated there.

[26] ". . . moralisch recht schlecht, unfügsam, launisch, boshaft, träge."

to drink water and quenched her thirst only by eating fruits and melons. She told Breuer that this symptom had started soon after she happened to observe a lady companion's dog drinking water from a glass. She had been disgusted at this sight, but had said nothing. Five minutes after telling Breuer the story she was able to drink water and the "drinking inhibition" (*Trinkhemmung*) disappeared forever. Breuer found that certain other *caprices* could be traced back simply to some "fantastic thought" that the patient had imagined. Such, for instance, was her refusal to eat bread. The next step in the progress of the treatment was Breuer's discovery that not only *caprices* but seemingly neurological symptoms could be made to disappear in the same way.

The end of the case history is disappointing. Breuer states in a few lines that Bertha came back to her mother in Vienna at the beginning of November 1881, so that he was able to give her the talking cure every evening. However "for unaccountable reasons" her condition became worse yet again in December. At the end of December, during the period of the Jewish holidays, she was agitated. During that whole week she told Breuer every evening the fantastic stories that she had imagined at the same period of the preceding year. They were, day by day, the same stories.

The report unfortunately contains nothing about the "fourth period" of the illness, although it is stated at the beginning of the report that it extended from December 1881 to the middle of June 1882. It ends with the enigmatic sentence: "After termination of the series, great alleviation."[27] It should also be noted that there is nowhere any mention of a hysterical pregnancy and that the word *catharsis* appears nowhere in the report of 1882.

The Follow-Up Report of the Bellevue Sanatorium

The copy of Breuer's long handwritten report is immediately followed on its last page by an additional 2½-page follow-up report, obviously written at the end of Bertha's sojourn by one of the staff physicians of the Bellevue Sanatorium. This report bears the title "Evolution of the Illness during the Sojourn in Bellevue from July 12, 1882, to October 29, 1882." This follow-up is in many regards very instructive, in other regards uninformative. Someone who knew of Anna O. only what Breuer related in the *Studies on Hysteria* would hardly guess that it is an account of the same patient just after she had undergone Breuer's "cathartic cure." The follow-up report consists of a long enumeration of medications given to the patient on account of a severe facial neuralgia. We learn that the facial neuralgia

---

[27] "Nach Beendigung der Serie grosse Erleichterung."

.

had been exacerbated during the past six months (that is, during the "fourth period" of her illness) and that during that period large amounts of chloral and morphine had been prescribed. Upon her admission, the amount of morphine was reduced to seven to eight centigrams in two daily injections. But the pains were at times so intolerable that one had to administer ten centigrams. When Pappenheim left the sanatorium, she was still receiving injections amounting to a total of seven to ten centigrams *pro die*. The follow-up report also contains mention of "hysterical features" (*hysterische Merkmale*) in the patient, her "unpleasant irritation against her family,"[28] her "disparaging judgments against the ineffectiveness of science in regard to her sufferings,"[29] and the "lack of insight into the severity of her nervous condition" on the part of her doctors.[30] She often remained for hours under the picture of her father, and she told of visiting his tomb in Pressburg. In the evening, she regularly lost the use of the German language as soon as she put her head down on the pillow. She would even terminate in English a sentence that she had begun in German. The follow-up report ends with this sentence: "Here, she did understand and speak French, although it was difficult for her on certain evenings." There is no mention of where the patient went after leaving the Bellevue hospital.

Commentary

The time has not yet come for a complete and truly objective appraisal of Anna O.'s story. However, these two newly discovered documents may shed some important light upon a few points. We know now that when Breuer published Anna O.'s story in 1895 he had under his eyes a previous report he probably had written in 1882 (entire lines of the two sources are sometimes almost identical). This report, however, relates the story of the patient until December 1881 and leaves out the "fourth period" of her illness. On the other hand, it seems that during the period when Breuer treated his patient he did not write daily notes about her. There are good reasons to think that the 1882 report was written from memory, because there appear no precise dates, aside from those of the father's death and of Bertha's transfer to the country house. (Breuer does not even mention the date of his first visit to Bertha, nor that of the consultation with Krafft-Ebing.) This might also be the reason why Breuer tells in 1895 of his "incomplete notes" when referring to the "fourth period" of the illness.

Breuer's report of 1882 brings a more complete picture of the patient's family and environment. Breuer draws a connection between the fact that

---

[28] ". . . geradezu unliebenswürdige Gereiztheit gegen Angehörige."

[29] "So beurtheilte sie in abfälliger Weise die Unzulänglichkeit der Wissenschaft gegenüber ihren Leiden."

[30] "Die fehlende Einsicht in die Schwere ihres Stat. nervosus."

Bertha had never been in love and her "truly passionate love for her father." We learn of her difficulties with her "very serious mother" and her quarrels with her brother. There is also a passing mention of an aunt.

Bertha's stubborn character is also emphasized in the 1882 report, including her "childish opposition" to the doctors. Unexpected is the fact that Bertha was "thoroughly unreligious" in the midst of her strictly orthodox Jewish family. One would wish to know when she returned to the faith of her ancestors and how she became the ardent religious personality of the later years. We also learn of Bertha's visits to the theater and of her interest in Shakespeare's plays.

Medically, the problematic features of the "first period" of Bertha's illness appear more clearly in the 1882 report than in the 1895 case history. Breuer did not see Anna O. during the first period, and he emphasizes that her illness went completely unnoticed by her family. The patient did not remember her symptoms of that period and knew about them only what Breuer had learned from her under hypnosis and told her afterwards. One may wonder how Breuer could take at face value all the revelations of the hypnotized patient when he expressly notes that—on the conscious level— she "gave distorted accounts of what had irritated her during the last days."

In the report of 1882, the course of Bertha's illness appears as having been somewhat stormier than in the narrative of 1895. We learn why the father's death came as such a severe psychic trauma for the patient. We see more plainly that there was a succession of ups and downs in her case, with at least four periods of worsening: (1) after the father's death; (2) after the transfer to the country house; (3) during Breuer's vacation of July–August, 1881; and (4) "for unaccountable reasons," in November 1881. We see more clearly the origin and development of what was called later the "cathartic" treatment. At first, and for a long time, the "chimney-sweeping" merely meant that Bertha unburdened her mind of the stories she had imagined during the past days. But there came a time (in August 1881) when her fantasizing was exhausted, and she then started to talk about the events that had been the starting point of her (quite conscious and voluntary) *caprices*. Later, she extended this procedure to the more serious, seemingly neurological, symptoms. It is also noteworthy that the neurological symptoms, particularly the facial neuralgia, stand out more prominently in the report of 1882 than in the later published case history.* Breuer's concern with the brain-anatomical seat of the illness is noted in two places in the earlier report.

*[*Editor's note*: Subsequent medical historians have also placed greater emphasis than Breuer and Freud on the neurological symptomatology of Pappenheim's case. See above all Alison Orr-Andrawes, "The Case of Anna O.: A Neuropsychiatric Perspective," *Journal of the American Psychoanalytic Association*, 35 (1987), 387–419, which builds directly on Ellenberger's findings in this article.]

Unfortunately, the "fourth period" of Bertha's illness still retains its mystery entirely. The case history of 1895 tells of a strange, indeed unique, condition, and of two personalities, one living exactly 365 days before the other, and of the extraordinary therapeutic method of curing the illness by having the patient tell in reverse chronological order all occurrences of a given symptom, whatever the number, until one came to the first manifestation or the circumstances of its appearance. But Breuer's report of 1882 is almost completely silent about these strange facts. Similarly, the Bellevue follow-up report does not mention anything of this and merely refers to the fact that the patient had gotten used to taking high doses of chloral and morphine. In this follow-up, Pappenheim is depicted mainly as a neurological case of a rather unpleasant nature also manifesting some hysterical features.

Thus, the newly discovered documents confirm what Freud, according to Jung, had told him: the patient Anna O. had not been cured. Indeed, the famed "prototype of a cathartic cure" was neither a cure nor a catharsis.* Rather, by the end of the treatment, Anna O. had become a severe morphinist and had retained a part of her most conspicuous symptoms. Further, Jones's version of the false pregnancy and hysterical birth throes cannot be confirmed from these documents and does not fit into the chronology of the case.

In *The Discovery of the Unconscious*, I proposed the hypothesis that Anna O.'s illness was similar to one of those great "magnetic diseases" of the early nineteenth century, such as that of Justinus Kerner's "Seeress of Prevorst." This would mean that the illness was a creation of the mythopoetic unconscious of the patient with the unaware encouragement and collaboration of the therapist. However, there must have been in Bertha's case more than just a "romance of the subliminal self" (to use Frederick Myers' terminology). Anna O.'s illness was the desperate struggle of an unsatisfied young woman who found no outlets for her physical and mental energies, nor for her idealistic strivings. Much time and effort were required before she succeeded in sublimating her personality into that respectable figure of a pioneer of social work and fighter for the rights of women and the welfare of her people—Bertha Pappenheim.

* [*Editor's note*: It needs to be observed at this point that Ernest Jones, writing in 1953, had acknowledged that the patient fared worse than stated in Breuer's published case, with relapses and a later institutionalization. See Ernest Jones, *The Life and Work of Sigmund Freud*, 3 vols. (New York: Basic Books, 1953–1957), 1:225. In this instance, the reformation of a historical "legend" began within the psychoanalytic establishment.]

10

The Story of "Emmy von N.": A Critical Study with New Documents

[1977]

EVERYONE who has read the *Studies on Hysteria* (1895) by Josef Breuer and Sigmund Freud knows that this work begins with the detailed story, reported by Breuer, of the illness and treatment of a young hysterical woman, "Anna O.," whose real name was Bertha Pappenheim.[1] The *Studies on Hysteria* then continues, under Freud's signature, with the clinical observations of four other hysterical women. The first of these patients is pseudonymously named "Emmy von N." In the intellectual history of psychoanalysis, Emmy von N.'s story marks the beginning of a long evolution that would lead the young Freud from Breuer's cathartic method to his own therapeutic method, the free associative technique of psychoanalysis. Her case is of interest and importance for other reasons, too.

Up until now, almost nothing has been published about this enigmatic case. The credit belongs entirely to Ola Andersson for first investigating the case, including questioning several witnesses who had known the patient personally and reconstructing other parts of her life story following her treatment by Freud. But Andersson, out of respect for the patient's family, did not actually reveal Emmy von N.'s name, but only informed a small group of psychoanalysts of the results of his investigation in a report that has remained unpublished.[2] Since Andersson's work, however, the identity of Emmy von N. has been widely diffused.[3] The patient in real life was Fanny Moser, the widow of a great industrial businessman of Schaffhausen, Switzerland. In this article, I will continue from the investigations of Ola Andersson. I will begin with a summary and critical examination of the case-historical account of Emmy von N.'s neurosis, according to the

"L'histoire d'"Emmy von N.': Étude critique avec documents nouveaux," *L'évolution psychiatrique*, 42, no. 3 (July–September 1977), 519–40.

[1] Josef Breuer and Sigmund Freud, *Studien über Hysterie* (Vienna, Deuticke, 1895), 37–89.

[2] Ola Andersson, "A Supplement to Freud's Case History of 'Emmy von N.' in *Studies in Hysteria*, 1895" (Unpublished essay obligingly provided by the author).

[3] See notably Karl Schib, "Heinrich Mosers Briefwerk," *Schaffhauser Beiträge zur vaterländischen Geschichte*, 47 (1970), 80.

way that Freud recorded it in 1895. Then I will place this medical episode within the chronological course of events of the patient's life. Finally, I will attempt to sketch the distinctive familial, social, and cultural environment of the patient in order to make more comprehensible her particular neurosis.

Among the materials I will use, special attention will be paid to two unpublished documents. The first one is Fanny Moser's guest book. This is a beautiful album, made of fine-quality paper with a spun leather binding and metallic fasteners, decorated with fancy armorial bearings. It contains many signatures and inscriptions written by Fanny Moser's guests at one of her villas, in Au, close to Wädenswil, on the shores of Lake Zurich.[4] The first inscription in the guest book is dated 1888 and the last one September 10, 1924. The second source consists of the detailed autobiography of Mentona Moser, Fanny Moser's younger daughter. Unfortunately, this autobiography, a copy of which is housed at the Schaffhausen Archives, remains unfinished.[5]

Freud's Account of the Case in 1895

Freud's professional discretion compelled him to label his patient with a pseudonym and to make her place of residence Livonia, instead of Germanic Switzerland. He may also have changed the chronology of the case for the same reason. Freud's report begins on May 1, 1889. Emmy von N. had spent six weeks in Vienna, where she was undergoing a treatment with one of the best-known physicians in the city. At one point, this doctor referred her to Freud for further treatment. Emmy von N. was 40 years old at the time, although she looked younger. She had a strained appearance, and she spoke with difficulty, in a low voice, with pauses in her speech. Freud also noted the continuous mobility of her fingers and the frequent twitches of her face. Every few minutes, her face momentarily took on an expression of horror and disgust, and she would exclaim, "Keep still. Don't say anything. Don't touch me," as if she were defending herself against some fear or hallucination. Nonetheless, Emmy von N.'s speech was coherent. The patient reported that she was the thirteenth of fourteen children. Her mother, she said, had brought her up with severity. At 23, she had married a very rich industrial businessman, much older than herself, who had died shortly thereafter, which was now fourteen years ago. Since that

---

[4] *Gästebuch der Fanny Moser-von Sulzer Wart*, Schaffhausen Archives.

[5] *Lebensgeschichte von Mentona Moser* (typescript). The copyright to this document belongs to Mr. Roger Nicholas Balsiger of Zurich, who has kindly allowed me to cite extracts from it.

time, she had been almost continually ill. She was currently living on a beautiful and very exclusive property in Switzerland near a large town. She had two daughters, ages 16 and 14, both of whom also suffered from nervous troubles. Upon his first examination, Freud immediately required the patient to enter a sanatorium, during which time her two daughters were committed to the care of a governess.

According to his published account, on the next day, May 2, Freud prescribed for the patient baths and massages for the whole body twice a day. He gave the massages himself. Also twice a day he conducted with her long, unstructured conversations followed by a session of hypnosis. Freud was struck by the facility the patient showed in being hypnotized, even though she said that she had never been hypnotized before. After a week of treatment, there was some amelioration in Emmy von N.'s condition; however, on May 8, Freud again found the patient in a state of extreme fright. She said that the evening before she had read in the *Frankfurter Zeitung* the story of an apprentice worker whose mates had put a mouse in his mouth and who had actually died of fright from the incident. Freud discovered that the newspaper report had actually only talked about a bad treatment inflicted on some worker, but without reference to mice or death. On the same evening, the patient under hypnosis listed a series of emotional traumas suffered in her childhood. When she was 5, she stated, her brothers and sisters had thrown dead animals at her. When she was 7, she saw the body of one of her sisters in a coffin. At 8, one of her brothers dressed up as a ghost to frighten her. At 9, as one of her aunts was lying in a coffin, she thought that she saw the jaws of the dead move. While telling Freud about these scenes, the patient was reliving them with intense emotion.

On May 9, Freud found the patient terror-stricken. She had seen among the illustrations of a book some Indians dressed up as animals; also, she had recalled to memory visions from when she was 19 and one of her brothers had died. That day, Freud also learned from Emmy von N. that her strange facial twitches had started some five years previously, when she was taking care of her younger daughter, who was then ill. Under hypnosis, a second series of associated traumatic memories brought up the story of a cousin who had once been taken off to an insane asylum. Moreover, Emmy von N. often talked about asylums, and she revealed that her mother had spent some time in such an institution. A maid of hers had told her horrible things about what supposedly occurred in mental hospitals. At 15 years old, she had seen her mother struck down by an apoplectic stroke. At 19, on returning home one day, she had found her mother dead. During the same year, she had been desperately scared by a toad found by lifting up a stone. On May 10, she told Freud of yet another succession of traumatic events. Her stammering had started after two distressing incidents: one day, while driving along the road, the horses had bolted with the children in the carriage; on another occasion, while she was riding through the forest with children, a thunderstorm broke out, and a tree just in front of the carriage was struck by lightning. Among other traumatic experiences related to Freud by the patient that day was the irruption into her bedroom one night of a lunatic woman during one of her stays in a health resort.

The next day, May 11, under hypnosis, Freud asked Emmy von N. to recall her most traumatic memories. She then told Freud that her husband had died of a heart attack (he had already had one attack some time earlier on the Riviera) and that for six months their newly born child had been very ill. Under hypnosis, she also then began to complain vehemently about this child: her physical and mental development had been delayed so that she had been believed to be an imbecile; she cried almost all the time and never slept; she had once been paralyzed for a period. Emmy von N. then spoke again about the atrocities that occurred in asylums, with patients receiving ice-cold showers on the head or being placed in turning machines to subdue them.

On May 12, the patient talked about her private estate and the many celebrities that she received there. But she also lapsed again into reminiscences about snakes, wild animals, mice, and a big toad. Then she completed the narration started the day before concerning the misfortunes that followed her husband's death. She hated her younger daughter, she said bluntly. Further, she reported that she had been accused of poisoning her husband and had been snubbed socially on every side after his death. From this experience, she developed a hatred for other men.

On May 13, Freud questioned Emmy von N. about the origin of her fear of animals. To this, she simply answered that one day she had witnessed a huge lizard at the theater. She also said that she had fought very much to overcome her lack of love for her younger daughter. On May 14, other traumatic memories appeared. In Rügen, two men had insulted her. In Abbazia, she had been terribly frightened when confronted by a harmless lunatic. And one night, her estate had been broken into by trespassers. On May 15, she became fearful at the idea of using the elevator in the hotel in which her children were staying. She also mentioned again a toad, a sick person who had to be confined in a mental hospital, and a rebellion in Santo Domingo where one of her brothers was living. On May 16, she discussed a day when she had thought she was seeing mice everywhere in the trees. In Rügen, she was chased by a bull. Under hypnosis, she talked about more horrible animals. And on May 17, she dreamt that she was walking barefoot on leeches, which brought her to evoke still another series of incidents referring to animals: there had once been a bat in her wardrobe; she had walked on a path edged with toads; a pin cushion that she received as a present happened to be filled with small worms. She did not dare hold out her hand, fearing that it would turn into some monstrous animal.

The published case history of Emmy von N.'s illness stops on the eighteenth day, although Freud states that the patient received his care for a total of seven weeks. At the end of the treatment, she declared that she had never felt so well since her husband's death, and based upon this optimistic feeling she left Vienna to return home.

It is not Freud but Breuer who received some news from the patient seven months later. Her elder daughter had undergone a gynecological treatment and was suffering from nervous troubles. Emmy von N. became so agitated that she had to be admitted again to a sanatorium; but there she exhibited behaviors of violent opposition, and, with a friend's help, she had finally escaped. A short time afterwards, and exactly a year after her first meeting with Freud, she came back to Vienna to undergo further treatment with him.

According to Freud, this second period of therapy lasted eight weeks. Generally speaking, Emmy von N. was not as ill as she had been the first time. She mostly complained about frequent attacks of mental confusion, of insomnia, and of crying spells that could last for hours. One day, Freud found out that after her meals she would sometimes throw the food she didn't eat out the window, that she was drinking only thick fluids (milk, coffee, cocoa), and that she refused water and minerals. Under hypnosis, she said that in her childhood her mother had forced her to eat foods she disliked very much. Sometimes, she was even obliged to consume two hours later and from the same plate the meat she had refused after the meal. Her hatred for ordinary and mineral water dated back to her childhood to a stay in Munich, when the running water had been badly purified and had provoked gastric troubles for almost every member of the family. This second period of treatment by Freud seems to have produced excellent results.

Freud writes further in the *Studies on Hysteria* that in the spring of the following year, Emmy von N. asked him to come to her chateau, this time in order to examine her older daughter, whose behavior had grown intolerable. The girl was even becoming violent toward her mother. As for Emmy von N., Freud found her at this time in better health than before, even though she tended to fret about frivolous matters. At the time, she was also suffering from a railway phobia, which Freud suspected represented an unconscious refusal to make a new journey to Vienna.

In a note added to the book in 1924, Freud mentions that, some years after Emmy von N.'s treatment, he encountered a psychiatrist who told him that he also had hypnotized her successfully; however, at a still later date, the patient had suddenly turned against him and had relapsed into a pathological mental state. A quarter of a century later, the patient's older daughter requested that Freud report officially on her mother's mental state. She wanted her mother to be placed under tutelage, and she described Emmy von N. as a parent who had been odiously tyrannical, who had rejected her two daughters, and who refused to assist them in the difficulties they later had to face.

Some Remarks about Freud's Account of the Case

In the published version of Emmy von N.'s case, several points seem to be worthy of some remarks. First, we can only wonder to what extent the patient was Freud's or Breuer's. The prominent Viennese clinician who had treated Emmy von N. for six weeks before committing her to Freud is not named in the case, but could very easily have been Breuer. Breuer's name appears no fewer than eleven times in Freud's narrative. Freud expressly says that he was applying Breuer's therapeutic method; he mentions an unexpected visit from him, and the patient writes to Breuer some time after the first treatment to complain about Freud. Furthermore, the parallels between the cases of Emmy von N. and Anna O. are striking: Freud observes of Emmy von N. that she is very intelligent and that sexuality plays no role for her, just as in the case of Anna O. according to Breuer. Just like Breuer and Anna O., Freud spent an enormous amount of time treating Emmy von N., encouraging her to talk in a waking state and under hypnosis twice a day. Like Breuer, Freud was looking for the psychological origin of each of the patient's symptoms; he made a connection for each of the symptoms with an initial trauma, and he made them disappear from the memory afterwards under hypnosis. Emotional abreactions at this stage were out of the question, and the method he used sounds very much like Janet's method. Otherwise, Freud, unlike Breuer here, immediately required his patient's admission to a sanatorium, and he massaged her in person twice a day. But Freud, like Breuer with Anna O., also says that he learned a great deal from this patient. Above all, Emmy von N. made Freud understand that he should ask fewer questions during their therapeutic discussions and instead let her talk more and that once a story was started under hypnosis, he should let it go naturally to its end, for it was harmful if it went unfinished.

Second, the chronology of Emmy von N.'s story is not very clear, and various hypotheses have been suggested to explain the discrepancies in it. If Freud had been so struck by Breuer's story of Anna O., as he stated, why did he wait from 1882 to 1889, that is, seven years, before starting to apply a similar therapeutic method to a patient himself? The chronology of the treatment of the case is also confusing. Freud declares that he saw the patient for the first time on May 1, 1889, six weeks after she arrived in

Vienna. He treated her for seven weeks, that is, roughly until June 20, 1889. One year later, she came back to Vienna to undergo Freud's treatment for eight more weeks (therefore, during May and June 1890). This means that it was in the spring of the following year that Emmy von N. would have contacted Freud for a consultation about her older daughter, that is, roughly in March 1891. However, in another place, Freud places this visit to see the daughter in May 1890. The publishers of the *Standard Edition* of Freud's works formulated the following hypothesis: the first period of treatment occurred in 1888, and the second in 1889, which would place Freud's consultation at Emmy von N.'s home in 1890, which would then fit the date Freud indicated for this event.

Certain unpublished documents, however, do not confirm this hypothesis. In her unfinished *Autobiography*, Mentona Moser declares that her mother, her sister, and herself spent the winter of 1888–1889 in Abbazia and that it was here, on January 30, 1889, that they heard the news about the so-called Mayerling tragedy, in which the Crown Prince Rudolf was found dead in his hunting lodge in the town of Mayerling. Also, according to the autobiography, they arrived in the beginning of spring in Vienna, where her mother was treated for six weeks by another doctor before he committed her to "his first assistant" (that is, to Freud). All of this confirms the date Freud indicates as the beginning of the treatment, namely, May 1889, and not 1888. But otherwise, we find Freud's signature in Fanny Moser's visitors' book dated July 19, 1889, that is, hardly a month after the end of the first period of treatment in Vienna. The only possible explanation, it seems, is that Freud was invited at least twice to the Moser chateau, the first time in July 1889 and the second time at a later, undetermined date when he saw the daughter.

Third, when we read the long recital of Emmy von N.'s complaints and symptoms, we are struck by the great number and diversity of the traumas suffered. One would think a priori that her husband's death and the sensational accusations of having poisoned him would occupy the primary place among her sources of unhappiness; but in fact we find only two explicit references to these events, on May 11 and May 12. Rather, she attributed her illness much more often to difficulties she met with her two daughters. Among her innumerable fears, she talked most frequently about dead persons, animals, and ghosts. The terror that she felt for animals is the most striking association. Mice, rats, toads, worms, leeches, snakes, and bats, not to mention various imaginary animals, appear constantly in her remarks. We also learned that Emmy von N. talked often about mental hospitals. Apparently, her mother, as well as a cousin, had been confined to such institutions. She imagined them as horrifying places where patients were tortured. This obsessive fear is all the stranger given that Fanny Moser, it turns out, had donated in 1875 a sum of 10,000 Swiss francs (a considerable amount of money at that time) to the construction of a mental hospital in Schaffhausen.[6]

The Biographical Context: Who Was Fanny Moser?

Fanny Moser was the widow of an extremely wealthy industrial business-man of Schaffhausen, Heinrich Moser; but she belonged herself to an old patrician family from Winterthur, Switzerland, the family of von Sulzer-Wart. The Sulzer genealogy and story have been studied in detail in a large work from which I borrow some information.[7]

Fanny's grandfather, Johann Heinrich von Sulzer-Wart (1768–1840), was a prodigiously active man, gifted in business matters. His great services to the Bavarian king during critical circumstances allowed him to be raised to the peerage and to receive the title *Freiherr* (baron) while remaining strongly attached to his native Swiss country. Grandfather Sulzer-Wart purchased the castle of Andelfingen, where he spent the later years of his life. One of his sons, Heinrich von Sulzer-Wart (1805–1887), Fanny's father, although not as brilliant as his father, was also a very energetic man who divided his time between Switzerland and Bavaria and also bore the title of baron. These details explain why Fanny, brought up in such a family environment, aspired always to an aristocratic way of life and later tried to be introduced to the European courts.

Fanny Louise von Sulzer-Wart was born on July 29, 1848. Very little information exists about her childhood. According to what she reported to Freud, her mother was an excessively strict and rigorous person. Her father probably did not have much time to pay attention to her, since there were fourteen children in the family, of which Fanny was the thirteenth. One of her brothers, Heinrich Jr., founded a bank, fell into bankruptcy, was sentenced in absentia to hard labor, and escaped to Haiti (not to Santo Domingo, as Freud wrote) and then to New York City as a refugee. The youngest son in the family, Max, whom Fanny admired very much, had a military vocation and entered the Prussian army for some time, but came back to Switzerland when his father requested his return. Max was among the pioneers of automotive travel and aviation in Switzerland.

Fanny von Sulzer's wedding to Heinrich Moser, which took place on December 28, 1870, was a sensational, if not scandalous, event. This was not because it was an unsuitable marriage, since both families were equally

---

[6] Mr. Hans Lieb has verified for me the accuracy of this fact in the Cantonal Archives of Schaffhausen, where the donation is recorded in the Acts of the Cantonal Government of Schaffhausen on February 3, 1875. (See the *Regierungsratsprotokolle*, vol. 24, p. 94.)

[7] Alice Denzler, *Die Sulzer von Winterthur*, 2 vols. (Winterthur, 1933).

rich and belonged to upper society, but because of the age difference: she was 23 and he was 65. [. . .] Heinrich Moser (1805–1874) was a proto-type of "the self-made man."[8] He learned the profession of clock- and watchmaking in French-speaking Switzerland and then moved to Russia, where he established a factory. He perfected a certain kind of watch that was inexpensive but sturdy and of excellent quality, and he swamped the Russian market with it. His watches spread out to Persia and central Asia. In this fashion, he accumulated an immense fortune. While running this business in Russia, and a second factory in French Switzerland, he also set up a wagon and railroad enterprise in Schaffhausen as well as a number of other businesses. Eventually, he bought a magnificent estate, Char-lottenfels, overhanging the Rhine River. In his business and family life equally, he was considered a harsh and authoritarian man. With his first wife, he had five children—four daughters and a son, Georg Heinrich, who changed his name to Henri. Henri Moser (1844–1923), who was born in Russia and brought up in Switzerland, worked several years with his fa-ther, then revolted against his authority, entered the Russian army, traveled several times in central Asia, bred silkworms, served for a while in the Austro-Hungarian diplomatic service, and gave to the Bern historical mu-seum the magnificent ethnological collections he had acquired in central Asia.[9]

After his first wife's death, Heinrich Moser *père* remained a widower for twenty years. His remarriage with Fanny von Sulzer-Wart was very badly accepted by his children, especially by Henri Jr. In several letters published by Karl Schib, a local historian in Schaffhausen, Heinrich Moser talks about his happiness at home and about his wife's devotion to him; but he also mentions her constant nervousness. They traveled a great deal to-gether, because Heinrich had to visit his various enterprises, and they took numerous vacations in the town of Menton, along the French Riviera. Heinrich and Fanny had two daughters—Fanny, born on May 27, 1872, and Mentona, born on October 19, 1874.

Soon after his remarriage, Heinrich Moser wrote a will in which he bequeathed the lion's share of his fortune to his wife, so that after his death, she became, it was said, the richest woman in central Europe. But even before the will was opened, Henri Moser, the son, legally contested its validity. He also spread a rumor that his father had been poisoned by his second wife.

It was at this point that Fanny Moser's biography begins to read like a

---

[8] A biography, already rather dated, has been devoted to him: Adam Pfaff, *Heinrich Moser: Ein Lebensbild* (Schaffhausen, Brodtmann, 1875). See also Heinrich Moser, *Briefe in Auswahl*, compiled by Karl Schib (Schaffhausen, Verlag Peter Meili, 1972).

[9] Henri Moser has related some of his adventures in an amusing and well-written book, *A travers l'Asie Centrale* (Paris, Plon, [1885]).

detective novel. Apparently, Fanny, in an attempt to put an end to the rumors accusing her of murdering her husband, requested that his body be exhumed for the performance of an autopsy and a toxicological analysis. When this request was agreed upon, however, it was discovered that the children of the first marriage had already privately proceeded with an autopsy, under a secret agreement with the police. The additional examination found no indication of foul play, but stories about Fanny having poisoned her husband persisted, and Ola Andersson, during his investigations, was able to meet townspeople who still believed in the poison thesis. Apparently, this was also the reason why Fanny was later shunned socially by royal and aristocratic circles. In addition, she had to endure a number of trials about her husband's will. But this, unfortunately, is the most unknown part of her life, and we can only hope that further research based on the remaining judicial documents will someday be done.

At any rate, following her husband's demise, Fanny Moser attempted to reorganize her existence. From 1875 to 1887, she was in the habit of spending a part of the year in Karlsruhe and a part in Badenweiler, both in Germany. She also frequented the best-known European spas. With her great wealth, she had a large household staff and surrounded herself with a kind of court. In 1887, she bought a new beautiful chateau, often referred to as a "castle," in Au, near Wädenswil, not far from Zurich. She settled in at Au, and began extensively to entertain distinguished guests there. Andersson, who interviewed numerous people who knew Fanny, says that she gave the impression of a mixture of dignity and eccentricity and that she was excessively touchy. She had admirers, and lovers, including among the latter, it was said, several of her doctors. She tried to keep these relationships secret, but her daughters and her immediate circle knew about them.

Fanny's official guest book, signed by the many people who visited her castle, reflects her style of living. Among the famous names there we find those of the poet Friedrich von Bodenstedt, the geologist Albert Heim, the neuropsychiatrists Auguste Forel, Eugen Bleuler, and Otto Wetterstrand, and later the philosopher Ludwig Klages. When she took a dislike to one of her guests, she was in the habit of sticking a small piece of paper on the place where the person had signed. This is what she actually did beside Freud's signature, which appears on July 19, 1889. Also included in the book is a letter dated May 31, 1907, sent from a lawyer's office, along with letters of apology, from two men who had trespassed on her property without permission. One of them, as if making a joke, addresses his letter to "Hochwohlgeborene Freifrau von Sulzer-Wart auf Schloss Au," which seems to confirm what witnesses said about her extreme sensitivity and reputation for eccentricity. Of her later years, we know only a few facts. Evidently Fanny fell in love with a much younger man than herself. She was ready to marry him; however, he managed to extract a large portion of her fortune. Afterwards, she was haunted by the idea that she was living in penury, even though she still retained millions of her wealth. Fanny Moser von Sulzer-Wart died on April 2, 1925. She was buried in the cemetery of Kilchberg, near Zurich. Her grave is located close to that of Thomas Mann.

The Stories of the Two Moser Daughters

Fanny Moser's story would not be complete if it did not consider the destiny of her two daughters, Fanny and Mentona. In spite of Freud's unfavorable opinion of them, both women made remarkable careers for themselves.

The older daughter, Fanny (1872–1953), developed a passion for academic studies, but she inevitably came up against social obstacles and preconceived ideas which at the time made it almost impossible for women in Switzerland to gain access to higher education. In his narrative of Emmy von N.'s story, Freud referred to this older daughter and to some behavioral problems and intellectual ambitions he considered excessive. Therefore, it is strange to read in Mentona Moser's *Autobiography* that it was on Freud's private counsel that the mother decided to allow her older daughter to pursue formal studies. In the biographical résumé attached to her dissertation, the young Fanny states that she was 21 (that is, in 1893) when she left for Lausanne in order to study. She passed her examinations in Lausanne and obtained her baccalaureate degree in 1895. After a one-year stay at home, she then studied successively at the universities of Fribourg-en-Brisgau, Zurich, and Munich. At first she began medical studies but ended up devoting herself professionally to zoology. She wrote and defended a dissertation on "The Comparative Development of the Lungs of Vertebrates."[10] She then worked in Munich and in the zoological maritime stations of Villefranche, France, and Naples. She took a peculiar interest in jellyfish and wrote an exhaustive monograph on this subject.[11] When we read this work, we do not know what is more admirable: the immense quantity of scientific material gathered or the critical closeness with which

[10] Fanny Moser, "Beiträge zur vergleichenden Entwicklungsgeschichte der Wirbeltierlunge (Amphibien, Reptilien, Vögel, Säuger)," *Archiv für mikroskopische Anatomie und Entwicklungsgeschichte*, 60 (1902).

[11] Fanny Moser, *Die Siphonophoren der deutschen Südpolar-Expedition, 1901–1903* (Berlin, 1925), reprinted in Erich von Drygalski, ed., *Deutsche Südpolar-Expedition* (Berlin and Leipzig, Walter Gruyter, 1925). See also Fanny Moser, *Die Ctenophoren der Siboya-expedition* (Leiden, E. J. Brill, 1903); and idem, *Japanische Ctenophoren* (Munich, Beiträge zur Naturgeschichte Ostasiens, 1906).

the data are analyzed and classified. The foreword of the book indicates that it was finished in February 1914, but because of the First World War its publication was delayed until 1925.

We are almost entirely ignorant about young Fanny's personal life. We do know, however, that in 1903 she married a certain Jaroslav Hoppe, who died in 1927 after a long illness. Afterwards, Fanny settled in Zurich.

When we go through Fanny Moser's bibliography of writings, we see that her publications stop abruptly in 1925, with her copious work on siphonophores. They then begin again in 1935, with an equally substantial work about occultism or, as we would say today, parapsychology.[12] But where did this change of intellectual orientation come from? Fanny Moser explains it herself in the introduction to her book on the subject. It is not a question of a sudden mutation of interest but rather a gradual evolution, she explains. In 1890, she had once been surprised to hear the geologist Albert Heim declare that some water diviners had been more cunning than himself in detecting underground running water. Then, in 1895, she had come to Stockholm with "a relative who suffered from nerves" (read: her mother) to be treated by the celebrated Dr. Otto Wetterstrand. Wetterstrand, an excellent hypnotist whom her mother appreciated very much, spent several weeks before being able to hypnotize the patient. During one hypnotic session, young Fanny was stunned to see that, after Wetterstrand gave her mother the order to awaken from the trance twenty minutes later, she indeed came out of the hypnotic sleep precisely twenty minutes later, with no watch or clock in the room. Later, young Fanny heard Forel talk about experiences in which some burn marks had been provoked on a medium through hypnotic suggestion and about another patient who during hypnotic sleep had precisely described the interior of the hypnotist's house, without ever having set eyes on it. In 1898, during a talk about parapsychological frauds, she also heard Bleuler claim that many of these people first had been real psychics and had only later defrauded when they began to lose their genuine mediumistic abilities.

Fanny Moser-Hoppe also reports that for a long time, in spite of these opinions of Forel and Bleuler, she did not believe there existed any legitimacy in the work of so-called psychics. She was herself considered "anti-psychic," which means that her presence in a group of spirits would allegedly prevent any apparition of psychic manifestations. Her skepticism disappeared only in the beginning of 1914, when she met in Berlin a highly gifted male psychic. She was invited to a session where, after some laborious efforts, the psychic finally produced an apparition, the "spirit" of the socialist leader August Bebel, who declared that he was repudiating everything he had said and done during his lifetime. It was at this moment

---

[12] Fanny Moser, *Okkultismus: Täuschungen und Tatsachen*, 2 vols. (Zurich, Orell-Fussli, 1935).

that the wonder occurred: the table around which they were all gathered began to dance, to slope, and then to rise up almost to the ceiling three times. Once it fell down so abruptly that a leg broke. Then the psychic himself started to levitate. Fanny Moser-Hoppe was convinced that there could not be any fraud. This was for her a most striking experience, so much so that, while pursuing her zoological research, she began systematically to read the voluminous literature devoted to the mysterious phenomena of the mind, the soul, and the unconscious. Later on, she took part in some experiments with famous parapsychological subjects, like Rudy Schneider and Hanussen. She was always concerned to distinguish between the fraudulent and the authentic in these phenomena. This is a leading idea in her book on the subject, which represents a good synthesis of the parapsychological literature up until 1935 and is still interesting today as a critical collection of documents.[13]

This area of interest led her later to conduct research on the subject of haunted houses. For this work, young Fanny gathered written documentation as well as declarations by firsthand witnesses. It should be noted that one of the cases she reports was that of Carl Gustav Jung, who in 1920 had a brief personal experience of this kind during a stay in England. Jung also wrote the foreword to Moser's book. The first volume, devoted to an exposition of the facts, should have been followed by a second volume, which unfortunately never appeared.[14] Fanny Moser-Hoppe died in Zurich on February 24, 1953.

Such was the story of the first daughter. The life of the younger daughter, Mentona Moser, was even more exceptional. Born on October 19, 1874, in Baden-Weiler, in Germany, four days before the death of her father, Mentona was considered for a while a subnormal child. Her mother did not hide her hostile feelings toward her. Mentona revolted against her family background more openly than her sister, finding a way out through social and political activism. She became a member of the Swiss Communist party in 1919, and she set up an orphanage in the USSR in 1928. Her parents had chosen her first name in memory of happy days they spent together in Menton. It was said that she detested the name.

Mentona Moser's life and personality are partially known to us thanks to her lengthy autobiography.[15] Starting with her birth and her father's death, she related in this document this controversial family episode. She does not offer her own opinion about the matter but gives some rather bizarre factual information: rat poison found in the bedroom where her father had died; her dead father's nose having a strange white color; her

---

[13] See in particular the second volume of Moser, *Okkultismus*.

[14] Fanny Moser, *Spuk: Irrglaube oder Wahrglaube? Eine Frage der Menschheit*, with a Foreword by C. G. Jung (Baden bei Zurich, Gyr-Verlag, 1950), vol. 1.

[15] *Lebensgeschichte von Mentona Moser.*

mother announcing to her dying husband that the newly born child was a boy, and not a girl, in order to get him to bequeath to her a larger part of his fortune. The details that Mentona relates about the trials that came afterwards are also strange. Some of the most important evidence in her father's file, she writes, had disappeared, including the pages about the brain from the toxicological report. A box filled with documents about the case had accidentally been burned.

Offering a detailed account of her childhood, Mentona also writes in the autobiography about "the terrible melancholy of well-being" from which she suffered at home. Her mother used to spend summers in Baden-Weiler and winters in Karlsruhe; she made strenuous but always unsuccessful efforts to be introduced to the court. At home, she had organized her own court, which included her own "*Leibarzt*—private doctor," where they spoke French and later English, and where they affected to speak German with a foreign accent. Neither of the daughters was allowed to go to school, but they always had private tutors. Mentona found this fashionable life appallingly tedious. She also talks with horror about the way her mother treated the household staff as well as about her superficial charity acts toward the poor. Mentona's autobiographical account confirms what was said earlier about the property her mother acquired in Au, on the Zurich lakeside, and about the style of life of the place. However, the main estate did not prevent the family from traveling quite often to holiday resorts, for instance, to Abbazia in the winter of 1888–1889 and to fashionable beach resorts on the Adriatic coast. Mentona also talks about the famous professor her mother consulted in Vienna, but does not indicate his name. This professor soon committed her to "his first assistant," who, we have said, was Freud: "He was short and thin, he had blue-black hair, and big black eyes; he looked shy and very young. He made a deep impression on me."

It is interesting to compare the different ways in which the two daughters revolted against their mother. While Fanny, the older one, went on to higher education and devotion to science, the younger Mentona was attracted to social and political service. In 1903, Mentona published a booklet entitled "Feminine Youth of the Upper Classes: Considerations and Recommendations," which constitutes a vehement, at times sarcastic, critique of the education given at the time to young women of the wealthy classes.[16] Such women, Mentona writes here, inculcate the same set of preconceived ideas their mothers suffered from, which only produces a vicious circle of unhappiness from one generation to the next. At present, she adds, only one outcome is possible: to become the sort of spinster that the entire world ridicules, pities, and despises. What is required, according

---

[16] Mentona Moser, *Die weibliche Jugend der oberen Stände: Betrachtungen und Vorschläge* (Zurich, Schulthess, 1903).

to Mentona, is that these women develop the courage and the self-confidence necessary for living. As the example of Florence Nightingale shows, other careers are open to them, such as medical care for patients and social service. Two years later, Mentona published a second booklet with additional practical advice and recommendations.[17] Efficient and successful work by women in these fields, she writes here, requires caution, single-mindedness, and systematic application. Material help to social groups has to come from specialized organizations rather than individuals with goodwill.

Based on a reading of these two significant booklets, we are not surprised to learn that Mentona eventually became a militant member of left-wing political parties. In 1919, she joined the Swiss Communist party, and in 1926 she traveled to Soviet Russia. In 1928, she set up an international children's institution in Ivanovo for the care of abandoned children from any country. It was said that in so doing, she was attempting to give back to Mother Russia a part of the money that her father had once earned there in such large amounts. Later in life, she returned to central Europe and settled in East Berlin.

One other biographical fact about Mentona remains to mention. In 1941, she published a popular collection of animal stories entitled "Learn to Know Them."[18] The book is mostly about birds, but also horses, donkeys, dogs, cats, mice, rabbits, and squirrels. Mentona writes that her book has been examined and corrected by a professional zoologist from Zurich, a reference probably to her sister. The book is nicely printed and well illustrated. A few years later, another edition was published in Berlin with the identical text but different illustrations.[19] Again, we know almost nothing about Mentona Moser's private life, except that she got married, had two children, and divorced. She died in East Berlin, on April 10, 1971, at the age of 96.[20]

Reflections on the Facts

The critical commentary about the case of Emmy von N. has up until now hardly surpassed the level of nosological diagnosis: Was hers really a case of hysteria, as Freud said, or rather of schizophrenia? But I think that

---

[17] Mentona Moser, *Beiträge zur Wohltätigkeit und sozialen Hilfeleistung in ihrer praktischen Anwendung* (Zurich, Schulthess, 1905).

[18] Mentona Moser, *Lernt sie kennen*, with woodcuts by Remi Nüesch (Zurich, Büchergilde Gutenberg, 1941).

[19] Mentona Moser, *Lernt sie kennen*, with illustrations by Kurt Kranz (Berlin, Verlag Lucie Groszer, 1949).

[20] See the necrological notice, Roger Nicholas Balsiger, "Wesen und Wirken einer ungewöhnlichen Frau: Mentona Moser," *Schaffhauser Nachrichten*, 8 (June 4, 1971), 17.

to fully understand the complexity of the case, we should have more information at our disposal than we do currently. For instance, it would be most helpful to have access to the judicial records pertaining to the accusations of Fanny Moser's poisoning of her husband and to Heinrich Moser's will. Above all, Emmy von N.'s story requires placement in the familial, social, and cultural contexts in which the patient lived as well as in the framework of the three generations embracing her parents, herself, and her children.

Central Europe in 1889, when Freud first met Emmy von N., was a wholly different world from ours, so that it is difficult for us today to imagine it. That world was experiencing a rapid demographic, industrial, and commercial expansion and was engaged in an unrestrained exploitation of global natural resources, which then seemed inexhaustible. The intellectual atmosphere was dominated by Darwinism (or pseudo-Darwinism), and the idea of a fight for life had resulted in a wild competition between the five or six greatest military and economic powers. The general public mentality of the time was aggressive but optimistic and forward-looking. Bold and assertive men, starting with nothing, could become very rich not only in America but also in the Russian Empire.

Switzerland in particular was a country from which many of its citizens traditionally went away to foreign countries, either to make their fortunes or simply to earn a living, while remaining strongly attached to their homeland. It was not extraordinary to see a Swiss decorated or raised to the peerage in a foreign country; but it was generally badly received to avail oneself of these titles or decorations once back in the native country.

Europe was then still in many ways an aristocratic world where the monarchies set the fashion. And all European countries, with the exceptions of France and Switzerland, were monarchies; and, even in a country as fundamentally democratic as Switzerland, the aristocratic style of life exerted a certain hold over the imagination. Fanny Moser's biography, with her claims to nobility and her tireless efforts to be introduced to a princely court, represent an involuntary caricature of these contemporary values, which, incidentally, her brother, Max, and her husband's son, Henri Moser, managed to fulfill.

Also, the world at that time was made by men, and for men, with women, even in the upper classes, occupying a secondary position. A rich young woman, however clever and talented, was in effect exposed to the double psychopathology of extreme leisured wealth and cultural and intellectual frustration. The results of this frustration on women in these circumstances have been described in detail by Pierre Loti, after the turn of the century, in his novel *Disenchanted*; but it was not necessary to travel to Turkey to see examples of it.[21] In 1889, the Viennese physician Moritz

---

[21] Julien Viaud (pseud. Pierre Loti), *Les désenchantées; roman des harems turcs contemporains* (Paris, Calmann-Lévy, 1906).

Benedikt related that he was called to examine a young woman suffering from intolerable headaches that were feared to indicate a case of meningitis. Benedikt took the patient aside, and she told him in confidence that her family would not allow her to pursue her studies in spite of her very strong desire to do so. With her consent, Benedikt explained the situation to her parents. The young woman was then allowed to study and her symptoms, as if by magic, disappeared.[22] A very similar situation pertained for Anna O., for the daughters of Emmy von N., and for many other women of the time who have not met with a biographer. The fate of these young persons in fact was even further aggravated by an extremely severe and rigorous moral education.

At the same time, and reinforcing this position of women in society, there was a psychopathology centered around "the terrible melancholy of well-being," as Mentona Moser called it aptly. A neurosis determined by this destructive boredom can also be found in Freud's report of the case of "the Wolf Man." Actually, it seems that the neurosis of the Wolf Man was a specific case of this strange neurosis among the great idle and listless land-owners of Russia—the *oblomovchtchina*—who have been captured so well by the novelist Ivan Goncharov.[23] Wealthy and idle women of the same period, compelled to so many repressions, could vent their anger on their domestic staff, which was numerous, badly retributed, and devoid of legal protection. In her *Autobiography*, Mentona describes the severity, even cruelty, with which her mother treated the servants. But these channels of expression were obviously insufficient, which explains the resort of many women to a fashionable neurosis: hysteria. In my view, the diagnosis of hysteria was fully justified in Emmy von N.'s case, as well as in Anna O.'s; but it was a particular kind of *sociogenic hysteria* that we no longer know today.

It is in this light that we should finally judge the attempts at self-healing among patients in this category. The case of Bertha Pappenheim represents the story of a person who, after a long and debilitating illness, managed to free herself from her social circle, and from her doctors, in order to write a pamphlet ridiculing the education given to young upper-class women and then to devote herself, in an almost religious fashion, to social work.[24] In the process, she realized what Leopold Szondi has called a "socialization," or sublimation, of neurotic energies into work. In Emmy von N.'s case, this same sublimation was made, but not by the patient herself, but rather by one of her daughters, Mentona, who, once emancipated from her familial

---

[22] Ellenberger, "Moritz Benedikt (1835–1920)," *Confrontations psychiatriques*, 11 (1973), 183–200.

[23] Ivan Aleksandrovich Goncharov, *Oblomov* [1859], translated from the Russian by Natalie A. Duddington (London, G. Allen and Unwin, 1929).

[24] Bertha Pappenheim, "Zur Erziehung der weiblichen Jugend in den höheren Ständen," in *Ethische Kultur* (1898).

heritage, also went on to write a booklet denouncing the education received by upper-class women and then to involve herself, again like Pappenheim, in social work. As for her older sister, her sublimation took a different form, a "socialization" devoted to academic science.

Moreover, it seems that these patterns of sublimation were made in meaningful detail. It might be recalled that Emmy von N. abhorred animals, especially small, crawling ones. Now, her older daughter, it turns out, spent many years in her adulthood studying jellyfish, while the younger daughter chose to write a popular children's book in order to help young people to identify and love animals. Also, Emmy von N. had a morbid fear of sudden apparitions, and young Fanny Moser explored in great detail, and with a rational methodology, the mysterious world of occultism.

Finally, the process of this emotional and social sublimation appears to have taken place differently in different families. While the sublimation of Anna O. was realized in an individual lifetime, the case of the Mosers required two generations to complete. In fact, if we consider it closely, we see that Emmy von N.'s case has to be considered within the framework of three, if not four, generations. The generations of her parents and grandparents were made up of daring and assertive men, like Heinrich Moser, who first accumulated their fortunes and who, like grandfather Heinrich von Sulzer-Wart, acquired for themselves courtly positions and noble titles. The second generation of these European families profited from the fortune and the new high social and material status earned by the previous one. This second generation willingly adopted an aristocratic style of life, as the examples of Max von Sulzer-Wart and Henri Moser illustrate. Fanny Moser von Sulzer-Wart was desirous of doing so, too, but powerful obstacles stood in her way. Instead, she was reduced to leading a kind of pseudo-aristocratic life, which no doubt contributed to her eccentric, if not hysterical, nature. The third generation of family members, however, inherited the problems created by the second. They felt the need to break with what they perceived as a boring and frivolous way of living and to liberate themselves, in different ways, from "the terrible melancholy of well-being." As Julien Green has expressed so well in the foreword to his novel *Varouna* (1940), "A life does not seem to be enough for the accomplishment of a destiny. . . . Our life is only enlightened in its link with the previous and the following ones."[25] In much the same vein, all of this also calls to mind the well-known aphorism of Jung: "Nothing influences children more powerfully than the lives that their parents did not live. . . . The entire life of some individuals is sometimes only a search for an answer to a question posed by their parents."

[25] Julien Green, *Varouna* (Paris, Plon, 1940).

11

C. G. Jung and the Story of
Helene Preiswerk: A Critical Study
with New Documents

[1991]*

THE STORY of the young woman Helene Preiswerk reveals once again the role that certain patients have played in the history of dynamic psychiatry. The origin of Carl Gustav Jung's theoretical teachings cannot be understood without reference to the experiments he made in his student years with a young medium, Helene (known as Helly) Preiswerk, as reported by him in his medical dissertation.[1]

Let us remind ourselves that any historical event can be approached from three different viewpoints: (1) The current version, based mostly upon family tradition and hearsay. Relatives, friends, and colleagues make incomplete, inaccurate, and sometimes fictitious statements. Not infrequently, a joke is taken at face value and will later become a historical fact. (2) Corrected findings based on documents and the testimony of reliable persons that may fill gaps, correct inaccuracies, and dispel a few legends, but that generally still cover only fragments of the whole story. The picture remains incomplete and distorted. (3) The unknown history: that side of

---

*[Editor's note: This essay was written by Dr. Ellenberger specifically for the present volume at a time when his physical mobility was severely limited. Upon completion, the essay was published immediately in History of Psychiatry, 2, no. 5 (March 1991), 41–52. Dr. Ellenberger is aware of the fragmentary nature of the documentation and the argumentation in the article but believes that the historical information it contains is important. The essay also nicely illustrates the author's continued interest in the history of Jungian psychology as well as in writing medical history from the perspective of the patient. In a number of places, I have integrated into the account factual material from an earlier essay by Ellenberger that appeared under the title "Carl Gustav Jung: His Historical Setting," in Hertha Riese, ed., Historical Explorations in Medicine and Psychiatry (New York, Springer, 1978), 142–49.]

[1] This essay has been completed with the help of numerous persons. I am immensely indebted to Mrs. Stephanie Zumstein-Preiswerk, who gave me a wealth of information about her aunt, Helene Preiswerk, as well as unpublished letters of C. G. Jung pertaining to his youth. My sincerest thanks also go to Mr. Beat Glaus, of the Eidgenössische Technische Hochschule, Zurich, who sent me photocopies of precious documents. I am also grateful to the librarians of the Basel University Library who facilitated my research in heaps of old newspapers and magazines.

an event or biography which escapes our awareness and which we often do not even suspect. The veil of oblivion drops rapidly upon a man after his death. Certain events are deliberately concealed by the individual or the family.[2]

In the present essay, we will first follow Jung's version of the story of Helene Preiswerk as recorded by him in his M.D. dissertation in 1902.[3] Second, we will take into account the recent biographical and historical researches on this subject of Stefanie Zumstein-Preiswerk, a member of the Preiswerk family. In addition, we will consider the sociocultural context of the case as providing the means for making an indirect approach to the unknown history of the case.

The Traditional Story

According to Jung's dissertation, the story of his encounter with Helly Preiswerk began in July 1899 and lasted approximately a year and a half. Jung was a 23-year-old medical student at the time, deeply interested in parapsychology, but without practical experience in that field. Then he happened to learn that a 15-year-old girl, whom he designated with the initials "S.W.," was a member of a small group who played table-turning and that she manifested mediumistic capacities. Jung joined the group, eager to utilize these sessions as a means of exploring the human mind.

Jung depicted "S.W." as a sickly person. She had a somewhat rachitic skull, a pale complexion, and dark eyes with a peculiar piercing glance. She was a mediocre schoolgirl, not gifted, devoid of musical sense, interested more in needlework than in books, absentminded. She was treated harshly by her mother and was looked down upon by many of her numerous brothers and sisters.

Nor is Jung's description of her family flattering. The grandfather on the mother's side, a Protestant minister, claimed to be visited frequently by spirits, and he experienced visions. One of his brothers was tainted with imbecility and also had visions. One of his sisters was also abnormal. The grandmother on the father's side suffered hysterical and somnambulistic fits, during which time she prophesied. The medium's father and two of his brothers were also characterized as eccentric. The medium's mother showed mental abnormalities, too. Two of the medium's sisters were plagued with hysterical symptoms. There was also much strife between the family children, and their education was deficient.

---

[2] See Ellenberger, *The Discovery of the Unconscious* (London, Allen Lane, 1970), 657–741.

[3] C. G. Jung, *Zur Psychologie und Pathologie sogenannter occulter Phänomene: Eine psychiatrische Studie* (Leipzig, Mutze, 1902).

During the weekly table-turning sessions, Jung watched the medium closely and kept a record of everything that took place. It was not clear to what extent "S.W." remembered what she had said during her somnambulistic states, but she always maintained that it was truly spirits of the dead who spoke through her mouth. In sharp contrast to her often silly behavior in daily life, she now attracted respect and admiration from several relatives and friends who asked for her advice. For some time, "S.W." 's guiding spirit was her grandfather, Reverend Samuel Preiswerk. She had never known him but spoke with his solemn voice. She had chanced to read Justinus Kerner's *The Seeress of Prevorst* (1829), with its remarkable story of Fredericke Hauffe.[4] Following the example of the Seeress in Kerner's book, "S.W." started to magnetize herself, and she allegedly spoke in foreign languages. New spirits appeared to her, among others a most talkative and stupid one who called himself Ulrich von Gerbenstein.

Later, a new guiding spirit, Ivènes, came to the fore. Ivènes was supposed to be a very sensitive Jewish woman of small size with black hair who spoke the language of the spirits. Her task was to encourage and forward good spirits and to teach and correct black spirits. Such an activity entailed frequent journeys on and between the stars, including the planet Mars, of which she described the inhabitants and civilizations. "S.W." then started to tell the stories of her previous incarnations. She claimed to have been a young woman seduced by Goethe. Earlier, she had been none other than Friedericke Hauffe, the Seeress of Prevorst; in the fifteenth century she had been Madame de Valours, burnt at the stake as a witch. Still earlier in Rome she had been a Christian woman martyr at the time of Nero. In her remotest incarnation, she had been loved by King David. In each one of these previous lives, she had numerous offspring. "S.W." wove an immense network of imaginary genealogies that made her the ancestor of most of the people she was acquainted with.

According to Jung's printed accounts, a further step in "S.W." 's revelations was the teaching of a mystical science of Nature. Jung gave a detailed account of her revelations concerning the secret structure of the mystical world with its seven circles, its original force in the most central place, matter in the second circle, light and darkness in the third one, and so on. Bizarre names emerged: Magnesor, Cafar, Connesor, and the like.

During the course of his experiments, Jung observed changes in the medium's personality. Among the spirits who assailed her, some were rather dour, others exuberant. Jung noticed that these features reflected the

---

[4] Justinus Kerner, *Die Seherin von Prevorst: Eröffnungen über das innere Leben und über das Hineinragen einer Geisterwelt in die unsere*, 2 vols. (Stuttgart and Tubingen, J. G. Cotta, 1829); *The Seeress of Prevorst*, translated by Mrs. Crowe (London, J. C. Moore, 1845).

two aspects of her personality, between which she constantly oscillated. Ivènes, a serious and balanced personality, was none other than the adult personality in the process of being elaborated in the medium's unconscious. It is not clear at what point in time Jung began to realize that the young girl he referred to as "S.W."—who, in fact, turns out to have been his cousin—was in love with him and that she multiplied her mediumistic revelations in order to please him. However, he states that the medium's romances abounded in stories about overt or secret love affairs and illegitimate births. He suspected the existence of secret dreams of sexual gratification.

And how did Jung's encounter with "S.W." end? Jung states that "S.W." 's revelations gradually became less vivid and more repetitive, until one day she was caught red-handed attempting to defraud. Then Jung ceased to participate in the sessions.[5] One and a half years later, he learned that she had developed a pleasing personality and was now working in a business. As we shall see, this story is somewhat different from Zumstein-Preiswerk's revised version.

The Revised Story

It was given to Stefanie Zumstein-Preiswerk, a niece of the medium, to write in 1975 a corrected account of this important story.[6] Zumstein-Preiswerk's book relies on original, printed documents (unfortunately not always specified) and on the memories of Emmy Zinsstag, Helly's intimate friend. From Zumstein-Preiswerk's account, there are many significant differences in the chronology of the events. The succession of mediumistic phases is seen in closer connection with events in the Preiswerk and Jung families.

Stefanie Zumstein-Preiswerk found that Jung, in his printed account, changed the chronology of the experiments, concealed important facts, and modified the order of the mediumistic manifestations. According to Jung, the experiments started in July 1899 and ended in the fall of 1900. Stefanie Zumstein maintains that they began as early as June 1895 and went on, with several interruptions, until September 1899. Jung also said that he had joined an already organized group; but Zumstein-Preiswerk contends that he was the initiator. The location of the séances was the mansion of Klein-Huningen, the parish of which Reverend Paul Jung was the pastor. Reverend Paul Jung was at the time lying severely sick in bed and

---

[5] Jung, *Zur Psychologie und Pathologie sogenannter occulter Phänomene*, 57–58, 107.
[6] Stefanie Zumstein-Preiswerk, C. G. *Jungs Medium: Die Geschichte der Helly Preiswerk* (Munich, Kindler, 1975).

was not told of the experiments, which would have displeased him; his wife, however, encouraged them. The five initial participants in the session were Carl Jung (the only man), his mother Emilie Jung-Preiswerk, Helly Preiswerk, her sister Louise (called Luggy), and Helly's inseparable friend Emmy Zinsstag. Nobody's father was told about the experiments. Carl was then 20 years old; Louise, 21; and Helene, only 13½. From the start, Helene showed remarkable mediumistic abilities.

In the very first session, old Reverend Samuel Preiswerk, in a mediumistic communication, urged the participants to pray for Bertha. Bertha was the third oldest child of the fifteen children of Rudolf Preiswerk, Samuel's son. Two years before, Bertha had emigrated to Brazil and since then had sent little news. Grandfather Samuel explained that she had committed a sin, but that the family should forgive her. (Actually it turned out that she had given birth to a Negroid baby, and it was revealed later that she had married a mulatto two years before.) In the second session, Grandfather Samuel was again the one to speak while Grandfather Jung was invisibly present but kept silent. (One may sense here an intimation of rivalry between the Preiswerk and Jung families.) The third session, which took place sometime in July 1895, again had a dramatic character. This time, the scandalous event concerned Celestine (called Dini), the second-oldest Preiswerk child, who was soon to give birth to a child somewhat too soon after her marriage. The gloomy forebodings seem to have borne fruit later. The baby was physically abnormal and died soon after its birth. It was later revealed that the mother was infected with syphilis, but she pretended to have been bewitched by her mother-in-law.

The regular table-turning experiments of the Preiswerk family were then interrupted for two years (1896–1897). Helly was undergoing religious instruction, which was incompatible with such practices. During that period, both fathers, Paul Jung and Rudolf Preiswerk, died. When the sessions resumed, great changes had occurred in the utterances of the medium. In the meantime, Helly had been presented by Carl with a copy of Justinus Kerner's book, *The Seeress of Prevorst*. The guiding spirit was no longer old grandfather Samuel but a female spirit called Ivènes who was a sensitive Jewish woman with whom Helly gradually identified herself. For this part of the story, the reader is referred to Jung's dissertation.

When we come to the concluding phase of the experiments, there are wide discrepancies between Jung's version and Stefanie Zumstein-Preiswerk's account.[7] Zumstein-Preiswerk explains that Dini became se-

---

[7] In 1970, in my *Discovery of the Unconscious*, I cited *Notes on the Seminar in Analytical Psychology, Conducted by Dr. C. G. Jung, Zurich, 23 March–6 July 1925* as a private publication sent to me by Dr. D. A. Meier with Jung's permission, in which Jung recounted how he came to a session at which the collaborators proved that Helly was cheating, and which led to the sessions being stopped. See now the recent publication of this seminar: C. G.

verely psychotic and that she instilled delusions in Helly. It seems almost to
have been a case of *folie à deux*. Dini's mother-in-law was said to be the
reincarnation of a certain Madame Voisin, a celebrated poisoner of the
seventeenth century. Dini called Helly for help. Helly desperately tried to
respond. One evening, Helly returned home from the séance totally exhausted. Her mother was upset and forbade her any further pursuit of these
practices. She accused Carl and his mother of being responsible for Helly's
state. It came to a *Familienkrach*, that is, a dispute within the family.[8]
Reverend Samuel Gottlob Preiswerk severely condemned the spiritistic
séances. Helly was ashamed of these developments and took to her bed for
several days, refusing to eat or do anything. Life in Basel became intolerable for her. Her mother arranged for Helly to learn dressmaking in Basel,
but she then canceled the arrangement. Helly instead went to Montpellier
to an aunt of her friend Emmy Zinsstag. She spent two years in France,
learning dressmaking, first in Montpellier, and later in Paris. Carl too left
Basel, but for other reasons. Carl and Helly were to meet again briefly two
years later.

The Sociocultural Background

The story of Helly Preiswerk and her mediumistic performances can be
better understood if placed in the unique sociocultural context of the city of
Basel in 1895 to 1900. Basel is not an ordinary city. It is a rare example of a
self-contained political unit with its own government, administration, and
ministerial departments. Although in the late nineteenth century, Basel had
110,000 inhabitants, and was not yet the industrial center it became in the
twentieth century, it boasted a strong cultural tradition. Among the great
men who had lived there were Erasmus, Vesalius, and, in recent times,
Bachofen and Nietzsche. The population of Basel was made up of stern,
serious workers, but once a year the Carnival was the occasion for an
outburst of tumultuous enjoyment with dancing and singing in the streets,
unlike anywhere else in Switzerland. The Basler were also known for their
sarcastic witticisms.

Political power in Basel resided in the hands of the men "vom Teig," that
is, the old patrician families. Armed warfare between country and city had
ended in 1833 with the splitting of the canton into two political units: Basel
City and Basel Land. However, the half-canton of Basel City still included

---

Jung, *Analytical Psychology: Notes of the Seminar Given in 1925,* edited by William
McGuire (Princeton, Princeton University Press, 1989).

[8] Zumstein-Preiswerk, C. G. *Jungs Medium,* 90.

fringes of the countryside, including the above-mentioned village of Klein-Huningen, where the Preiswerk parapsychological sessions took place.

The old families were small societies in their own right. Each was proud of its name, history, genealogies, coat of arms, traditions, and legends. There were sometimes rivalries between the older and the newer families. The domination of children by parents was strong as well as the domination of women by men. The pervasive family spirit explains why tuberculosis and mental illness were so much feared, since these were believed to be hereditary evils. Even worse was the shame whenever an unmarried girl was found to be pregnant or the firstborn child followed on the heels of a wedding. If a son were constantly misbehaving, he might well be expelled from the family or sent to America by being given money for the fare or a one-way ticket. Sometimes an errant family member would mend his ways and become prosperous; sometimes he disappeared without a trace.

Religion also played an essential role in the old Basel families. Protestantism was a state religion. Pastors and ministers were poorly paid but highly respected. It was the rule to attend religious services, undergo religious instruction for two years, and thus prepare for receiving the First Communion by the age of 16. It would have been out of place to go to a dance party or to the theater during those two years. One typical feature was the belief in a guardian angel protecting everyone, especially little children. Sometimes, a child would build a strong relationship with his angel, who became a sort of imaginary companion. In this regard, Helly Preiswerk was no exception. She believed that her guardian angel, clearly identified for her as Ivènes, acted as an intermediary between herself and her deceased grandfather Preiswerk. She entrusted Ivènes with messages for her grandfather, who supposedly gave her advice through the angel.

Another belief that was current among certain pietist and fundamentalist circles was that of the impending end of the world. Among the forewarnings of such a development would be the return of the Jews to Palestine. As we have seen, one firm believer in this eventuality was Reverend Samuel Preiswerk. It is perhaps no mere coincidence that the First Zionist Congress took place in Basel at the end of August 1897. A perusal of the Basel press of that year shows that the First Zionist Congress was favorably received by the population. One can imagine how proud the Preiswerk family felt when Theodor Herzl, the chairman of the congress, evoked the memory of Reverend Samuel Preiswerk as one of the precursors of Zionism. This memorable event was also reflected in Helly's mediumistic utterances. Grandfather Samuel entrusted her with the mission of bringing the Jews back to Palestine and converting them to the Christian faith.

A picture of that time would not be complete without a mention of spiritism. The great wave of table-turning that had originated in the United

States in 1847 swept over Europe in 1852, manifesting itself in countless small groups of people calling forth spirits of the dead by means of table-turning, automatic writing, and mediumism. There was considerable diversity in the interpretation of the supposed messages from the world beyond. Many people were skeptical, but practiced turning tables as a kind of parlor game. Staunch believers turned spiritism into a religion of its own. Some religious-minded people saw in it the work of the devil. However, Samuel Preiswerk entered into long conversations with the spirit of his deceased wife.

Pathological manifestations during the episodes were not infrequent, extending from acute hysterical reactions to chronic hallucinatory delusions. Aside from spiritism there was much interest at the time in occultism. Among best-selling books at this time were Justinus Kerner's *The Seeress of Prevorst* and Carl du Prel's *The Riddle of Man*.[9] To these should be added the works of Camille Flammarion, especially his *Astronomie populaire*, of which the family of Rudolf Preiswerk treasured a copy.[10] Flammarion and some of his colleagues believed they had seen a network of canals on Mars and drew the conclusion that our sister planet was inhabited by intelligent beings. "We are not alone in the universe," they proclaimed. Mars and Martians played a great role in the imagination of many people in the late nineteenth century, including mediums.

The spirit of the time was also influenced by contemporary literature for children and youth. Here we should mention the name of Ottilie Wildermuth, the author of numerous novels for young ladies. Wildermuth was sufficiently famous for her to have biographies written about her, and for her statue to have been erected in Tubingen, Swabia. She was a distant relative of the Preiswerks, and a younger sister of Helly was named Ottilie in her honor. Stefanie Zumstein-Preiswerk asserts that several of Helly's mediumistic characters were inspired by Wildermuth's novels.

A Story of Two Families: The Preiswerk Family

The story of Carl and his medium Helly may be interpreted as an episode in the rivalry of two major Basel families: the Preiswerks and the Jungs. In reality, there was no overt hostility, and the rivalry did not extend much beyond a kind of boasting on both sides.

The Preiswerks were one of the most ancient families in Basel, as evi-

---

[9] Kerner, *The Seeress of Prevorst*; Carl du Prel, *Das Rätsel des Menschen: Einleitung in das Studium der Geheimwissenschaften* (Leipzig, Reclam, n.d.).

[10] Camille Flammarion, *Astronomie populaire* (Paris, Marpon & Flammarion, 1881).

denced by their history, genealogy, coat of arms, and family folklore.[11] By the end of the nineteenth century, their great hero was the pastor Samuel Preiswerk (1799–1871), who was a poet, an author of religious hymns, and a professor of Hebrew, and who also wrote a grammar of that language. Samuel Preiswerk had become the *Antistes*, that is, the president of the Company of Pastors in Basel. He created and directed a magazine, *Das Morgenland*, which published articles about the history, geography, and literature of the Middle East with particular emphasis on the Jewish people.[12] Samuel Preiswerk maintained that the Jewish nation was the only one that had received its name personally from God.[13] He also advocated the return of the Jews to Palestine, and he went so far as to rebuke the Jews for their supposed lack of interest in their promised land.

Old Samuel Preiswerk was also a strong believer in the existence of spirits. The story circulated that once a week he had a talk with the spirit of his first wife, to the sorrow of his second. He promoted the teaching of Hebrew on the grounds that it was the language spoken in Heaven; rumor had it that he was looking forward to talking with the Prophets of the Old Testament in their own language. From there it was not far to assume that he occupied an important position in Heaven. Little Helly could not have chosen a better intermediary between herself and God.

Samuel Preiswerk had one child by his first wife and eleven by his second. The son by the first marriage, Pastor Samuel Gottlob Preiswerk, was much respected in the family. In contrast to his father, he was opposed to spiritism. Helly was the eleventh of fifteen children of another son of old Samuel Preiswerk, Rudolf, who was the founder and owner of an ironmongery. A photograph taken at a family gathering in 1891 with the two parents and fifteen children shows Helene, at the age of 10, isolated at one end of the lowest row, in the pose of a little Cinderella, looking straight ahead, whereas most of the others are looking at the photographer.

The Jung Family

Among the great and illustrious men of the city of Basel was another striking figure, Carl Gustav Jung the Elder (1799–1864). Few characters in the history of dynamic psychiatry have been more endowed by legend. C. G. Jung the Elder was a typical representative of that generation of

---

[11] Ernst Schopf-Preiswerk, *Die Basler Familie, Preiswerk* (Basel, Verlag Freidrich Reinhard, 1952), including fifty genealogical tables, with supplements in 1961 and 1979.

[12] *Das Morgenland* (1838–1843).

[13] Gen. 33:26.

German romantic youth that was enthusiastic about democratic ideas, but became victims of political repression. He had been personally acquainted with several of the major figures of philosophical and literary Romanticism; but he had composed patriotic songs, and at one point he was arrested and arbitrarily thrown into prison for thirteen months. Eventually, he was expelled from the country and fled to France. The story had it that on a certain evening he was sitting, half-starving, on a bench in a Paris street when he was engaged in conversation by an unknown gentleman who invited him to come and see him the next day. This gentleman was none other than Alexander von Humboldt, who commended him to the Basel city authorities. He was appointed in 1822 to a professorship of anatomy, surgery, and obstetrics in the medical school in Basel. Jung the Elder gradually restored the school, which had fallen into a pitiful state of decay, to its previous fame. He was finally elected rector of the university, wrote a few scientific treatises, and became a sought-after consulting physician.[14]

Psychiatric observations and insights abound in Jung the Elder's writings. Given his definition of mental illness borrowed from Ideler—"the loss of the power of directing oneself according to one's own determination"— he believed in the efficacy of psychic therapy. When it was decided to create an asylum in Basel, he took a firm stand in favor of a hospital where patients would be treated instead of receiving merely custodial care. This principle was no matter of course at that time. In addition, he founded an institute for mentally retarded children. In an article on nostalgia, he claimed that it is not a mental disease as such, but can become one if the patient keeps his suffering a secret. This emphasis upon the deleterious effect of secretiveness anticipates his grandson's future concept of the pathogenic secret. The psychiatric principles of Jung the Elder thus provide one of the many intermediate links between the Romantic psychiatry of Ideler and the later dynamic psychiatries of Freud, Bleuler, and Jung.

By most accounts, Jung the Elder was a man of irresistible charm, kindhearted, tactful, and humorous. He had a certain inclination for the mysterious. He wrote two theater plays, which he published under a pseudonym, and he became head of the Swiss Freemasons. According to a widespread legend, he was an illegitimate son of Goethe. Scholarly inquiry, however, shows this rumor to be totally unfounded.[15] His famous grandson did much to propagate this legend in his youth but denied it later. The semi-legendary figure of the grandfather had a powerful impact upon his grandson, even though the latter was born eleven years after his grandfather's death. Although his first name was spelled "Karl" in city records, the

[14] Ernst Jung, *Aus meinen Leben* (Winterthur, Selbstverlag, [1909]).
[15] Zumstein-Preiswerk, *C. G. Jungs Medium*, 113–19.

psychiatrist adopted the antiquated spelling of "Carl" as if to identify himself with his illustrious grandfather.

C. G. Jung the Elder was apparently not happy in his personal life. His first wife, Virginie de l'Assault, died from tuberculosis at the age of 24, leaving four children, of whom three also died from the disease. His second marriage with Elizabeth Katharina Reyenthaler gave rise to a new legend. It was said that Jung the Elder went to the mayor of Basel, asking for the hand of his daughter, Sophie Frey. The mayor turned down his request; thereupon he went straight to a local tavern and asked a waitress if she wanted to marry him. She accepted at once and the marriage, to the consternation of many people, took place immediately. According to Stefanie Zumstein-Preiswerk, Jung the Elder's second wife entered his house at the age of 15 to take care of the children of his first wife. He married her three years later and had three children by her. She died giving birth to her third child. This time, the Mayor Frey granted him his daughter. She in turn gave him six children.

Of the thirteen children from the three marriages of Carl Gustav Jung the Elder, two deserve special mention. One, also named Carl Gustav, the third child of the second wife, was born on January 5, 1833, the day of his mother's death. Obviously, she died in childbirth, a circumstance that necessarily impeded the emotional development of the child. For some reason the young boy became a *Sorgenkind* ("child of sorrow"), a rebellious child who seemed unable to put himself to rights. In the end, the father resorted to a desperate measure: in 1853, at the age of 20, the son was exiled to America.[16] There were rumors that the son married, had four children, and had become a medical doctor. Eventually, on July 4, 1888, the brothers and sisters of the Jung family went to the *Zivil Gericht*, where they declared under oath that they had no news of him.[17] Thereupon he was officially declared to be dead since January 20, 1873. This was recorded in the *Verfallbuch*, that is, the register of people who disappeared, in which his name was followed by the letters "M.D." This would suggest that he had found a protector, studied medicine, and became a physician. The rest remains a mystery.

The second noteworthy child of Carl Gustav Jung the Elder was Paul Achilles (1842–1896), the fifth child of Sophie Frey. Paul Achilles' life is devoid of romantic features. He displayed a strong scholarly interest in classical and Oriental languages. He completed a Ph.D. dissertation, which dealt with a "Commentary on Solomon's Song," written in Arabic

---

[16] Ernst Jung, *Aus den Tagebüchern meines Vaters C. G. Jung* (Winterthur, Selbstverlag, [1912?]).

[17] I am grateful to Mr. Beat Glaus for providing me with a photocopy of the corresponding page of this official record.

by a Jewish scholar in the tenth century A.D., and could have been an
opening to a career as an Orientalist. However, for unknown reasons, Paul
Jung took up theology instead and spent the rest of his life as a modest
country minister.[18] According to most accounts, he was a good man, well
liked and respected by his parishioners.

In his *Memoirs*, Jung complains that his father (Paul Achilles Jung)
dissipated himself in futile activities and that his personal development had
ceased with his student years. Jung also had doubts about his father's
religious faith. He felt that his parents' marriage was not a happy one. One
of Jung's aphorisms was that "nothing is more important for the destiny of
a man than the life his parents have not lived." This undoubtedly applied to
Jung himself. He compensated in his life for the lack of ambition he had
sensed in his father. Jung's wide erudition in the history of religions was
more like that of a theologian than a physician; it is as if he had taken over
these studies at the very point at which his father had given them up.

The link between the Preiswerk and the Jung families of Basel was forged
by the marriage of Paul Achilles Jung to Emilie Preiswerk, the youngest
daughter of his professor of Hebrew. Extant descriptions of Emilie Jung
Preiswerk (1848–1923) are somewhat contradictory: she was described as
a capable and sociable lady, but also as a fat, ugly, authoritarian, and
haughty person afflicted with depressive moods. Like her father, she believed fully in the existence of spirits and is said to have had parapsychological experiences about which she kept a diary. The couple had two
children: Carl Gustav, the psychologist, and Gertrud, who was nine years
younger. Both were on good terms with the family of uncle Rudolf Preiswerk. Uncle Rudolf was the godfather of Carl Gustav, who often spent time
in his workshop. One of Helly's sisters, Louise (known as Luggy), one year
older than Carl Gustav, often did housework for Aunt Emilie. Later, in a
letter to his friend Andreas Vischer, Carl Gustav wrote that Luggy had been
his first love. She had also been an assiduous participant in the mediumistic
sittings of the 1890s, although she did not believe in spirits.

The End of the Story

After the painful termination of the mediumistic experiments, Helene
Preiswerk and her friend Emmy Zinsstag went to Montpellier, where
Emmy had relatives. There, Helene began an apprenticeship in dressmaking. One year later, the two friends moved to Paris. They lived in Versailles,
and they worked in the big city. One of Helly's sisters, Valerie Preiswerk,

---

[18] Paul Achilles Jung, *Über des Pharisäers Jophet arabische Erklärung des Hohen Liedes*
(Göttingen, 1868), 30.

decided to join them. She arrived sometime in October 1902. There was no question that a 19-year-old girl would travel alone from Basel to Paris by railway, so Carl acted as chaperon. His biographers explain that he had taken a leave of absence from the Burghölzli Hospital in order to come to Paris and to study with Pierre Janet.

Meanwhile, during the previous two years, Carl had passed his final medical examinations, had joined the staff of the famous University Mental Hospital Burghölzli in Zurich, and had completed a period of military service. He had also written his medical dissertation, in which he related in detail the story of Helene Preiswerk. Apparently Helly did not yet know that her story would be publicized in such a way.

Both Jung and his biographers have always chosen to remain reticent about this episode in his life. However, some recently discovered and un-published letters throw light upon Jung's sojourn to Paris. In a letter writ-ten to his friend Andreas Vischer, Carl goes into great detail about his current occupations.[19] He is enthusiastic about the beauty of the French capital but deplores the laxity of mores. He gets up late in the morning and spends hours rambling through the streets. He frequents the marvelous museums where one can buy reproductions of etchings at fair prices. He devotes two hours a week to Janet's lectures, with no further comment, unfortunately, about either the lectures or Janet. Every day he takes a lesson of English at the Berlitz School. He also reports that he writes a long letter to his bride-to-be every third day. Curiously enough, he does not mention a word about his visits to his cousins and her friend in Paris. But Stefanie Zumstein-Preiswerk has discovered three letters that Jung wrote to Helly toward the end of his stay there. On November 15, 1902, that is, on Helly's birthday, Jung had invited her and Valerie to the theater. In his last letter, dated January 11, 1903, he tells of his leaving Paris to spend a dozen days in England and how he would then return to Switzerland to get married on February 14.

Back in Switzerland, Jung's dissertation had appeared in print under the title *On the Psychology and Pathology of So-Called Occult Phenomena*. The thesis won an enthusiastic review by Théodore Flournoy, the man who had studied another medium for several years.[20] However, in Basel specifi-cally, the reception was different. Although he had used pseudonyms and altered the chronology, the identities of the characters were soon recog-nized. Some of his descriptions were rather unflattering, and many Preis-werk relatives were deeply hurt. In those days, considerable stress was placed on heredity, and the whole maternal side of the family appeared now to be tainted with insanity. (Later, rumors circulated that the younger

[19] C. G. Jung to Andreas Vischer, December 14, 1902.
[20] *Archives de Psychologie*, 2 (1903), 85–86.

Preiswerk daughters could not find husbands because of Jung's dissertation.) Publication of the dissertation in fact aroused a storm of indignation among the Preiswerk family and their numerous relatives and friends.
Carl Gustav complained about the narrow-mindedness of the "Preis-
werkerei."[21] It is even quite probable that the publication of the story of
Helene Preiswerk and the family séances cost him a career in Basel and
contributed to his move at this point to Zurich.

This makes one wonder further what was the objective result of these
experiments. Carl Gustav was convinced that he was opening a new path in
the study of the human soul. He understood fully that he was not dealing
with the voice of the disembodied in these séances, but rather with projections of unconscious material, that is, with what he called "psychological
realities." Furthermore, he studied the development of the medium's personality and understood that she was struggling against barriers that impeded the development of her personality. This was the early formulation
of the process the mature Jung would call "individuation."

Today, in retrospect, we are drawn to consider another facet of Carl
Gustav's relationship to Helene Preiswerk. At first, it seems that Jung was
not much interested in Helene's personality; she was only the subject of an
intellectual inquiry. Gradually, in fact, he became bored with her, the more
so when he perceived that she was in love with him. The picture he gave of
her in his dissertation is one governed by contempt. Later, when he saw her
again in Paris, he realized that Helene was a sensible and charming personality. He was attracted to her, but she was reserved. This is quite plainly
stated by Emmy Zinsstag, who observes that "the roles were reversed."[22]
This psychological situation created a pattern that was revived later when
Carl Gustav Jung met Sabina Spielrein, the young Jewish woman who
became in turn his analysand and his mistress.[23] The similarity was soon
understood by Jung. Jung went so far as to show to Sabina an excerpt of his
own diary in which he says that he once had a vision of Helly, clad in a
luminous white robe. He had identified Helly with her guardian angel,
Ivènes, and projected this vision onto Sabina. This may well have been the
origin of Jung's concept of anima.

As for Helly, we do not know what her reaction was when she saw her
painful story printed for all the public to see or when she read of Carl
Gustav's negative judgment of her character. In late 1903, Preiswerk left
Paris and with her sister Valerie returned to her hometown of Basel, where
she opened a dressmaker's shop. According to Jung, she made dresses of

[21] Jung to Vischer, August 22, 1904.
[22] Quoted in Zumstein-Preiswerk, C. G. Jungs Medium, 100.
[23] Aldo Carotenuto, A Secret Symmetry: Sabina Spielrein between Freud and Jung (New
York, Pantheon, 1982).

rare elegance. In 1911, at the age of only 30, Helene died of tuberculosis. Jung said that during the last few months of her life she underwent a process of slow emotional disintegration and fell to the level of a 2-year-old child. Stefanie Zumstein-Preiswerk, however, has maintained that Helene was entirely clear-minded until the end and declares instead that "she died of a broken heart."[24]

[24] Zumstein-Preiswerk, C. G. *Jungs Medium*, 110.

Part Four

THEMES IN THE HISTORY OF
PSYCHIATRIC IDEAS

12

The Fallacies of Psychiatric
Classification

[1963]

THE PRESENT ESSAY is not designed to evaluate the respective merits of different schemes of classification of mental illness. Nor does it aim to propose a new system of classification. Rather, its goal is simply to bring to attention several historical points that seem thus far to have escaped the attention of the authors of psychiatric nosologies.

In order to achieve its goals, any body of organized knowledge has to establish a system of methodological rules; but it must also set down the errors of methodology to avoid. When the ancient Greeks first formulated the fundamental rules of logic, they also gave their attention to defining the diverse types of sophisms. After stating the principles of scientific research, Francis Bacon in the early seventeenth century also described the numerous "idols" that the scientist had to avoid (such as prejudice, the uncritical admission of tradition, the romance of words, and so on). When René Descartes wrote about "the guidelines for the direction of intelligence," Spinoza soon thereafter directed a treatise to "the purification of understanding." In the time of Bacon, Descartes, and Spinoza, it was primarily a matter only of conscious, *intellectual* errors in thinking. However, with the publication in 1947 of Gaston Bachelard's study of scientific epistemology, with its emphasis on the disruptive role that emotional and unconscious factors may play in scientific research, a new factor was introduced into this question.[1] In the present essay, I would like to take Bachelard's work as the starting point from which to inquire specifically into the problem of psychiatric classification. What irrational factors and unconscious motivations have played a role in the creation, elaboration, and selection of systems of psychiatric classification in the past? Before proceeding to the

"Les illusions de la classification psychiatrique," *L'évolution psychiatrique*, 28, no. 2 (April–June 1963), 221–42; "Le aberrazioni della classificazione psichiatrica," in Ellenberger, *I movimenti di liberazione mitica*, 79–99.

[1] Gaston Bachelard, *La formation de l'esprit scientifique: Contribution à une psychanalyse de la connaissance objective* (Paris, Vrin, 1947).

subject itself, I should briefly sum up some features of psychiatric nosologies in general.[2]

Scientific Nosologies and Their Problems

Nearly all contemporary psychiatric nosologies rest more or less tacitly on the belief that mental illnesses constitute specific pathological entities that may be meaningfully gathered into a natural classification, comparable in this regard to classificatory systems in botany and zoology. In other words, the "principle of specificity" which, Armand Trousseau observed, "dominates the whole of medicine," and which established its greatest successes in the field of infectious illnesses, is extended also to psychiatry. The discovery of general paralysis of the insane in 1822 served for generations of physicians as an irrefutable demonstration that this medical principle could be applied equally to psychiatry. From the early nineteenth century onward, then, most authors believed that the insufficiencies of psychiatric classification came either from a defective delimitation of "nosological entities" or from the inaccurate selection of classificatory criteria. When these two sources of difficulty were eliminated, it was believed, the perfect system of classification could be achieved and would be agreed upon permanently by everyone, as was the case in botanical and zoological science.

In erecting their systems, past nosologists have begun by choosing between three fundamental approaches, which reflect their views of the nature of mental illnesses. These approaches are those of natural classification, artificial classification, and no classification at all. The first solution, the utilization of natural classification, has a very long lineage. The Roman physician Galen described this approach appreciatively in the work of Mnesithius, an Athenian physician: "Mnesithius thought that one should begin with the most general classes of things, to establish progressively species, genders, and varieties. After these divisions, others could be made, and again still others, until one finally comes to obtain an indivisible unity."[3] Classifications of this sort abounded above all during the nineteenth century. The work of nosologists in this mold consisted, as I have said, in isolating specific morbid entities and then in locating some criterion of classification based on clinical characteristics, on projected etiology, or on some other principle.

---

[2] I will not address here the philosophical and epistemological aspects of classification in regard to the mental sciences. For this subject, refer to Jean Piaget, *La genèse du nombre chez l'enfant* (Neuchâtel and Paris, Delachaux, 1941); and idem, *Introduction à l'épistémologie génétique*, 3 vols. (Paris, Presses Universitaires de France, 1950).

[3] Galen, *Oeuvres anatomiques, physiologiques et médicales de Galien*, translated from the Latin by Charles Victor Daremberg (Paris, Baillière, 1856), 2:707.

A second approach to the challenge of classification is through artificial classifications. The most common artificial methods are based on statistics of some sort. Let us imagine that in a group of patients we are looking for the symptoms a, b, c, d, e, f, and g. In some patients, we will find a constellation characterized by symptoms a, b, and c in an average degree of intensity, e in a mild form, and no sign of f and g. According to classifications of this sort, these cases will be gathered into category I. All of the other cases differing from this group in only one or two symptoms will be gathered into a second category, and so on. A notable modern-day attempt of this type was made by Carlos Seguin and his collaborators and was reported in a preliminary presentation to the World Congress of Psychiatry in 1961.[4] In a random selection of 1,000 psychiatric patients, Seguin identified after observations 530 different symptoms. With the help of electric calculators, he then tabulated and classified patients based on their symptom profiles. Patients with only one or two symptoms were eliminated. Seven symptoms predominated, and most patients revealed three, four, five, six, or seven symptoms in different combinations. The challenge was then to organize these patients into clinical categories—ninety-nine categories in all—based on the patterned combination of the symptoms. According to Seguin's team, there emerged nine statistically meaningful groups that could be said to constitute "clinical pictures."

A third approach to psychiatric classification is pursued by those authors, such as Heinrich Neumann, who asserted that all psychiatric classification is meaningless and should be discarded.[5] According to Neumann, "there is no mental illness; there are only patients." If we desire to find some order in the multiplicity of clinical cases, we need only place these cases in a continuous series. The difficulty here is to arrive at some meaningful serial principle. In Spain, Bartolomy Llopis has adopted a clinical continuum based on the phenomenology of states of consciousness, ranging from the clearest to the darkest consciousness.[6] In the United States, Karl Menninger uses a continuum based on the degree of disorganization of the self under the influence of progressively increasing stress.[7] This method implies a notion of the psychological self as a homeostatic system and of psychological problems as the result of environmental anxiety.

In addition to natural and artificial classifications, as well as the nosologies of the anticlassifiers, there have been intermediate systems, such

[4] Carlos Seguin, Renato Castro, Oscar Valdivia, and Sergio Zapata, "Cuadros clínicos y cultura: Sobre un nuevo método de agrupación nosográfica en psiquiatría," Congrès mondial de psychiatrie, held in Montreal, June 1961.

[5] Heinrich Neumann, *Lehrbuch der Psychiatrie* (Erlangen, F. Enke, 1859), 75–76, 167.

[6] Bartolomy Llopis, "La psicosis única," *Archivo de neurobiología*, 17 (1954), 1–39.

[7] Karl Menninger et al., "The Unitary Concept of Mental Illness," *Bulletin of the Menninger Clinic*, 22 (1958), 4–12.

as the well-known system of Henri Ey, but these will not be examined here. My goal, again, is only to point out certain persistent sources of errors that classifiers have been open to in the history of psychiatry. The examination of over a hundred psychiatric nosological structures reveals three general recurrent sources of error.* These fallacies concern: (1) incomplete or inaccurate conceptions about the basic nature and the function of classification; (2) the extrapolation of a classificatory schema from other branches of science or medicine to psychiatry; and (3) the unconscious expression or projection of the personal affective characteristics of the author onto a nosological structure.

The Fallacies of Clinical Pragmatism and Philosophical Idealism

The first category of error results from a classificatory orientation that is directed too exclusively toward either the concrete and practical or the abstract and philosophical. The process of classification belongs to that class of mental procedures that Pierre Janet called "double operations— *conduites doubles*." The act consists in coordinating the dual operations of specification and abstraction. The French language clearly differentiates between the concrete action of *classement* and the abstract operation of *classification*. In this view, classification is the larger plan according to which each individual classing or filing is made while filing is the material work that, without a guiding plan of classification, would be incoherent.[8]

Occasionally, we find that a psychiatric nosologist has restricted himself to one of these two procedures or that he accentuates too much one of them. This results in one of two errors, which we will call, for lack of better terms, the *pragmatic fallacy* and the *idealist fallacy*.

The *pragmatic fallacy* appears in those nosologists who seek to reduce the classification of mental and nervous illnesses to an immediate, useful, and clinically practical procedure. Every other concern is secondary or superficial to them. An example of this phenomenon may be found in Joseph Daquin's system of classification. At the end of the eighteenth century, Daquin proposed to classify the insane according to the follow scheme:

---

*[*Editor's note*: The great number of psychiatric nosologies that Ellenberger gathered and examined in preparation for this essay were later published, with commentary, by his former colleagues at the Menninger Clinic. See Karl Menninger, with Martin Mayman and Paul Pruyser, *The Vital Balance: The Life Process in Mental Health and Illness* (New York, Viking, 1963), Appendix, 419–89.]

[8] On this difference, see Thérèse Leroy, *La technique du classement: La science de la classologie* (Paris, Guy le Prat, 1945).

1. Raving lunatics (or maniacs)
2. Quiet lunatics (to be confined without being tied up)
3. Eccentrics (to be watched over constantly)
4. The insane (with unpredictable behavior)
5. Imbeciles (to be directed like children)
6. Demented lunatics (to be cared for physically)[9]

Another example may be found in the classification of the early-seventeenth-century English forensic lawyer Sir Edmund Coke, who distinguished four main groups of abnormal psychological subjects:

1. Natural fools (irresponsible from birth)
2. The insane (at one time normal but now insane)
3. Lunatics (who occasionally recover their reason)
4. Normal individuals (who only occasionally and momentarily lose their reason, for instance, during a drunken spell or a seizure)[10]

Classificatory schemes such as those of Daquin and Coke are actually only filing systems designed to meet an immediate and practical need. The director of a mental hospital may need to decide quickly in what part of the institution new patients are to be placed; or a lawyer may require a practical means to describe the degree of responsibility of an accused person suspected of having psychiatric problems. Very probably, such classifications have occasionally played a role in the history of full-scale psychiatric nosologies. For instance, Philippe Pinel's classification in the second edition of his great treatise on insanity presents a system that is even more summary than Daquin's ("manias," "melancholias," "dementias," and "idiotism") and that has such a utilitarian aspect.

The *idealist fallacy* represents the contrary of the pragmatic one. Nosologists falling into this trap replace an overemphasis on the real with an accent on the "idea" of mental illness. They reduce classification to an abstraction. There is nothing easier than to erect a system of classification that ignores the clinical facts themselves. Ancient Greek and Indian mythologies, for instance, offer examples of hierarchies of gods, demigods, heroes, nymphs, monsters, and dragons that were carefully classified according to their species and genres. Unfortunately, some designers of psychiatric nosologies have not done much better than this.

---

[9] Joseph Daquin, *La philosophie de la folie ou essai philosophique sur le traitement des personnes attaquées de folie* (Paris, Cléaz, 1792): "1) Fous furieux (ou 'fous à lier'); 2) Fous tranquilles (à enfermer sans les attacher); 3) Extravagants (à surveiller constamment); 4) Insensés (à comportement imprévisible); 5) Imbéciles (à conduire comme des enfants); 6) Fous en démence (ayant besoin de soins physiques)."

[10] Cited in John C. Bucknill and D. Hack Tuke, *A Manual of Psychological Medicine*, 4th ed. (London, Churchill, 1879), 25.

Some, for instance, have sought to synthesize all preceding terms and doctrines. Robert Burton, the famous author of *The Anatomy of Melancholy* (1621), was not a physician; but he seems to have read every medical and literary work about this subject from his time.[11] For Burton, the word *melancholy* had a very imprecise meaning and applied to any and every kind of mental disease and intellectual defect. Therefore, Burton had to divide and subdivide melancholy into countless varieties. Burton himself claimed that this classification, which attempted to reconcile and integrate the opinions of all preexisting authors, was "a labyrinth of uncertainties and errors." The result was an extremely heterogenous system as well as a very dense book that is saved from oblivion only by its literary qualities.

Other authors through the generations have ignored their predecessors' proposals and have built totally a priori psychiatric nosologies. Immanuel Kant, who had no personal or clinical experience of mental illnesses, nevertheless described their diverse forms, which he thought could be deduced from the normal functions of the mind. In an appendix to his *Anthropologie* of 1798, Kant in this way published a classification of mental diseases which, to say the least, fell down in its excessive abstraction.[12]

Pragmatic and idealist fallacies belong to that category of error that Bacon called "the idols of the cave," that is, fallacies issuing from the author's personal intellectual viewpoint. In the first case, a practitioner is too absorbed by his clinical and administrative work and fails to perceive the need for a theoretical perspective. In the second, the abstract thinker remains remote from the human reality of his subject. The most readable chapter in *The Anatomy of Melancholy* remains the one in which Burton describes the pains of "scholar's melancholy," from which he suffered himself.

The Projection of Faulty Intellectual Models

Another group of sources of error in psychiatric classification results from the existence of particular intellectual habits or assumptions in the mind of the classifier which, without his knowledge, exert a directing influence on both the form and content of the nosological conceptions. Such are the *numerical*, the *linguistic*, and the *sociocentric* fallacies, as well as the fallacy of what we might call *disciplinary projection*.

[11] Robert Burton, *The Anatomy of Melancholy* (Oxford, John Lichfield, 1621).

[12] Immanuel Kant, *Anthropologie in pragmatischer Hinsicht* [1798], edited by J. H. Kirchmann, 3d ed. (Leipzig, E. Koshny, 1880), Appendix.

The Numerical Fallacy

It has often been noticed that individuals tend to have a conscious or unconscious predilection for a certain number or numerical system. Such individuals tend to organize or classify everything by 2, 3, 4, or some other number. As Théodore Flournoy has observed, "every individual has a marked predilection or aversion for some numbers without knowing it. These idiosyncrasies are permanent and were found again after a lapse of time of four years."[13] The most frequent predilections are for the numbers 3, 5, and 7. We do not know, however, if the "favorite numbers" expressed under experimental conditions are the same ones that have exercised so much influence on the theoretical conceptions of nosologists.

The number 2, for instance, was exalted by German Romantics, either as complementary notions or as systems of polarities or as sets of antagonists. In this regard, Freud resembles the Romantics. Ernest Jones asserts of Freud that "he felt completely unfamiliar with any kind of pluralism."[14] Mental life, according to Freud, was dominated by polarities, such as subjects–objects, pleasure–displeasure, activity–passivity, Eros–Thanatos. Jones adds that some people said jokingly that Freud had never learned to count further than the number 2.

Other theorists have tended to employ a binary system that in turn is divided by 2, and then by 4, and so on. Michael Balint notes that, in Leopold Szondi's system, everything can be divided by 2 and its multiples, but nothing by 3 or 5. So, Szondi distinguishes two classes of reactions subdivided into four forms; there are then four vectors, eight factors, sixteen impulsive classes, and so forth.[15] In Galenic doctrine, everything goes by 4. There are four physical qualities, four matters, four elements, four humors, four degrees, four natural functions, four ages of life, and so on. There also exists the peculiar phenomenon of "quatromania": the number 4 is represented by a square the sides of which constitute two sets of polarities. This was the case in Jean Fernel's system of the humors of the body; today, C. G. Jung's theory of psychological functions is another example of this.

Many fields of thought have privileged ternary systems. In his treatise

---

13 Théodore Flournoy, "Sur l'association des chiffres chez les divers individus," *III Internationaler Congress für Psychologie*, Munich, August 4–7, 1896 (Munich, J. F. Lehmann, 1897), 221–22.

14 Ernest Jones, *The Life and Work of Sigmund Freud*, 3 vols. (New York, Basic Books, 1953–1957), 2:318.

15 Michael Balint, "On Szondi's *Schicksalsanalyse* and *Triebdiagnostik*," *International Journal of Psychoanalysis*, 29 (1948), 240–49.

On Celestial Hierarchy, Denys l'Areopagite divided the angels into three orders, each of which is subdivided into three classes to make a total of nine classes. Dante's *Divine Comedy* gives another good example of a ternary structure. Ternary psychiatric classifications were frequent in Germany at the beginning of the nineteenth century, the most famous being that of Johann Christian Heinroth.[16]

The phenomenon of the "favorite number" does not occur only on the individual level. It also happens collectively, either as a sacred number (or number having a magical meaning) or simply as a basic number for many other numerations and classifications. We know that the number 7 was very important for the ancient Babylonians, as our seven-day week testifies today. Among North American Indians, the number 4 played a great role. Ethnologists have gathered abundant documentation of this fact.[17] I might also mention the use of the number 10 in the *quipous* of the ancient Peruvians.[18] These small cords, the *quipous*, were used for very complex countings and relied on a system of decimal classification. This is an example of a very rational artificial classificatory system, comparable to the universal decimal classification, created in 1873, as we know it, by the American librarian Melvil Dewey.

Flournoy observed that the number 1 hardly ever appeared as a favorite number in his experimental evidence. However, on the collective psychological level, several observers have noticed its importance in the United States. "It's one world" is a popular American saying that reveals this mentality, which aspires to a single, unified, even homogenized society in which distinctions of origins, nationality, and language tend to be erased. It is striking for a foreigner to see how vigorously American sociologists deny the notion of social class and replace it with that of a "continuum" of degrees of material wealth and social welfare. Is it just a coincidence that it is precisely in America today that the notion of psychiatric classification is resisted and replaced by that of a "continuum" and a "unitary theory of mental illnesses"?

In conclusion, the phenomenon of the "favorite number," whether on the individual or collective level, can be the object of a conscious or unconscious projection producing a kind of numerical fantasy for the classifier. When we see Heinroth dividing all mental illnesses into three orders, each of which had three types, and each of them four species, for a total of nine

[16] Johann Christian Heinroth, *Lehrbuch der Störungen des Seelenlebens*, 2 vols. (Leipzig, Vogel, 1818).

[17] See the work of the German mathematician Karl Menninger, *Zahlwort und Ziffer: Eine Kulturgeschichte der Zahl*, 2 vols. (Göttingen, Vandenhoeck & Ruprecht, 1958).

[18] L. Leland Locke, *The Ancient Quipu or Peruvian Knot Record* (New York, American Museum of Natural History, 1923).

types and thirty-six species, we can only marvel at how geometrical nature is!

The Linguistic Fallacy

In 1836, Wilhelm von Humboldt published a famous work on the structure of the varieties of human language.[19] Humboldt claimed that language was "the constructive organ of thought" and that the highest function of language was to generate thought through the combination of concepts, which in turn depended on the structure of the language used. These ideas have recently been repeated and elaborated by two American researchers, Edward Sapir and Benjamin L. Whorf. Sapir and Whorf have tried to define the ways in which the dominant philosophy of a given population is structured by its language, that is, the ways in which language constitutes in itself the first system of classification.[20]

For their part, historians of philosophy and science have also shown the ways in which the development of scientific disciplines depends upon the language employed. For instance, F. M. Cornford asserts that Greek philosophers, knowing no other language than their own, believed that the structure of the Greek language reflected directly the structure of the universe itself. As Cornford writes: "Plato wrote a dialogue, *Cratylus*, in order to refute the belief that everything has a name which naturally belongs to it. . . . Aristotle resolved several problems by showing that a given term had several meanings."[21] However, grammar and logic were first established in India and in Greece most likely because their thinkers had at their disposal languages of rare perfection, Sanskrit and ancient Greek, which operated in themselves as excellent tools for the analysis and constitution of thought. It is very unlikely that the same sort of work could be accomplished using a language without grammatical structure, such as Chinese (whatever the literary qualities of the language of Confucius may be).

These psycholinguistic considerations can enlighten the study of psychiatric nosologies in two important ways. First, the words that are to designate the diseases themselves are necessarily borrowed from the vocabulary of the classifier's language. Now it is well known how difficult it is to

19 Wilhelm von Humboldt, *Über die Verschiedenheit des menschlichen Sprachbaues* [1836], reedition (Darmstadt, Claassen & Röther, 1949).

20 Edward Sapir, "The Nature of Language," in *Selected Writings*, edited by David Mandelbaum (Los Angeles, University of California Press, 1951); Benjamin L. Whorf, *Language, Thought and Reality*, edited by John B. Carroll (New York, Wiley, 1956).

21 F. M. Cornford, *The Unwritten Philosophy* (Cambridge, Cambridge University Press, 1950), 43.

communicate from one country to another the meaning of words, not only of words that are colloquial (for example, *Sehnsucht*, *spleen*, or *cafard*) but also those that are more scientific, such as *melancholy*, *paranoia*, *psychopathy*, and the like. The difficulty increases when the communication occurs between countries of very different cultures. A psychiatrist from Tokyo, Dr. Takeo Doi, has demonstrated, for instance, the way in which Japanese psychological terms, such as *toraware* and *amaeru*, could not be meaningfully translated into European languages. The word *shinkeishitsu*, Doi adds, even though it is derived from the German *Nervosität*, has acquired such peculiar connotations that it again is effectively untranslatable.[22] If we consider populations whose mentalities are even more remote from ours, it then becomes nearly impossible to overcome this obstacle, which concerns not only individual terms but basic concepts of mental illness as well. In 1936, Hans Koritschoner published a curious study about the organization for forms of *sheitani*, or mental diseases, as taught by healers in certain areas of East Africa.[23] Koritschoner recorded the name and a brief clinical description of twenty-two different *sheitani*, each of which was designated as a differentiated disease, even though both, in name and clinical phenomenology, failed to correspond to entities in any Western nosology. The native healers classified these *sheitani* in two groups: one contains nine forms of *sheitani ya pwani*; the other contains thirteen *sheitani ya bara*. The native physicians all agreed among themselves on the groups to which each *sheitani* belonged, but Koritschoner admits that he remained completely mystified about the principle of classification.

Perhaps even more than the vocabulary, it is the grammatical structure of a language that imparts its basic principles to nosology. Our modern European languages are analytical. They distinguish categories of words (verbs, nouns, adjectives, pronouns); their verbal morphology differentiates persons, tenses, and moods; and their syntax distinguishes the subject, the verb, and the extension. Even the slightest variation in these structures of language may be reflected in systems of psychology and psychopathology.

It has been asked why the problem of the Self hardly appeared in European thought before the seventeenth century. Could this be in part a matter of linguistic usage? When Descartes said "Cogito, ergo sum," what was emphasized was the act of thinking and the facts of being themselves. But when Descartes translated the maxim into French, "Je pense, donc je

---

[22] L. Takeo Doi, "Morita Therapy and Psychoanalysis" (Unpublished essay obligingly communicated by the author).

[23] Hans Koritschoner, "Ngoma ya Sheitani: An East African Native Treatment for Psychical Disorders," *Journal of the Royal Anthropological Institute of Great Britain and Ireland*, 66 (1936), 209–19.

suis" ("I think, therefore I am"), the subject of the verb was stated separately and the problem of the Self appeared. Within modern European
languages, the differences between the pronouns alone provoke notable
conceptual variations. Let us recall how difficult it has been to transpose
the *Es* ("Id") of Freudian psychoanalysis into French. The *Ich und Du* of
Martin Buber proves just as difficult to translate. In English, should we say
"I and Thou," when English does not know the concept of the familiar
"Du," or rather, only use it when speaking in antiquated terms to God? In
Latin, will it be "Es et tu," when in this language everyone is indis-
criminately referred to with the familiar "you"? Even between French and
German, the use of this familiar "you" differs in subtle ways. Almost the
entire vocabulary of European existential analysis (*Daseinsanalyse*), copied directly from the structure of the German language, presents major
difficulties in translation.

The examination of the verbal structure of languages and its influence
upon psychiatric nosologies would be of considerable interest; but this
subject has hardly been explored. One of the very few and most original
attempts in this direction was made by the American psychiatrist Ernest
Southard earlier in the century.[24] In 1916, Southard claimed that delirious
ideas could be defined more rigorously and classified more meaningfully in
terms of their grammatical than their logical categories. Relying on the
close grammatical analysis of speeches by a number of delirious patients,
Southard found that the active voice predominates in cases of delusions of
grandeur, the passive voice in cases of persecution mania, and the reflexive
voice in manias of self-accusation. The persecution mania can be expressed
either in the first person or, more often, in the second and third persons,
differences that also correspond to other clinical distinctions. (Let it be
recalled that in chronic alcoholic hallucinosis, the patient hears himself
being mentioned in the third person.)

Southard proceeded to explore other diverse "verbal aspects" of psychopathology. There exist other capital differences, he found, between two
categories of persecution mania. In one type, the patient relates his or her
story in the perfect tense (corresponding with the Greek Aorist); in the
other type, the patient uses the imperfect, which indicates unfinished or
iterative action. As for sentence forms, Southard indicated that the imperative form is the most psychologically primitive, corresponding with the
mind of the savage or small child and with the belief in the omnipotence of
thought and language. The indicative mood little by little replaces the
imperative, just as in the life of the child the pleasure principle is replaced

---

[24] Ernest E. Southard, "On the Application of Grammatical Categories to the Analysis of
Delusions," *Philosophical Review*, 25 (1916), 424–55. I thank Dr. Karl Menninger for
bringing this article to my attention.

by the reality principle. As for the subjunctive form, it is the form for the divided or differentiated will, while the optative form is that of desire. Southard concluded by asserting that what he calls *pragmatic mania* is a "precipitate of the subjunctive form" and that *fantastic mania* is an "optative precipitate."

Southard's work, conducted over a half-century ago, does not seem to have been noticed up until now. Perhaps the recent progress of psycholinguistics will revive this line of inquiry. It would be very interesting to determine to what extent the clinical frameworks of our nosologies derive from the structures of our languages. It would also be interesting to know what kinds of nosological conceptions correspond with linguistic categories of idioms that are the most unlike the Indo-European languages, such as the Polynesian and the American-Indian languages.

The Sociocentric Fallacy

In a report written at the turn of the century that has since become a classic, the French sociologists Émile Durkheim and Marcel Mauss studied the origins of early systems of classification.[25] Durkheim and Mauss observed in that study that "every classification implies a hierarchical order for which neither the sensible world, nor our consciences, determines the pattern." Where, then, does this pattern, this hierarchy, come from? Is not an important source here the surrounding social structure? Indeed, it is noteworthy that past classifiers have spoken regularly of "affinities" (that is, "kinships") between categories, about "families," and about "genera" (words that etymologically express the idea of a familial group or genus). To highlight this problem, Durkheim and Mauss began by studying certain Australian systems of classification, which are the most primitive that are known today.

Australian tribes, Durkheim and Mauss noted, are all divided into two "phratries," which in turn are generally subdivided into two "matrimonial classes," which often include several "totemic clans." "In other words, every member of a tribe is categorized into well-defined classes which cohere closely within the society. Now, the system of the classification of *things* in these societies reproduces this classification of men." In the simplest tribes, which know only a bipartite division of two phratries, the natural world too—stars, plants, animals, and so on—is distributed between two phratries: for instance, between the sun and the moon in one

---

[25] Émile Durkheim and Marcel Mauss, "De quelques formes primitives de classification: Contribution à l'étude des représentations collectives," *L'année sociologique*, 6 (1901–1902), 1–72.

category, and the wind and the rain in another. In other tribes in which human beings are distributed into two phratries and four classes, we move beyond a simple dichotomy of the natural order. Here, we find a more hierarchical conception of the universe. In more complexly organized tribes, classified into phratries, matrimonial classes, and clans, the world becomes comparable to a large, heterogeneous tribe. "If totemism is in certain ways the gathering of men into clans according to the natural objects associated with totemic practices," Durkheim and Mauss conclude, "then it is also on the contrary a gathering of natural objects according to the dominant social structure."

Moving from Australia to North America, Durkheim and Mauss found more elaborate systems of classification. Among the Zunis, for instance, "the notion that society maintains of itself and the representation it has constructed of its surrounding world are so interconnected that one can very accurately describe their organization as mytho-sociological." Animate and inanimate creatures, natural phenomena, and the elements are classed into a single, interdependent system "whose parts are all coordinated and subordinated to each other according to the degrees of kinship in the society." The universe is divided into seven regions—North, West, South, East, Zenith, Nadir, and Center—and every being, animate and inanimate, and every kind of human activity is classified into one of these seven regions.

With one more degree of complexity, Durkheim and Mauss reach the astrological Chinese system, which results, the authors tell us, from the combination of several previous systems. One system is based on the division of space into four regions and eight subregions or "powers"; the other one is based on the distinction between five elements of the world. Two cycles, then, follow these two systems, and, through a combination of elements and cycles, the Chinese calendar is formed. In this way, every being, living or inert, as well as many abstract concepts, is incorporated into a highly artificial but comprehensive system of classification. According to Durkheim and Mauss, the origin of this system is undoubtedly sociological, particularly with regard to the divisions of space, which originally paralleled social subdivisions. In the end, then, "the starting point of the first schematizations of nature was not the individual but the social."

The report of Durkheim and Mauss has been criticized over the years on points of fact by specialists.[26] But, coming back to the subject of this essay, we can only wonder what role the "sociocentric fallacy" has played in determining the nature and structure of psychiatric nosologies. The proclivity of certain Hindu civilizations for very clear-cut, rigid, and artificial systems of classification, in their nosologies, philosophies, and myth-

---

[26] Claude Lévi-Strauss, *La pensée sauvage* (Paris, Plon, 1962), chap. 2.

ologies, has been observed by many people. And American society, as mentioned before, is diametrically opposed to the idea of systems of immutable casts or hierarchies. The phenomenon of the American "melting pot" occasionally seems to be reflected in nosology, for instance, in a marked preference for unitary systems of conceptualization and classification.

Other, more specific correspondences can be found, too. In antiquity, with the birth of the first great political states, complex and hierarchical systems of classification appeared in many areas of culture and human activity: within the nobility and the military, in provincial and administrative governments, and so on. It was said that the scientific treatise *On Celestial Hierarchy*, by Denys l'Areopagite, attributed to the celestial powers a hierarchy that reflected that of the Imperial Court's dignitaries of Byzantium.

Another example of the phenomenon, closer temporally and perhaps less questionable, concerns the famous naturalist Carolus Linnaeus. Linnaeus's system of nature is striking because of its sociomorphic nature. Linnaeus considered the world of nature a large empire divided into great realms or "kingdoms": animal, vegetable, and mineral. At the very bottom of the scale were the countless living creatures whose nomenclature was very confused. Linnaeus first attributed to all life forms a double name. This binary system of designation paralleled the nomenclatural system, which had just been adopted by society at large, and consisted of a family name preceded by a first name. Linnaeus had brought order to the chaos of the botanical world. According to Louis Agassiz's history of zoological classification, Linnaeus, good classical Latinist that he was, transposed the divisions of the Roman political, military, and administrative systems into the field of plants.[27] Linnaeus is even said to have used the following system of equivalences:

Botany:	Classis	Ordo	Genus	Species	Varietas	
Roman Army:	Legiones	Cohortes	Manipuli	Contubernia	Miles	

It is well known that Linnaeus then applied his system of botanical classification to the field of zoology, and from there to medical nosologies, which of course includes psychiatric nosology.

Fallacies of Contemporaneous Disciplinary Models

When we examine the history of psychiatric classifications as well as of botanical and zoological ones, we are often struck by the curious "family

[27] Louis Agassiz, "Essay on Classification," in *Contributions to the Natural History of the United States of America* (Boston, Little, Brown and Co., 1857–1862), 1:189–90.

resemblances" between different systems from the same period. For example, we know that the eighteenth century was a time when detailed and highly systematic classificatory systems met with great success. In medicine, zoology, and botany, these systems often seem to be copied one from the other. This was often quite literally the case, and in some instances, the authors of the systems were the same. François Boissier de Sauvages, for instance, in his *Traité des classes de maladies*, distinguished ten classes, subdivided into four orders and twenty-three types. One of his disease types, melancholy, included fourteen species. Obviously, Boissier de Sauvages was adapting here the principles of Linnaean systematics to a branch of medicine. Conversely, Linnaeus, we know, imitated Boissier de Sauvages when he wrote his treatise on nosology, the *Genera Morborum*, in which he revised Boissier de Sauvages's classification and terminology. Throughout the eighteenth century, there arose across Europe systems of classification in which animals, plants, physical and mental illnesses, even chemical bodies, were classified minutely into classes, orders, genera, species, and varieties.

The French Revolution at the end of the eighteenth century brought a revolution in classificatory science, too. The best illustration of this sudden change is in the work of Philippe Pinel, who, in 1798, published his *Nosographie philosophique*, a complex and highly detailed schema for classifying mental illnesses in the mold of earlier botanical classifications. But, only three years later, in 1801, Pinel published his *Traité médico-philosophique de la folie*, in which he proposed no more than four major types of mental illness: mania, melancholy, dementia, and idiotism. Can it be purely coincidental that Georges Cuvier, the great French naturalist, had at this exact same time thrown the previous systems of zoological classification into confusion with his new, radically simplified classification of animals into four great "embranchments" (Vertebrates, Molluscs, Jointed or Segmental Animals, and Radiata or Zoophytes)?

At roughly the same time in Germany, philosophical Romanticism was influencing natural science and medicine, including psychiatry. We can get a glimpse of this tendency by comparing two characteristic classifications of the time. Lorenz Oken was one of the most eminent German naturalists of the nineteenth century. Oken considered man the highest being in the creation, the key to the entire animal kingdom, and the stage of perfection toward which all other species strove. Everything that existed in the animal world, he found in correspondence in man. Oken classified animals into five "cycles" and thirteen "classes":

Cycle I: Digestive Animals
  Class 1: Infusoria
  Class 2: Polyps

    Class 3: Acalephas
Cycle II: Circulatory Animals
    Class 4: Acephals
    Class 5: Gasteropods
    Class 6: Cephalopods
Cycle III: Respiratory Animals
    Class 7: Worms
    Class 8: Crustaceans
    Class 9: Insects
Cycle IV: Fleshy Animals
    Class 10: Fish
    Class 11: Reptiles
    Class 12: Birds
Cycle V: Sensorial Animals
    Class 13: Mammals[28]

We can see that Oken's zoological groups appear like "disjecta membra" of the human organism, that is, they seem to be reduced to the organ system believed to be the most perfected.

We might now briefly consider Heinroth's contemporaneous classification for mental illnesses. Heinroth first discerned three fundamental faculties in the human mind: affectivity, intellect, and will. According to him, any mental disease consisted either of a depression, an exaltation, or a mixed state of depression and exaltation, of one of the three faculties. This resulted in nine basic forms of mental dysfunction:

	Exaltation	Depression	Mixed State
Affectivity	Wahnsinn	Melancholia	Wahnsinnige
Intellect	Verrücktheit	Blödsinn	Verwirrtheit
Will	Mania	Willenlosigkeit	Scheue

Heinroth then subdivided each of these nine categories into four species, whose specific nomenclature is not important here. We can already see from this schematization that, to Heinroth, mental illness was identified in some ways with a single great function of the human mind. Since it is highly improbable that Heinroth and Oken inspired one another directly, we are led to suggest that both men created their respective theories according to a common conceptual schema at the time, as was the case for Pinel and Cuvier, and Linnaeus and Bossier de Sauvages.

[28] Cited in ibid., 212–13.

The Unconscious Motivations of the Classifier

Finally, two kinds of psychiatrists may be said to exist. The great majority of psychiatrists do not pay much attention to the business of classifications, or they merely use the system that is most convenient or official at the time. However, a small category of other psychiatrists place great importance on the problem of classification and in the end may devote their entire lifetimes to it. Concerning this second group, the questions arise: Where does this pressing and endless need for classification come from? And how do these individuals decide upon the universal validity of one classificatory system over all others?

When we consider a figure like Robert Burton, the unfortunate Oxford "scholar" who devoted his lifetime to studying the hundreds of medical doctrines available to him and to synthesizing them into a single doctrine, we cannot but wonder if the "melancholy" he suffered personally is not sufficient explanation. Unfortunately, we know almost nothing about Burton's life. Or we might consider the case of Emil Kraepelin. Throughout his career, Kraepelin continually expanded and refined his system of classification, so that his students were always anxious for the next edition of his *Lehrbuch* to appear in order to see what changes in their practice it would bring. What mysterious factors motivated Kraepelin in this lifelong preoccupation? (Some of his contemporaries used to accuse him of directing psychiatric nosology the same way that Bismarck maneuvered the political parties of the Prussian Parliament.) Unfortunately, the known biographical details about Kraepelin too are insufficient to enlighten us on this point.

With three other cases, however, we can at least hypothesize. Few medical figures are as well known in Switzerland today as the Basel physician Felix Platter (1636–1714). Platter was a pioneer in anatomy, epidemiology, medical teaching, and psychiatry. Today, we have Platter's many publications, his administrative papers, his autobiography, a detailed journal that he kept for many years, his correspondence, full catalogues of his collections, and the writings of many of his students and friends. We possess many more documents about the life and personality of Platter than of Burton or Kraepelin. J. Karcher has written a reliable biography of him, and Hans Christoffel has produced a brief psychoanalytic study.[29]

One of Platter's main characteristics, as revealed in these sources, was his passion for order, precision, and minute detail. Another feature was his

[29] Johann Karcher, *Felix Platter: Lebensbild des Basler Stadtarztes* (Basel, Helbing & Lichenbahn, 1949); Hans Christoffel, "Psychiatrie und Psychologie bei Felix Platter," *Monatsschrift für Psychiatrie und Neurologie*, 27 (1954), 213–27.

intense activity as a collector. Platter gathered a large collection of medicinal drugs, a voluminous herbarium, medals, engravings, musical instruments, minerals, a private botanical garden of specimens, and even a small zoological collection! He left behind minute, up-to-date records and inventories of all his collections. Among his medical records are meticulous case observations on certain patients. It is quite certain that Platter's entire nosological system arose from his passion for collecting and from his interest in and need to order and classify all materials. Relying on an examination of numerous aspects of Platter's life, Christoffel concludes that Platter was affected by an "obsessional neurosis with disguised aggressivity and misogyny." Platter also presented a certain misoneism, which could explain why, once the main outlines of his classification were settled, he never made major alterations but spent much time refining the minute details of the system. Platter's eminent historical role as a pioneer in psychiatry is clear; but it is difficult not to agree with Christoffel's diagnosis and not to admit that this particular system of classification was closely linked to the personal neurosis of its author.

Paracelsus (1493–1551) is another major early figure in the history of psychiatry, including psychiatric nosology. Paracelsus's life, which for a long time was obscured by legends, is less well documented than Platter's. Some people at the time said that Paracelsus was a genius while others called him a charlatan, a mystical philosopher, and a precursor of modern-day psychiatry. Certain aspects of his personality have been illuminated by biographers.[30] Today, we can see that Paracelsus's life and medical doctrines represented in part desperate attempts to unify the two very different worlds that he was born into. Paracelsus's father, born into the noble family of Bombast von Hohenheim, was an illegitimate child, who as a result was rejected by his family and reduced to the model role of a practitioner in a small town. Paracelsus's mother worked as a servant at a rich and powerful monastery in Einsiedeln, a place of pilgrimage, it was said, for local people and a site of many miraculous cures. His mother's early death was accompanied by the departure of his father for Villach in Austria, where he worked in the business of mines and metallurgy. The young Paracelsus, uprooted at an early age, became a physician, like his father. He felt that he was destined for great honors, but he was usually condemned everywhere. He felt solidarity with the popular classes of his mother. He hated the world of nobility as well as the university, where an ineffective medicine was still taught in Latin at the time. In contrast, Paracelsus wanted to bring the people a new medicine, in a vernacular language, that was founded both on experience in the natural world and on faith in miracles. We can

[30] The most recent monograph is Walter Pagel's *Paracelsus* (Basel and New York, S. Karger, 1958).

speculate that Paracelsus's constant efforts to build and rebuild new psychiatric classifications were, unconsciously, attempts to resolve on the theoretical level the internal contradictions that he had to confront throughout his lifetime.

Finally, we can also suspect that a similar psychodynamic occurred with Bénédict-Augustin Morel (1809–1873). Morel was a French citizen, born in Germany, and brought up in the bilingual setting of Luxemburg. He was a Catholic by upbringing, who had intended to work in the priesthood; but Morel, while he remained a pious man, passed through the medical, materialistic world of Paris and became, among other things, a friend of Claude Bernard. Morel without doubt had many difficulties to surmount before he could reconcile the cultural and intellectual contradictions in his background, and his work reflects clearly his efforts to reconcile science and theology, psychiatry and biology. Morel's great and prolonged effort to create a new psychiatric classification, in his theory of mental degeneration, may well be explained in part as an attempt to solve his own internal contradictions.

Conclusion

The purpose of this study has not been to discuss the validity or invalidity of extant psychiatric classifications but rather to draw attention to the various and recurrent unconscious, irrational factors that have influenced the work of classifiers in the past and present. Some of these classifiers, owing to a flawed or imperfect concept of the nature of scientific classification, have attempted to elaborate exclusively practical or exclusively abstract classifications. Other authors have unconsciously projected into their classifications various kinds of numerical, linguistic, sociological, or cultural patterns. Finally, others have yielded to an unconscious personal dynamic that has led them unknowingly to attempt to gratify some emotional tendency or to solve some personal problem through their theoretical work.

13

The Concept of "Maladie Créatrice"

[1964]

THE CONCEPT of creative illness seems to have been anticipated by Novalis, the German Romantic poet and philosopher. In his *Fragmente über Ethisches, Philosophisches und Wissenschaflisches*, Novalis observed, "Illnesses are certainly an important matter for humanity, since they are so numerous and because everyone has to struggle against them. But we know only very imperfectly the art of putting them to good use. These are probably the most important materials and stimulants for our thinking and activity."[1] Elsewhere, Novalis declared that hypochondria in particular is a very remarkable illness: "There is a petty hypochondria and a sublime hypochondria. It is through the latter that one should attempt to find an access route towards the soul." These sentences seem to indicate that according to Novalis there exist certain illnesses of superior essence that are, so to say, more wholesome than health, and, in reverse, that one can speak of the false appearance of health due to illness, for instance, in the case of a nation in the state of revolution: "There is an energy caused by illness and weakness which appears to be stronger than real energy, but which, when disappearing, leaves the person in a state of weakness that is still greater."

These reflections of an original thinker (who, moreover, through personal experience was well acquainted with mental and physical illness) have generally been regarded as empty dreams of a Romantic poet. With the mid-nineteenth-century advent of positivism, the utilitarian, materialistic notion came to prevail that illness is simply and exclusively a disorder of physical origin to be cured or prevented by scientific methods. The old moral that taught "the good use of illnesses" was later considered a consoling fiction or even "moral masochism." The twentieth century

"La notion de maladie créatrice," *Dialogue: Canadian Philosophical Journal/Revue philosophique canadienne*, 3, no. 1 (1964), 25–41; "The Concept of Creative Illness," *Psychoanalytic Review*, 55, no. 3 (1968), 442–56.

[1] Novalis (Friedrich von Hardenberg), *Fragmente über Ethisches, Philosophisches und Wissenschaftliches*, vol. 3, *Sämmtliche Werke*, edited by Carl Meissner (Florence, E. Diederichs, 1898), 164, 169, 170.

added only one corrective to the positivistic and scientific concept of illness: it admitted the possibility of the psychogenic origins of certain physical illnesses and granted recognition to "psychosomatic medicine," a new name for a very ancient concept.

So far as I know, it has occurred to only a single psychosomatician to invert this theory: if misdirected emotions or ideas can be transformed into illness, why could not illness disappear through a transformation into an idea? This is the concept of *logophania* proposed by the mid-twentieth-century physician–philosopher Viktor von Weizsäcker.[2] Weizsäcker maintains that he has seen cases in which the disappearance of a physical symptom was followed by the appearance of an idea, even of philosophical notions in the mind of the patient. Von Weizsäcker illustrates this notion with an example taken from a novel by Jean-Paul Sartre, *La nausée*. Sartre's novel presents itself as the personal diary of an intellectual engaged in some boring historical research; as a result, the figure becomes a neurotic who takes a dislike to the entire world and to himself. However, in the last pages of the book, the nausea disappears and is suddenly replaced by the idea of a new philosophy which our hero develops and which, as is noted by von Weizsäcker, in some respects resembles the existentialist philosophy that Sartre himself was later to present.

In the view of von Weizsäcker, logophania seems to represent the reverse of the current psychosomatic illness and the spontaneous equivalent of a psychosomatic cure. But could we not go a step further and try to find out whether, in certain historical cases, there may not be something of a creative process hidden under the appearance or disappearance of a neurosis or psychosomatic illness? I do not know if this subject has ever been treated in its entirety, but it seems to me that sufficient data exist to allow us to present a broad outline of it in the hope of opening a dialogue that might prove fruitful. Creative illnesses indeed have existed in several domains of thought and have played a particular role in the history of religion, literature, philosophy, and psychiatry.

How, then, does a creative illness manifest itself? At times, as an ordinary neurosis, or sometimes altogether differently, according to the current psychiatric concepts. Symptoms of depression, exhaustion, irritability, insomnia, headaches, and neuralgia may develop; sometimes it takes on the character of a serious psychosis or it may assume the form of a psychosomatic illness. However, in all cases it exhibits the following distinguishing characteristics:

---

[2] Viktor von Weizsäcker, *Der kranke Mensch: Eine Einführung in die medizinische Anthropologie* (Stuttgart, K. F. Koehler, 1951), 322–27. See also Weizsäcker's *Körpergeschehen und Neurose. Analytische Studie über somatische Symptombildungen* (Stuttgart, E. Klett, 1947).

1. The beginning phase of the illness appears generally right after a period of intense intellectual effort, long reflection and meditation, and perhaps also after some work of a more technical nature, such as the research and accumulation of empirical material. The German word *studieren* (to study) as it is used colloquially in the German-speaking parts of Switzerland, with the meaning of "to make oneself sick through study or worry," expresses rather well the relations between the intense effort of the mind and the appearance of the nervous disorder.

2. During the illness, the subject is generally obsessed with an intellectual, spiritual, or aesthetic problem that is dominant, which he will sometimes display publicly, but which he often hides. The individual is preoccupied with the search for a thing or an idea the importance of which he sets above everything and never loses sight of completely.

3. The termination of the illness is experienced not only as the liberation from a long period of psychological suffering but as an illumination. The mind of the subject is possessed by a new idea which he regards as a revelation or a series of revelations. The cure is often so sudden that the subject cannot give the exact date of occurrence. It is generally followed by a feeling of exultation, euphoria, and enthusiasm so intense that the person may feel compensated in one stroke for his past suffering.

4. The cured illness is then followed by a lasting transformation of personality. The subject has the impression of entering into a new life. He has made an intellectual or spiritual discovery that he will now try hard to develop. He has discovered a new world that he will devote the rest of his life to exploring. If it is an idea or theory, he will now tend to present this as a universal truth. Often, he will do so with such conviction that he will succeed in having the idea or theory accepted by others in spite of many difficulties. Such is the general picture of a creative malady. Now let us review some cultural domains in which creative illness may be observed in the past.

Religions of Primitive Peoples

Among many primitive peoples there is a strange individual, the "shaman," who plays a fundamental role in the life of the tribe. Intermediary between the world of men and the world of spirits, the shaman exorcises, prophesies, watches over the life and the prosperity of the people, and cures certain illnesses, not to mention many secondary functions. Ethnologists today no longer simply discuss shamans as quacks or madmen. Rather, they stress the curious relationship between the profession of shaman and the aptitude for preventing psychopathological manifestations. From this point of view, Erwin Ackerknecht distinguishes three types of shamans: those who can become shamans only after a long period of mental illness, such as Siberian shamans and those of certain South African and Indonesian tribes; those who practice ritual possession, a psychopathological state comparable to autohypnosis, or to the trances of our Occidental mediums; and those whose psychopathological troubles are purely subjective, sometimes provoked by artificial means, such as fasts, alcohol, or drugs.[3]

Only the shamans of the first category interest us here. Russian anthropologists, such as Georg Nioradze, have described in detail how the adolescent who feels he is destined to become a shaman withdraws from the company of men, observes periods of fasting, sleeps on the bare ground or even in the snow, experiences a multitude of sufferings, and communicates sometimes with the spirits. A European or North American observer today would not hesitate to take him for a mental patient.[4] However, Nioradze adds, the shaman himself considers this period as an illness, the cure of which coincides with the beginning of his public activity as a shaman.

But, one will ask, is this not a case of simple schizophrenia as well as an example of the custom of reserving the profession of shaman for former schizophrenics? The answer is that this strange psychosis sets in at the precise moment when the young man begins to follow the call to become a shaman, an idea that will not leave him from that point onward. Moreover, throughout the duration of this psychosis, the patient or shaman-in-training, under the direction of an old shaman, pursues the professional initiation that will come to an end at the same time as the illness and that will be sanctioned by a public ceremony during which the title of shaman is finally conferred upon him.

We cannot meaningfully compare such an illness to ordinary schizophrenia. In the latter, the fixed idea to attain a certain aim is absent and so is the relationship with a master who guides the efforts. Add to this the fact that the schizophrenic who is cured finds himself weakened physically and mentally for some time and experiences difficulty recovering his past equilibrium whereas the shaman, once cured, enters a new, higher life, as we see most clearly in the "initiating" illness of the Siberian shaman. The

[3] Erwin Ackerknecht, "Psychopathology, Primitive Medicine and Primitive Culture," *Bulletin of the History of Medicine*, 14 (1943), 30–67.

[4] Georg Nioradze, *Der Schamanismus bei den sibirischen Völkern* (Stuttgart, Strecker & Schröder, 1925).

shamans of Alaska, who show some essential resemblances to those of Siberia, subject themselves, according to Ivan Lopatin, to a very hard life. "They go through periods of severe fasting and of absolute chastity. They live in isolation, without friends, exposed to the jealousy of their rivals."[5] What prompted them to choose such a difficult and austere profession? Is it because of the real prestige or the prerogatives attached to this dignity? Perhaps both; but Lopatin believes that there is a more important reason, namely, the exaltation of a supernatural life, for "in his imagination the shaman invents a fantastic world in which he lives constantly."

Religious Mystics

I hope that someday the affinities between the inner sufferings of the great past mystics of various religions and the development of creative illness will be studied closely. Let us limit ourselves now to one example, that is, "the dark night of the soul" of which we find a description in the works of the Spanish mystic poet Juan de Yepis (St. John of the Cross).[6] The religious mystic who decides on this course will have to cope with hardships so numerous and severe "that it is beyond the power of human science to understand them and to experience or to expose them." During the first phase of the experience, there exists a fear of having gone astray or of having been forsaken and an inability to fix one's mind in meditation. In a subsequent phase, the mystic experiences the feeling of having been rejected by God and the impossibility of finding any satisfaction in things divine or in God's creatures. Now how do we know that this too is not an ordinary state of mental depression in which the preoccupation of a mystic character dominates for the simple reason that the person who experiences these depressions is a monk? St. John of the Cross indicates again and again the characteristics that make it possible to recognize whether we have to do here with a truly "dark night," or with the effects of religious imperfections, or with a melancholia.[7] In the state of authentic mystic aridity, the soul is not in search of, nor does it find, any comfort in tangible things. And it does not allow itself to be diverted from constant preoccupation with God, even if it feels forsaken or rejected by Him. Rather, we find here a long, haunting, and uninterrupted search, which is one of the fundamental characteristics of creative illness. The other essential features are present as well. The beginning of the experience is linked with a specific point of

[5] Ivan A. Lopatin, *Social Life and Religion of the Indians in Kitimat British Columbia* (Los Angeles, University of California, Social Science Series, No. 26, 1945), 63–80.

[6] Saint Jean de la Croix, *Oeuvres spirituelles*, translated by R. P. Grégoire de Saint Joseph (Paris, Seuil, 1947), 19.

[7] Ibid., 512.

departure, namely, the choice of an ascetic and mystic life aiming at a transformation of the soul by means of a mystical union. Let us note also that the mystic accepts the direction of a spiritual guide and that allusions are made to useless sufferings brought about by inexperience or by the errors of certain directors. All this reveals the essential differences between the long "dark night" of the mystics and the evolution of a mental illness, such as depression or schizophrenia.

In the vast domain of mysticism and religious psychology there are countless other facts to be noted but that I am unable to discuss here. Creative illness no doubt takes on multiple other forms, too, such as the extraordinary trials of the ascetics, which have found their literary expression in the temptation of St. Anthony and the periods of anguish preceding conversions at the time of the Anglo-Saxon revivalist movements.

The Phenomenon of Literary Aridity

There has been an enormous amount of discussion over the years about poetic inspiration; but there has been far less consideration of its opposite, the aridity of the poet who, in spite of desperate efforts, fails to create. It is curious that writers should have shown so little interest in a question that concerns them directly. I have found only two serious studies of this subject.

One writer, who hides his identity under the pen name of "Nicias," has written a short but interesting article on the artistic exhaustion of the novelist.[8] The facts reported by Nicias "reveal the existence of an unknown patient, namely, the author in travail of gestation." This class of individual, while moving around society, "is radiant with health, kind, sometimes witty, often gay." But as soon as they sit down at their desks and take pen in hand, "they break down and their minds are swallowed up in the abyss of impotence. . . . In a few seconds their brains are in darkness, in fearful darkness. They run away from their desk, saddened, wondering whether they will ever be able to write again." Nicias attributes the illness of the novelist to exhaustion. Every writer has at his disposal, he believes, a certain quantity of nervous energy to be used in literary creation; through overwork, he exhausts this reserve of energy. This is "the drama in the life of the intellectual creator who conceives a work that is always more powerful than the one he is able to achieve." The remedy here, then, would be to limit one's ambitions and to spare one's strength. According to this concept, the creative barrenness of the writer is a particular form of exhaustion through overwork, similar to physical and emotional strain.

[8] Nicias, "L'épuisement du romancier," *L'orientation médicale*, 4 (1935), 25–28.

But might there not be other forms of literary aridity, some more directly linked to the creative procedure? The second statement on the subject, Edmond Jaloux's remarkable article of 1937, supplies a fundamental contribution.[9] According to Jaloux, infertility and inspiration are two aspects of the same phenomenon or process, which is emotional in nature. He compares both phenomena to the experience of Marcel Proust's hero, who, having lost his grandmother, felt no grief for a full year, until some unforeseen happening caused him to realize his loss and suddenly to be overcome by sorrow. "Nothing compares better to aridity than this indifference with regard to grief." Jaloux cites some examples taken from literature (among them a very beautiful passage from Hofmannsthal) and from his personal observation:

> I have happened to see inspiration taking hold of a writer in whose presence I was during a voyage and then in his office. There is an evident transfiguration. The expression of his face becomes peaceful and is radiant at the same time. His features relax. The eyes become illuminated with a particular light, with a kind of strange desire aiming at nothing real. There is here an unmistakable physical presence. But during the period of aridity, the appearance of a man changes, too. His complexion may grow sickly and livid, his eyes, dull, his face, frowning, his expression, sullen. Whereas in the first instance the person seems to surpass himself, in the second instance, he is inferior to himself.

These crises of noncreativity, says Jaloux, happen without warning, and do not seem to involve health or illness or the events of the person's emotional life. Rather, "we have here to do with a particular vitality, with a force that is little known and which remains to be fully identified."[10] One thing is clear: Jaloux does not doubt that this aridity is nearly always productive in the long run, and he compares it to the earth's rest that follows autumn. Whether it be long or short, it is only an intermediary period that separates the writer from an improvement or a deepening of his talents. Attributing this phase of barrenness to mere fatigue does not seem satisfactory. It is rather due to an inner process through which are torn apart "these icy partitions which separate the deep self from the superficial self, and which prevents them from joining together." We may conclude that, in at least some cases, the state of poetic aridity is caused by something other than mere exhaustion; it is a development through which the writer succeeds in bringing to the surface of his mind a world of images and thoughts buried in the depths of the unconscious. This development may be terribly painful and thus constitutes the creative illness.

[9] Edmond Jaloux, "L'inspiration poétique et l'aridité," *Études Carmélitaines: Illuminations et sécheresses*, 22e année, 2 (1937), 31–45.
[10] Ibid.

The History of Philosophy

Has creative illness played a role in the development of the work of certain philosophers, that is to say, in the history of philosophy? To answer this question, it would be necessary to know a great deal more about the lives of the major philosophers than I do. [. . .]

It would serve a useful purpose if somebody attempted to collect the scattered data that are available on this subject. Until such a work is achieved, however, the most satisfactory example I have been able to find of a creative illness concerns the life of a philosopher, that of Gustav Theodor Fechner (1801–1887). We know that Fechner first studied medicine, then physics and chemistry, all with success, while writing textbooks and encyclopedias in order to make a living. In 1833, at the age of 32, Fechner finally was appointed professor of physics at the University of Leipzig; but from that time onward he began to suffer mysteriously from exhaustion, which was attributed to continuous overwork. In 1840, at the age of 39, his health broke down, and he was forced to cease all activity during a period of three years. The strange illness that Fechner went through at that time is known to us primarily from an autobiographical report that was used by his biographer, Johannes Kuntze.[11]

In modern psychiatric terminology, this illness would be diagnosed as a serious neurotic depression with hypochondriacal preoccupations, rendered more complicated, perhaps, by the effects of a lesion of the right retina as a result of a physical injury. (Fechner had once looked straight at the sun in order to study visual postsensorial images.) During most of the time of his illness, Fechner lived in complete isolation in a dark room surrounded by black walls, wearing a mask or an occlusive apparatus over his eyes. He could hardly take any food, and people worried about his physical condition. [. . .] Fechner eventually undertook to force his mental faculties to function again, an effort that exhausted him and that he compared to the attempt of a horseman to break in a rebellious mount. After one year, he saw in a dream the figure "77" and concluded that he would be cured on the seventy-seventh day, which indeed happened. But this protracted period of depression was followed by a burst of intellectual excitement and euphoria that lasted a few weeks. Fechner then experienced ideas of grandeur, feeling capable of solving all the enigmas of the world. This state of hypomania (in today's psychiatric language) eventually disappeared, too, but Fechner was convinced at this stage that he had discovered

[11] J. E. Kuntze, *Gustav Theodor Fechner (Dr. Mises): Ein deutsches Gelehrtenleben* (Leipzig, Breitkopf & Härtel, 1892). An abridged account of Fechner's illness is found in English translation in Walter Lowrie, ed., *Religion of a Scientist: Selections from Gustav Theodor Fechner* (New York, Pantheon, 1946), 36–42.

a universal principle comparable in importance to Newton's principle of universal gravitation. He called his new theory the "pleasure principle" (*Lustprinzip*).

We find here a typical example of *logophania*, in which hypomanic euphoria was replaced by the appearance of a philosophical idea. Moreover, at the moment when Fechner for the first time after three years opened his eyes in his garden, he had been startled by the beauty of the flowers, which he now perceived had a soul. This experience provided the impetus to his book *Nanna, or the Soul of Plants*, a curious piece of work that examines from all angles the problem of "vegetal psychism." After his cure, Fechner remained in good health for the rest of his life, but he had gone through a strange metamorphosis. The physicist had become transformed into a philosopher, and Fechner now exchanged his university chair in physics for that of philosophy. His first course was now devoted to the pleasure principle, and some time later he achieved fame through his research in psychophysics. Let us recall that it is from Fechner that Freud, by his own admission, borrowed not only the notion of the pleasure principle but also the concepts of the economy and repetition of the "topographical" aspects of mental life.

What should we think of this rather mysterious illness? Doubtless, one could attribute it to overwork or nervousness, but neither of these explains the sudden halt of the illness, the resulting metamorphosis in Fechner's personality, or the sudden onrush of new ideas at the moment of recovery. We should note that during the entire course of the illness, Fechner's mind remained very active and that he spent the entire last year of the experience in a direct fight with his illness. Wilhelm Wundt was right in asserting that Fechner brought about his cure through a process of autosuggestion. For all these reasons, it seems appropriate to include Fechner's illness in the group of creative illnesses.

The influence of creative illness, in my opinion, is also very probable in the life of Friedrich Nietzsche. I do not have in mind the organic cerebral illness that over time incapacitated Nietzsche and caused his mind to give way entirely. I am thinking rather of the works he wrote during the years following his resignation from his professorship at Basel. It is to the credit of Lou Andreas-Salomé that she understood that the sufferings Nietzsche complained about almost continually during this period were part of a cycle including each time three phases: several months of suffering of a neurotic type, followed by a period of creative activity, followed by an intermediary period of relatively good health.[12] This cycle in fact is reflected in the titles of certain of Nietzsche's works, such as *Morgenröte* (*Dawn*), that is, the dawn of illumination that follows a long period of

[12] Lou Andreas-Salomé, *Friedrich Nietzsche in seinen Werken* (Vienna, Carl Konegen, 1894).

mental darkness and suffering; and *Die fröhliche Wissenschaft* (*The Gay Science*), or joyousness when one is in possession of oneself after long months of depression. It would be tempting also to examine the life of Descartes in order to ascertain whether the famous episode of his philosophical illumination, during which the principles of a universal science were revealed to him, was the outcome of a long and dark period of creative illness.

The History of Psychiatry

In a previous article written in 1961, I attempted to demonstrate that the decisive discoveries of dynamic psychiatry in the last century and a half were realized under the influence of two main factors: (1) the experience of the psychiatrist's personal neurosis accompanied by his own efforts to cure himself; and (2) the psychiatrist's ambiguous relationships with neurotic, often hysterical, patients whom he tried to cure, often without success, and yet with whom he makes unexpected discoveries during the treatment.[13] It appears to me today that the role of the psychiatrist's neurosis was more complex than first believed. Has it been a matter simply of an ordinary neurosis that the psychiatrist tries to eliminate in himself, that is to say, of an unfortunate obstacle that he succeeds in turning to his advantage, or has it been rather a matter of a full-fledged creative illness? Whatever the answer to this question, it seems clear today that we can recognize with certainty the direct role of creative illnesses in the genesis of at least two great systems of psychiatry, Freud's psychoanalysis and Jung's Analytical Psychology.*

The real origins of the fundamental concepts of psychoanalysis have remained mysterious for a long time. For many years, it was believed that Freud had discovered his ideas simply while examining and treating his neurotic patients. However, the appearance of the first volume of Jones's biography in 1953 and, even more so, the publication of a large part of Freud's correspondence with Fliess in 1955 have made it possible to become much better acquainted with the generative role of another fundamental episode in Freud's life at this time: the self-analysis of Freud to which Didier Anzieu has recently devoted a most interesting study.[14]

We now know that during the 1890s Freud suffered from an ill-defined

---

*[*Editor's note*: See Ellenberger's later elaboration of this point in *The Discovery of the Unconscious*, Conclusion, 889–91.]

[13] Ellenberger, "La psychiatrie et son histoire inconnue," *L'union médicale du Canada*, 90, no. 3 (March 1961), 281–89.

[14] Didier Anzieu, *L'auto-analyse: Son rôle dans la découverte de la psychanalyse par Freud, sa fonction en psychanalyse* (Paris, Presses Universitaires de France, 1959).

nervous disorder—what he often called his "neurasthenia"—and that in 1897 he began to treat himself through the method that he had invented a few years before of free association and the interpretation of dreams. In the course of this self-analysis, Freud discovered facts about his infancy that he had forgotten or half-forgotten: his amorous attraction to his mother, his rivalry with his father, in brief, those elements that he eventually combined and called the Oedipus complex. Further, Jones has told us that Freud emerged from his self-analysis in 1901 completely transformed. Freud's feelings of inferiority had disappeared and had instead now been replaced by a new and complete self-confidence. Also, he was now in possession of a doctrine, a new psychotherapeutic method, and in a position to become the leader of a school.

However, Freud's successful self-analysis was only one side of his experience during these years. The other side was constituted by the neurosis he had been suffering from for some years. We find in Freud in fact the essential characteristics of a major creative illness. The illness began at the moment when Freud got interested in the exploration of the mysteries of the human mind, which he never lost sight of during the time of his neurosis and self-analysis; and the end of the illness coincided with an intellectual illumination, a lasting transformation of the personality, the conviction of having made a permanent, epochal discovery. Indeed, all those who knew Freud have agreed that to him the universal existence of infantile sexuality and the Oedipus complex was certain and absolute—truths allowing no discussion.

Freud's biographers have termed Freud's self-analysis a heroic achievement, and they are surely right. But is it necessary to agree with them when they assert, as does Jones, that it is something radically unique in the history of humanity, that it constitutes an event that had no precedent, and that will never be paralleled? That would be to overlook the existence of a group of other individuals who have also experienced creative illnesses, a group that includes another pioneer of dynamic psychiatry, C. G. Jung.

The psychological and psychotherapeutic work of Jung is still very imperfectly known.[15] A historical legend represents Jung primarily as a rebellious disciple of Freud who subsequently lapsed into hazy mysticism. It is certain that the Jungian notions of the collective unconscious, archetypes, animus and anima, and others appear quite metaphysical when one has not studied Jung's doctrines in detail. But those who knew Jung personally remember that Jung spoke about these concepts with absolute conviction, as if through direct personal acquaintance, much in the same way that

---

[15] Carl G. Jung, *Erinnerungen, Träume, Gedanken*, edited by Aniela Jaffé (Zurich, Rascher, 1963). (The English translation of this source has unfortunately been abridged by several chapters and is not free of errors.)

Freud spoke about sexuality and the Oedipus complex. However, Jung did not in any way give the impression of being a mystic or a metaphysician; he was essentially a practical man who never lost sight of concrete reality.

In Jung's therapeutic activity, his first concern was to dissipate the patient's unconscious and to place the patient before the immediate and concrete reality of their life. Most people, he believed, live in their unconscious "a provisional life." He compared them to Tartarin, making a dangerous excursion in the Alps without experiencing any fear, who as soon as they become aware of the reality are seized with panic. To become conscious of reality was to Jung not only the crux of good psychotherapy but also the foundation of ethics. "*Unbewusstheit ist die grösste Sünde*—unconsciousness is the greatest sin," he said.

One wonders how a man as close to reality as Jung could have become so certain of the existence of the mysterious things he theorized about. It was believed for a long time that Jung too had discovered these notions during the psychotherapeutic treatment of his patients. But in 1925, in one of his "seminars" in Zurich, Jung explained how he had made his discoveries. For many years this course was never published and only a few persons were acquainted with it. However, the recent publication of Jung's autobiography allows us to see the matter in full light.* We know now that after his separation from Freud, Jung suffered from a kind of protracted neurotic disorder marked by anguish and feelings of loneliness and that in 1913 he undertook his exploration of the unconscious by means of his own self-analysis, but conducted in a way quite different from Freud's. (Probably Jung knew nothing about the latter's effort.) Jung's two main approaches to his self-analysis were the technique of forced imagination and of the "rêves dessinés." Jung's *Autobiography* relates the ways in which he explored the world of archetypes, became acquainted with his "anima," perceived the process of "individuation" and its consequences, and discovered the *Selbst* or "Self" (the inimitable and unconscious center of the personality). The essential features of Jung's teaching, therefore, are the result of his creative neurosis, just as early psychoanalytic theory is essentially the result of Freud's similar experience.

To these observations on creative illness many others could be added. In conclusion to this brief exposé, let me limit myself to two points. First, it is obvious that these illnesses take on a great diversity of clinical forms. They may be short or long, resemble a neurosis, a psychosis, or a psychosomatic illness. Sometimes they involve a unique or a single episode only, occurring in midlife and cutting the individual's existence, so to speak, into two distinctive parts, one preceding and one following the illness. In other

---

*[*Editor's note*: On this source, see Ellenberger's extensive review, "L'autobiographie de C. G. Jung," *Critique*, 20, nos. 207–8 (August–September 1964), 754–79.]

cases (as with Nietzsche, it seems) they involve a series of crises. One wonders whether creative illness with some people does not remain intermittent and spread out over the greater part of their existence. This would explain, for instance, Darwin's very singular neurosis, which puzzled his contemporaries as it continues to puzzle his biographers today—a kind of lifelong nontypical neurosis associated with an exceptional intellectual productivity.

It is also necessary to distinguish between planned, ritualized creative illnesses (such as the case of the shamans and the Christian mystics) and spontaneous creative illnesses, in which the patient is left to his own resources (as tends to occur with poets and philosophers). The examples of Freud and Jung prove that a creative illness, unique and spontaneous in its origin, may become, as it were, the prototype of a stylized creative illness and may be reproduced in many subsequent examples. Let us recall that it was Jung who, while working with Freud, first proposed the principles of didactic training analyses for all future analytical therapists. In Jung's opinion, this was a matter of apprenticeship through practice. Interestingly, the school of Jung later assimilated didactic analyses with the initiatory illnesses of the shamans. However, it is evident that no didactic analysis, be it Freudian or Jungian, can automatically lead the initiated or the apprentice to results that are comparable to those produced in the author of their prototype.

A second important and difficult problem concerns the heuristic value attributable to creative illnesses. Setting aside the case of the poet, what is the value of the discoveries made by the person who has successfully gone through such an experience? Fechner at once attributed a universal value to the "pleasure principle" and compared it to Newton's principle of gravitation. Freud accepted the universality of the Oedipus complex. Jung disputed this concept and asserted that, since Freud discovered the fact through self-analysis, the Oedipus complex holds true only for him and that it is improper to elevate it into a universal law. But the Freudians, in turn, may counter that Jung was wrong in generalizing the notion of anima, the discovery of Jung's self-analysis. Now, experience shows that people who are analyzed by Freudian analysts infallibly discover their Oedipus complex and have dreams of the "Freudian" type whereas those analyzed by a disciple of Jung discover their anima and have Jungian dreams. Genius, said the Frenchman Gabriel Tarde, has the ability to engender its own spiritual progeny. Let us conclude by expressing the hope that Novalis's wish may someday find its realization and that a study of "sublime hypochondria," as he called it, will offer the means to understand certain imperfectly known aspects of human creativity.

14

The Pathogenic Secret and Its Therapeutics

[1966]

THE PATHOGENIC effect of a heavily disturbing secret upon its bearer has been known from time immemorial as well as the healing action of confession under certain circumstances. In the following pages, I shall try to illustrate how from this very ancient notion a particular type of psychotherapy has evolved that eventually brought a noteworthy contribution to the origin of modern dynamic psychiatry.

The Concept of the Pathogenic Secret

The physical and mental manifestations of a pathogenic secret upon a person can be very different from one individual to another. Cases are known in which it can result in death in a dramatic fashion with accompanying physical symptoms unless a last-minute confession brings an immediate quasi-miraculous cure. A remarkable instance of this has been published recently in Germany by H. Aldenhoven.[1] Much more frequently, the pathogenic secret takes on the aspect of a chronic neurosis, which according to the place and time can be called melancholia, neurasthenia, hysteria, or even psychosis. Not uncommonly, it takes on the mild form of irrational or eccentric behavior.

The nature of the pathogenic secret can also differ widely. In certain patients, it is a matter of secret thwarted love or of some other suppressed passion, such as jealousy, hatred, or ambition. Sometimes it is a matter of a physical illness or infirmity, of which the patient feels ashamed. Frequently the secret is related to some kind of moral offense that can range from petty theft to murder, but frequently it is also of a sexual nature (adultery, incest,

"The Pathogenic Secret and Its Therapeutics," *Journal of the History of the Behavioral Sciences*, 2, no. 1 (January 1966), 29–42; "Le secret pathogène et son traitement," *Revue internationale de l'histoire de la psychiatrie*, 1 (1983), 5–22.

[1] H. Aldenhoven, "Klinischer Beitrag zur Frage der Todesahnungen," *Psychotherapie*, 2 (1957), 55–59.

abortion, infanticide, and so on). The secret can also involve painful re-
membrance of a traumatic event, sometimes connected with a secret of
another person (for instance, a young girl discovering her mother's
adultery).

In all cases the subjective experience is decisive; what really matters is
not so much the fact itself as the meaning that the patients attach to it
according to their personal scale of values. The pathogenic secret is not
necessarily connected with guilt feelings, but there is always an element of
hopelessness in it. In that regard, the main point is the way in which
patients view their situation and may believe it to be insoluble simply
because they do not realize that a solution could be found. In the present
essay, we shall try to trace as concisely as possible the successive steps in the
history of thinking about the pathogenic secret and its therapeutics from
primitive populations to modern times.

Primitive Psychotherapy

Rafaele Pettazzoni has written a well-documented survey on the practice of
confession among various populations of the world and throughout the
ages.[2] Among many past peoples, the occurrence of public calamities was
attributed to sins committed by unknown individuals, hence the resort to
collective confession in order to discover the doers and to perform expia-
tory ceremonies. Such sins could involve the infringement of a taboo either
known or unknown to the doer, but mostly not understood in the moral
sense of sin as present-day religion conceives it. The act of confession was
conceived as a magical procedure, confession was mostly public, and the
confessor was not bound to secrecy. But Pettazzoni also gives instances of
primitive populations among which certain illnesses were considered cured
by individual confession, particularly in cases of sterility or difficulties in
childbirth, and as a rule these were attributed to sexual sins. We thus
already find among primitive peoples the concept of the pathogenic secret
and of healing through individual confession.

Ancient Civilizations

Pettazzoni has also provided abundant information about the practice of
confession among ancient civilizations of the old and the new world.
Among ancient Mexicans, for instance, confession was obligatory, and

[2] Rafaele Pettazzoni, *La confessione dei peccati*, 3 vols. (Bologna, Nicola Zanichelli, 1929,
1935, 1936).

illness was often attributed to the commission of certain offenses, particularly adultery and other sexual sins and also inebriety. Among the ancient peoples of Mesopotamia the belief prevailed in the causal relationship between illness and sin. The same was true among the Hebrews, although the *Book of Job* makes an exception in that it defends the principle that disease is not necessarily the result of sin; this became also the viewpoint of the Gospels and of early Christianity. Nevertheless, the idea that illness is the result of sin survived throughout the centuries and found distinguished supporters among German Romantic physicians.[3]

Catholic Religion

Following a widespread and ancient tradition, the Christian religion established a systematic practice of confession that survives to this day in the Roman Catholic as well as the Eastern Orthodox church. This practice is considered an essentially religious act in connection with the sacrament of Penance. However, it was believed that confession and Penance could sometimes *also* bring forth the healing of a physical or mental illness. As to the difference from the practice of most primitive and ancient peoples, confession in the Christian church is a strictly private and individual matter, and the priest is bound to the utmost secrecy regarding anything that he has been told under the "seal" of confession.

There are good reasons to assume that the common practice of confession has exerted a significant influence upon the development of psychology. Its effect upon autobiographical literature is sufficiently illustrated by St. Augustine's *Confessions* and the subsequent literature in this tradition. The French Romantic poet Alfred de Vigny contended that the psychological novel owes its origin to the Christian practice of confession.[4] Furthermore, a certain body of psychological knowledge was acquired by the priests and to some extent systematized in textbooks of moral theology; but the very nature and rigidity of the priestly secret of confession made that systematized knowledge rather inaccessible.

The Protestant Religion

Protestant Reformers abolished compulsory confession, but it was among Protestant communities that a new practice and tradition arose, the "Cure

---

[3] Wolf Von Siebenthal, *Krankheit als Folge der Sünde: Eine medizinhistorische Untersuchung* (Hannover, Schmorl u. von Seefeld Nachf., 1950).

[4] Alfred de Vigny, *Journal d'un poète*, edited by Louis Ratisbonne (Paris, Michel Lévy, 1867), 172.

of Souls—*Seelsorge*." Certain Protestant ministers were considered to be endowed with a particular spiritual gift, which enabled them to find an approach to distressed souls, obtain a confession of a disturbing secret, and help these persons out of difficulties. These clerical men also maintained the tradition of absolute secrecy, though it was not imposed on them with the same rigidity as that of the moral theology of the Catholic church. For want of an authentic historical example of a healing of this kind, we will cite one provided in a novel of Heinrich Jung-Stilling, *Theobald oder die Schwärmer*, published in 1785.[5] In one of the main episodes of that novel, we find a detailed account of a "Cure of Souls," which most probably was inspired by a real occurrence that came to the attention of the novelist.[6]

A young unmarried woman, Sannchen, is afflicted with a peculiar kind of depression. Physicians attribute the condition to a "weakness of the nerves," diagnose it as hysteria, and treat the patient with medications without success. The anxious family then hears of a village pastor, Reverend Bosius, who is said to have a particular gift for "Cure of Souls," and they ask for his help. Reverend Bosius is described in the novel as a pious, learned, and unassuming man. As soon as he arrives he goes for a walk in the garden with Sannchen. His kindness impresses her favorably. He begins with a long, friendly talk about the love of God which is reflected in the whole of Nature, where every being is, as it were, a thought of God. Now, what is the most beautiful among all the thoughts of God? It is Love. And what is Love? It is the drive of the Lover to be united with the Beloved. This brings Sannchen to tell him of her secret and thwarted love for Theobald and of a transgression that she has committed. Having heard her confession, Reverend Bosius exclaims, "Good Souls! How little you know about Love!" Whereupon he starts to explain to her that under the guise of Love she has been deceived by passion. Passion is nothing but "natural sexual drive—*natürlicher Geschlechtstrieb*," that is, the natural instinct of animals to want to reproduce, however refined and sublimated it can look.

In the English translation, this sentence reads as follows: ". . . in reality, it is nothing higher than a mere natural instinct, the bare excitement of the animal principles which people may refine, sublimate, and raise to the most elegant Platonism, as they will; under all its sublimations it still remains the same gross, low, inferior principle notwithstanding." This is a somewhat refined translation of the plain language used by Reverend Bosius in the original text, and to which Sannchen answers with this exclamation: "Herr Pfarrer! Sie beschämen mich!—You make me feel

---

[5] Heinrich Stilling (Jung-Stilling), *Theobald oder die Schwärmer. Eine wahre Geschichte*, 2 vols. (Frankfurt and Leipzig, 1785).

[6] Heinrich Stilling, *Theobald, or the Fanatic: A True History*, translated by Reverend Samuel Schaeffer (Philadelphia, 1846). Schaeffer's translation is condensed and often inaccurate.

ashamed!" Following this first conversation, Reverend Bosius brings Sann-chen to accept her fate, and now, with her agreement, he explains the situation to her parents, and he talks Theobald into agreeing to marry her, so that the first part of the novel is concluded with a quiet wedding of Theobald and Sannchen.

This episode in Jung-Stilling's novel is worthy of comment. First, we note that the concept of sublimation, whose origin is sometimes credited to Novalis and Schopenhauer, is, in fact, older since in this novel published in 1785, it is mentioned as a current idea. However, what Reverend Bosius calls "sublimated" love was but a refined form of natural sexual instinct, in contrast to properly "spiritual" love, which was a gift from God. In that perspective, Sannchen's fault was not in having yielded to natural love, but in having confused that natural love with spiritual love, whereas marriage ought to be a fusion of the two. This concept of sublimation contrasts with that of Schopenhauer, followed later by Nietzsche and Freud, according to whom even the most spiritualized forms of love are nothing but the sub-limation of the sexual instinct.

As a second remark, we will note that the pathogenic secret that Rever-end Bosius came upon so rapidly was related to a love affair, and it looks as if he knew by past experience of the "Cure of Souls" that it must have been so. It is also noteworthy that Reverend Bosius did not consider that he had fulfilled his task once he had obtained the confession and given consola-tion. With the patient's permission he played an active role in bringing about solutions to the patient's distressing problems. If we now compare the Catholic practice of confession and the Protestant "Cure of Souls," we note that in the latter case the accent is more strongly on the psychological side and that the whole procedure is more reminiscent of present-day short-term psychotherapy.

The Pathogenic Secret in the First Laymen

There came a time when the knowledge of the pathogenic secret and its treatment fell entirely into the hands of laymen. When exactly this secular transition first occurred is not known, but we find evidence in a series of literary works throughout the nineteenth century.

In 1843, a novel was published in Switzerland with the title *Wie Anne Bäbi Jowäger haushaltet und es ihm mit den Doktorn ergeht*, by Jeremias Gotthelf, which was the pseudonym of Reverend Albert Bitzius.[7] In one episode of that novel a young man, Jacobli, the son of rich peasants, be-

---

[7] Jeremias Gotthelf, *Wie Anne Bäbi Jowäger haushaltet und es ihm mit den Doktorn ergeht*, 2 vols. (Solothurn, 1843–1844).

comes sick because he is secretly in love with a young servant girl, Meyeli, whom he feels his family would not accept for him because she is a poor orphan. This hopeless love is the secret of which the young man is slowly dying. The situation is even more serious because Jacobli's authoritarian mother has arranged a marriage with a rich and arrogant peasant girl, whom the mother likes but who is abhorrent to him. The passive father lets his wife decide everything. But Jacobli becomes increasingly sick, and because the physicians have been powerless, the parents resort to a fortune-teller, an experienced old woman who immediately guesses the secret. Following her advice, the engagement with the rich girl is broken, Jacobli is able to marry Meyeli, and from that moment onward he recovers rapidly. It would seem that the author, Reverend Bitzius, purposely did not attribute the patient's healing to a religious minister because it might have given the reader the impression that he was referring to a personal instance of his "Cure of Souls."

A few years following Gotthelf's novel, Nathaniel Hawthorne published his masterpiece, *The Scarlet Letter*.[8] Here, the terrible, destructive effect of a pathogenic secret is illustrated unforgettably. The bearer of the secret in Hawthorne's great novel is a Protestant minister, Reverend Arthur Dimmesdale, who had an adulterous relationship with a young woman, Hester Prynne, after her husband had disappeared and was believed to be dead. While Reverend Dimmesdale is abroad in England, Hester gives birth to a child, but refuses to betray the identity of the father. She is sentenced to be exposed for two hours on the pillory and for the rest of her life to wear a red "A" on her breast, which will stigmatize her forever as an adulteress. When Reverend Dimmesdale comes back, he at first wants to denounce himself, but he is dissuaded by Hester, and for several years he carries on with his pastoral ministry while suffering intensely with his secret. But Hester's husband, who had been held captive by the Indians, comes back and starts a kind of medical practice under the name of Roger Chillingworth. Through a series of small clues, Chillingworth guesses that the father of Hester's child is the Reverend. Here, Hawthorne's novel revealed a new facet of the problem. In contrast to the preceding novels, which illustrated how the pathogenic secret can be discovered in order to secure the patient's healing, *The Scarlet Letter* shows how it can also be exploited in a diabolical way to torture a man to death; and Hawthorne's book actually concludes with the Reverend Dimmesdale's self-denunciation and death.

We now turn from the United States to Norway and to the year 1888

---

[8] Nathaniel Hawthorne, *The Scarlet Letter*, The Centenary Edition (Columbus, Ohio State University Press, 1962).

when Ibsen wrote his celebrated play *The Lady from the Sea*.[9] A woman, Ellida, the second wife of a physician, Dr. Wangel, is suffering from a mysterious neurosis, which is a serious worry to her husband, her two adolescent stepdaughters, and her friends. Dr. Wangel invites a wise old friend, Arnholm, in the hope that he will be able to help the woman, and actually by talking first with Arnholm and then with her husband, Ellida gradually reveals the root of her illness. Meanwhile, the play shows admirably the ways in which the pathogenic secret manifests itself in symbolic ways. It obviously has some connection with the sea, because Ellida's thoughts constantly dwell on it, and she herself spends an abnormal amount of time bathing and swimming in the fiord, hence the nickname "The Lady of the Sea" which she has received. However, Ellida claims to hate the water of the fiord, which she calls a "sick and sickening water," in contrast to the vivid water of the open sea. Whenever one speaks of the sea and seafarers, she becomes startled and shows a deep interest. We learn at the beginning of the play that she has suggested to a local painter the idea of painting a Siren dying on the shore after the sea has receded. Later on, talking with a sculptor, she immediately thinks of modeling Tritons, Sirens, and Vikings. As the secret is revealed, its symbolic expressions become seemingly more disquieting. Speaking of the baby that she had with Dr. Wangel, and who died in infancy, she maintains that the color and glow of the child's eyes changed according to the various colors and aspects of the sea. She also holds a theory of her own that if mankind had chosen to live in the sea rather than on the earth, men would be better and happier; but mankind has taken the wrong way, and it is too late to go back to the sea.

Gradually the secret emerges. A few years before her marriage with Dr. Wangel, Ellida was attracted, or perhaps seduced, by a mysterious seafarer, with whom she allied herself symbolically. She and the stranger joined their rings on a single chain, which he threw into the sea. The stranger then disappeared, saying that he would come back soon to get her. Later, Ellida heard rumors that he had perished in a shipwreck. Parallel to the disclosure of the secret, an unexpected event occurs: the mysterious stranger turns out to be alive, and he now comes to demand of Ellida the fulfillment of her promise. Ellida is the prey of inner conflicts. Dr. Wangel, whose first thought was a forbidding attitude, decides to let his wife make the choice between himself and the stranger, although at the same time appealing to her sense of duty. Ellida chooses her husband, and the writer gives us to understand that this free and responsible decision will bring about her healing.

[9] Henrik Ibsen, *The Lady from the Sea* (*Fruen fra havet*, 1888), translated by Eleanor Marx-Aveling (London, Unwin, 1890).

Ibsen's play thus stresses two new aspects of the pathogenic secret concept: the many symbolic ways in which it may express itself involuntarily; and the fact that its healing may not depend solely upon the intervention of the therapist but on the free and responsible choice allowed the patient. Characteristic is the mixture of kindness and strength in the husband, so that at the end of the play Ellida tells him appropriately, "You have been a good physician for me, you have found the proper remedy, and you have had the courage to use it."

A few years following Ibsen's play, in 1893, Marcel Prévost published *L'automne d'une femme* (*The Autumn of a Woman*).[10] Marcel Prévost, whose writings are seldom read today, enjoyed in his time a reputation as a master of the psychological novel. This particular novel bears as a motto a verse of Alfred de Vigny: "Il rêvera partout à la chaleur du sein.—He will dream everywhere of the warmth of the breast." In Prévost's novel, a young man, Maurice, who had been unusually spoiled by and attached to his mother in his childhood, seeks women with motherly natures. He has a love affair with a frustrated woman who feels that she is getting old, and this love has a tragic quality because of Maurice's immaturity and because his mistress, Madame Surgère, as a religious woman, is torn with guilt feelings. At the same time, her adopted daughter Claire is deeply in love with Maurice; but Maurice, after a superficial flirtation with her, thinks of her as a future wife when he will be tired of his adventures. Meanwhile, the family has arranged an engagement between Claire and an older man whom she respects but does not love. As a result, Claire has fallen into a deep depression caused by this secret, which she does not want to reveal to anybody. Her condition worsens, and she is actually dying; however, there is one person who guesses her secret and obtains it from her, namely, Dr. Daumier, a young and brilliant neurologist at the Salpêtrière. An unusually skilled psychotherapist, Dr. Daumier handles the whole situation and makes each one of the characters aware of the basis of his or her troubles. He shows Maurice what the real situation is and appeals to his sense of responsibility. Maurice terminates the affair with his mistress and decides to marry Claire, who, as a result, is rapidly cured. In Madame Surgère's case, Dr. Daumier helps her to overcome the shock of the break from Maurice, and he refers her back to her priest, who will reconcile her with religion.

One remarkable feature of Prévost's novel is the picture of the psychotherapist, Dr. Daumier, with his acute perception of the situation, his skill in disentangling that emotional maze, and the tact he uses in talking with each one of the characters at the right moment. For those familiar with the

[10] Marcel Prévost, *L'automne d'une femme* (Paris, Lemerre, 1893).

personality and psychotherapy of Pierre Janet, it is highly probable that the writer used Janet as a model for the character of Dr. Daumier.

In *L'automne d'une femme*, yet another characteristic of the pathogenic secret is brought to light, namely, the fact that it can bring forth severe psychosomatic disturbances. Claire's illness begins in the form of an ordinary depression that gradually becomes worse and worse. She then has a severe hemorrhage, which brings her close to death. When comparing Prévost's novel with Jung-Stilling's *Theobald*, we also note that the treatment of the pathogenic secret, which previously belonged entirely to the realm of the religious "Cure of Souls," has now been fully secularized and has entered into the field of the physician. In Prévost's novel, the main therapeutic work is accomplished by Dr. Daumier. The role of the priest is maintained, but only insofar as the patient may have religious problems that cannot be solved by the psychiatrist. As mentioned, how and when the knowledge of the pathogenic secret entered into the medical field is not quite clear. However, this process was very probably helped through the progress of criminological theory on one side and of magnetism and hypnotism on the other.

The Pathogenic Secret in Nineteenth-Century Criminology

Throughout the nineteenth century, a number of judges and lawyers were increasingly interested in the psychological intricacies of the mind of the criminal. Paradoxically, certain criminals against whom insufficient evidence had been obtained and who were on the point of being released would unexpectedly give full confessions of heinous crimes. The reasons for such self-betrayals remained a mystery. Most authors explained them by assuming that for certain criminals the effort of keeping the secret of their crime causes such an inner tension that it comes to a breaking point.

In his *Philosophie pénale*, published in 1890, Gabriel Tarde described the feelings of certain criminals after their first crime.[11] According to Tarde, it is for the criminal as if a sudden abyss has been dug out between his fellowmen and the criminal; he feels a growing faith in his strangeness and superiority, and the thought of his crime becomes a fixed idea. "This incessant preoccupation betrays itself by a thousand indications; by drawings such as the one which Tropmann drew of one of his crimes . . . , or by the compromising words wherein is revealed the necessity of saying the thing which is still known only to oneself; by silence also, and even by sleep and dreams." The power of that secret is such that it brings the individual

[11] Gabriel Tarde, *La philosophie pénale* (Lyon, Storck, 1890).

to repeat his crime, either in imagination or in visiting the scene of his crime or even in repeating it in reality. "The propensity which drives a man to the repetition of a crime is thus a fatal one, still more fatal than the tendency to an amorous, artistic, or poetic repetition." Tarde has also described the transformation wrought in the mind of the criminal by the sudden disclosure of his crime. During this phase of his secret, he lived in a kind of daydream; now suddenly that feverish inner life in which he lived has disappeared and from that moment on he reflects into himself the disparaging opinion that his fellowmen have of him. What Tarde described from the point of view of a criminologist was also described by Dostoevsky in his celebrated novel *Crime and Punishment* (1866). A problem that seems to have attracted less attention is that of the long-range psychological effects of the burden of the secret upon the criminal, should his crime not be discovered. It would seem that the secret exerts a permanent and profoundly disturbing effect on certain criminals.

C. G. Jung tells the story of a woman, unknown to him, who came to his office, refusing to divulge her name, and told him how twenty years earlier she had poisoned her best friend in order to marry her husband.[12] But the husband died soon after she married him, and the daughter of this marriage disappeared in turn; even animals, she said, turned away from her so that she could no longer ride horses or own dogs. Finally she fell into an unspeakable loneliness; this was the reason why she felt that she must make a professional man share the knowledge of her crime. Jung never saw that woman again and wondered what happened to her. Actually the long-range disturbances caused by a secret of that kind in the mind of an undetected criminal constitute one of the least-known chapters of criminology.

Various aspects of the secret of the crime in the criminal's mind were discussed by the Austrian criminologist Hanns Gross in his textbook of criminal psychology in 1898.[13] Through Tarde and Gross, such problems began to be familiar in certain psychiatric circles.

Magnetism and Hypnotism

The notion of the burdening secret also became known to magnetists very soon after the discovery by A.M.J. Puységur of the state of "magnetic sleep," later known as "hypnosis." The very first patient in whom Puységur induced magnetic sleep in 1784, a young man named Victor Race, once

---

[12] Carl G. Jung, *Erinnerungen, Träume, Gedanken*, edited by Aniela Jaffé (Zurich, Rascher, 1963), 128–30.

[13] Hanns Gross, *Criminalpsychologie* (Graz, Langsehner & Lubensky, 1898).

told him in "magnetic sleep" about a conflict he had with his sister and about which he would never dare to speak in a normal state.[14] He asked Puységur for advice, which he followed in a waking state to his own satisfaction. In the early period of animal magnetism during the late eighteenth and early nineteenth centuries similar cases were reported everywhere. In 1786, the Count of Lutzelbourg published the story of one of his patients who was infatuated with a male friend, in whom he had the utmost confidence in the waking state.[15] However, in magnetic sleep he knew that his supposed friend was a traitor who harmed him and explained to the magnetist what he had to do in order to pass on this knowledge from his "sleep" to his waking state. Such occurrences in which magnetized patients related to the magnetist a pathogenic secret and the way to be relieved of it became less frequent in the second half of the nineteenth century when hypnotists began to use a more authoritarian approach toward their subjects and simply to give them orders to accomplish during and after the hypnotic session. It is probably for that reason that many hypnotists were frightened when their subjects began to tell them about painful, often intimate, secrets. DeMarquay and Giraud-Teulon described the case of a lady whom they had hypnotized and who had told them confidences so dangerous to herself that they hastened to wake her.[16] H.-E. Beaunis, one of Hippolyte Bernheim's associates at Nancy, relates that when he was a student he became acquainted with a young girl who told him in a somnambulic state that she had had a child, a secret that nobody around her was aware of; on waking she implored him never to reveal her secret.[17] In such occurrences, one has the feeling that later generations of hypnotists had forgotten much of what their magnetist predecessors knew and utilized to the benefit of their patients. Nevertheless, there were exceptions, and during the great wave of hypnotism of the 1880s and 1890s there were still hypnotists who knew how to relieve their patients of burdensome secrets related in hypnotic states. For instance, Dr. Bonjour, a Swiss psychotherapist, observed in 1895 that certain of his patients revealed under hypnosis allegedly painful things that they denied or pretended not to know in the waking state but later admitted that they always knew but did not dare to talk about.[18]

[14] A. M. J. Puységur, *Mémoires pour servir à l'histoire et à l'établissement du Magnétisme animal* ([Paris], 1784).

[15] Comte de Lutzelbourg, *Extraits des journaux d'un magnétiseur attaché à la Société des Amis Réunis de Strasbourg* (Strasbourg, Librairie Académique, 1786), 47.

[16] J. N. DeMarquay and Félix Giraud-Teulon, *Recherches sur l'hypnotisme ou sommeil nerveux* (Paris, Baillière, 1860).

[17] H.-E. Beaunis, *Le somnambulisme provoqué* (Paris, Baillière, 1887), 205.

[18] Dr. Bonjour, "La psychanalyse," *Bibliothèque Universelle et Revue Suisse*, 125e année, 97 (1895), 226–39, 337–54.

Moritz Benedikt

It seems that the first medical man who systematized the knowledge of the pathogenic secret and of its psychotherapy was the Viennese physician Moritz Benedikt (1835–1920) in a series of publications on hysteria and neurosis. As early as 1864 Benedikt contended that the root of hysteria was not in physical diseases of the genital organs, as was commonly believed in his time, but in functional disturbances of sexual life.[19] In his textbook on electrotherapy, published in 1868, Benedikt attributed the cause of hysteria to early psychic stimulation, notably from the sexual organs, and to abnormalities of sexual life, particularly to sexual frustrations.[20] Benedikt also told of four cases of male hysteria which he blamed on maltreatment during childhood and early disturbances in the patients' "libido," a term Benedikt used repeatedly. Although a practitioner of electrotherapy, Benedikt did not believe that this method could be effective with hysterical disorders, since their real causes rested in disturbances of sexual life that the woman keeps secret, thus making it difficult for the physician to uncover them.

In 1891, Benedikt restated his theory of hysteria. The basis of the disease, he now argued, consisted of an inborn or acquired vulnerability of the nervous system, but its actual cause was either a psychic trauma (which may occur in men as well as women) or a functional disturbance of the genital system or the sexual life, which a female patient will often keep secret, even from her nearest relatives and her family doctor.[21] Benedikt proclaimed the futility of a hypnotic treatment of hysteria and the necessity of psychotherapy on the conscious level.

In 1894, Benedikt elaborated on his idea of a "Second Life," which is the secret inner life of the healthy and sick individual.[22] Benedikt's "Second Life" originates from representative, imaginative, and creative activities that the individual keeps for him- or herself. Certain types of individuals are more inclined than others to develop such a "Second Life"—for instance, those sensitive men who have lacked recognition from their fellowmen, those whose personality forms a strong contrast with their environment, or those who have lacked the opportunity in life to develop their abilities. Benedikt described various types of this "Second Life" among eccentrics, gamblers, criminals, and neurasthenics. "Second Life," Ben-

[19] Moritz Benedikt, *Beobachtung über Hysterie*, reprinted from *Zeitschrift für practische Heilkunde* (1864), 27.

[20] Moritz Benedikt, *Elektrotherapie* (Vienna, Tender & Company, 1868), 413–45.

[21] Moritz Benedikt, "Über Neuralgien und Neuralgische Affectionen und deren Behandlung," *Klinische Zeit- und Streitfragen*, 6, no. 3 (1891), 67–106.

[22] Moritz Benedikt, "Second Life: Das Seelenbinnenleben des gesunden und kranken Menschen," *Wiener Klinik*, 20 (1894), 127–38.

edikt said, is far more prevalent among women than among men mainly because women are to a higher degree under the pressure of social conventions and must conceal emotionally and sexually much more than men. This is also the reason for the prevalence of hysteria among women. This inner life, Benedikt added, is a realm of the human mind that has been far too little explored by science, though it is of the utmost importance for psychotherapy. Its systematic exploration should be the first concern of the therapist in treating a depressed or hysterical woman.

In 1895, Benedikt also incorporated into a treatise on the human mind his previous publication on "Second Life," insisting upon the fundamental role it plays not only in hysteria and other neuroses but also in severe mental illness and in certain physical diseases.[23] He insisted again upon the great importance of thwarted love and sexual disturbances in the psychogenesis of neurosis, and particularly of hysteria.

In his autobiography of 1906, Benedikt came back to the topic of a psychological "inner life," which he obviously considered one of his most important contributions to medical science.[24] After restating all of his previous theories on neuroses and hysteria, he illustrated these ideas with cases from his former practice. In one case, for instance, he was called to see a young woman who had intolerable headaches which he feared indicated a case of meningitis. He found no physical illness, but he then took the patient aside and asked her about a secret love, which was not the case. She told him that her suffering was caused by the fact that she was taken out of school in spite of her burning desire to study further. Benedikt told her that he would arrange the matter with her parents on the condition that she would get out of bed, dress, and go to dinner with the family. He impressed the importance of her wish on her parents, who immediately acquiesced, so that when she appeared at dinner, her alleged meningitis had already disappeared, and she remained cured from that day on.

In most cases, however, Benedikt attributed the cause of the neurosis to a secret pertaining to the sexual life of the individual. There was, for instance, the story of a married woman who, it was feared, was also developing a meningitis. Actually, however, her husband was impotent, and the woman had some reason to fear an illegitimate pregnancy. As soon as a gynecologist had reassured her in that regard, the "meningitis" disappeared.

In still another instance, Benedikt was called as a consultant to see a woman who had repeated fits of coughing from morning to night. The patient received him with the words: "Herr Professor, you will not heal

[23] Moritz Benedikt, *Die Seelenkunde des Menschen als reine Erfahrungswissenschaft* (Leipzig, O. R. Reisland, 1895).

[24] Moritz Benedikt, *Aus meinem Leben: Erinnerungen und Erörterungen* (Vienna, Carl Konegen, 1906), 127–46.

me!" Benedikt suspected from the start that this remark meant that the woman was suffering from some secret, and he advised the family physician to try and discover it. The family physician found nothing, and the patient remained ill. Later, the parents brought the patient to Benedikt's office. Benedikt told the mother that experience had taught him that such young women as a rule suffer from a painful secret that they would not reveal even to their mothers. Had her daughter perhaps once been the victim of some kind of sexual abuse? The mother was at first indignant at the idea, but when she talked to her daughter alone she found out that at the age of 10 the girl had repeatedly been sexually abused by a man who was an acquaintance of the family and whom she still sometimes encountered at social gatherings. When Benedikt returned to the patient, she told him: "Now, Doctor, you will cure me!" The recovery actually happened rapidly, and some time later the woman was able to marry and have a happy life.

In still another case, the family of a young dressmaker was worried because of their daughter's increasingly eccentric behavior. The mother of the girl brought her to Benedikt, who immediately told the patient that she must be acting under the pressure of an internal secret, which it was now her duty to tell him. After insisting that there was nothing of the kind, the patient finally revealed that she was passionately attached to a woman friend, but a gypsy had told her that her friend would die if she, the patient, would not make a false confession every week. Out of concern for her friend, she did it, but as a Catholic she had guilt feelings. Benedikt showed the young woman the absurdity of her situation and convinced her to stop this silly behavior, after which time she gradually recovered. Benedikt cites several other instances of hysterical women cured by the confession of their pathogenic secrets and the practical and emotional working out of the related problems. Among such patients were allegedly paralyzed women who were rapidly enabled to walk. However, far from claiming to see psychogenesis everywhere, Benedikt also wrote of alleged neuroses that resulted from an ailment of a physical nature and that disappeared with the corresponding physical treatment.

Modern Dynamic Psychiatry

It is interesting to speculate to what extent the era of modern dynamic psychiatry was influenced by the accumulated century-old knowledge of the pathogenic secret and its healing. The theories of Pierre Janet and Sigmund Freud posit a specifically *unconscious* pathogenic secret, which the therapist has to unravel before being able to cure it. In contrast, Jung is concerned with pathogenic secrets of which the patient is aware (as in Benedikt's cases).

To our knowledge, the first published instance of a successful cathartic therapy was that of Pierre Janet's patient "Lucie" in 1886.[25] "Lucie"'s irrational fears resulted from a trauma that she had suffered in her childhood and that had then been forgotten; the symptoms of the case were eventually removed when the origins of the traumatic experience were brought to the patient's awareness. In 1889, Janet published the more complex case of "Marie," whose hysterical symptoms were found under hypnosis to have originated from three successive psychic traumas she suffered at different ages that manifested themselves independently in the symptoms of her crises.[26] Janet related how this patient was cured by the discovery and working through of her "subconscious fixed ideas." In publishing the cases of "Marcelle"[27] in 1891 and of "Madame D."[28] in 1892, Janet offered a more elaborate theory of "subconscious fixed ideas"—their origin, pathogenic effect, symptoms, and treatment. In a fifth case, published in 1893 and 1894, Janet tells the story of a man who came from a superstitious environment in a remote French province and was brought in 1890 to the Salpêtrière with manifestations of demoniacal possession.[29] "Achille" was in a state of furious agitation, proffering blasphemies, speaking sometimes with the voice of the devil and at other times with his own. Charcot asked Janet to treat the patient. The previous history of the illness indicated that Achille's problem had started rather suddenly six months before, after the patient had gone on a short business trip. After trying several devices, Janet succeeded in hypnotizing the patient and retrieving his real story. During his business trip, Achille had been unfaithful to his wife; he had tried to forget the incident but became more and more obsessed with guilt feelings and the fear of damnation, and then one day he suddenly felt himself possessed. Janet tells how he was able to work through the patient's fixed idea, first in hypnosis and then in a waking state, and how the patient afterwards remained permanently cured. In that remarkable story of Achille we find an instance of a pathogenic secret whose healing was not obtained with the old practice of confession, but with an elaborated new technique of dynamic psychotherapy. In later publications, Janet never lost sight of the notion of the pathogenic secret and its cure, although he unfortunately never fully systematized or theorized about the

[25] Pierre Janet, "Les actes inconscients et le dédoublement de la personnalité pendant le somnambulisme provoqué," *Revue philosophique*, 22 (1886), II, 577–92.

[26] Pierre Janet, *L'automatisme psychologique* (Paris, F. Alcan, 1889), 436–40.

[27] Pierre Janet, "Étude sur un cas d'aboulie et d'idées fixes," *Revue philosophique*, 31 (1891), I, 382–407.

[28] Pierre Janet, *Étude sur un cas d'amnésie antérograde dans la maladie de la désagrégation psychologique* (London, International Congress of Experimental Psychology, 1892), 26–30.

[29] Pierre Janet, *Contribution à l'étude des accidents mentaux chez les hystériques* (Paris, Rueff, 1893), 252–57; idem, "Un cas de possession et l'exorcisme moderne," *Bulletin de l'Université de Lyon*, 8 (1894), 41–57.

concept. From his point of view, this phenomenon belonged to the larger notion of "psychological" or "moral disinfection."

Next we come to Freud. In 1893, Freud published jointly with Breuer the important paper with the title "On the Psychic Mechanism of Hysterical Phenomena; Provisional Communication."[30] Two footnotes of that paper refer briefly to Janet and to Benedikt. In regard to Janet, Breuer and Freud recall his case of a hysterical girl who had been cured "through the application of a procedure analogous to our own." Another footnote reads as follows: "The closest approach to our theoretical and therapeutic statements, we have found in occasionally published remarks of Benedikt with which we will deal in another place."

This essay of Breuer and Freud came to the attention of both Janet and Benedikt. Janet simply stated that he was happy to see that "several authors, particularly Messrs. Breuer and Freud, have recently confirmed my already ancient interpretation of subconscious fixed ideas among hysterical patients."[31] Interestingly, Benedikt criticized Breuer's and Freud's concept of hysteria; obviously he did not believe that the traumatic pathogenic event in these cases had been unconsciously repressed by the patients.[32] At that time Benedikt no longer believed in the genuine character of the hypnotic sleep, and he thought that the patients just pretended to be in hypnotic sleep in order to please the physician. With the further development of psychoanalysis, the concept of the pathogenic secret became gradually absorbed into the wider frame of reference of traumatic reminiscences and of repression and later into the concept of neurotic guilt feelings. This is a significant but separate subject that cannot be explored in the present paper.

Among Freud's earliest followers was the Protestant minister Reverend Oskar Pfister of Zurich, who was the first figure to apply psychoanalysis to education and also—as can be expected from his profession—to the *Seelsorge*, or the "Cure of Souls." To those who knew Pfister personally as well as those who have read his writings carefully, it is clear that to him psychoanalysis was to a certain extent a rediscovery and perfecting of the traditional Protestant technique of the "Cure of Souls." Pfister saw in psychoanalysis a means of helping a greater number of suffering human beings; he always thought of his psychoanalytic practice as part and parcel of his own pastoral work, and for that reason many of his patients were treated gratuitously.[33] In Pfister's writings, it is also striking to see the great number of

---

[30] Joseph Breuer and Sigmund Freud, "Über den psychischen Mechanismus hysterischer Phänomene (Vorläufige Mitteilung)," *Neurologisches Centralblatt*, 12 (1893), 4–10, 43–47.

[31] Janet, *Contribution à l'étude des accidents mentaux*, 68.

[32] Moritz Benedikt, *Hypnotismus und Suggestion: Eine klinisch-psychologische Studie* (Leipzig and Vienna, Breitenstein, 1894), 64–65.

[33] Oskar Pfister, *Die psychoanalytische Methode* (Leipzig and Berlin, Klinkhardt, 1913). See also Pfister's many other writings.

accounts of short analytic therapies. One cannot help thinking that at times some of his patients pretended to have repressed unpleasant memories, in the same way that the patients of Dr. Bonjour pretended at first not to know in the waking state what they revealed in alleged hypnotic sleep.

Among the pioneers of modern dynamic psychiatry, the one who devoted the most attention to the concept of the pathogenic secret was Carl Gustav Jung. Is it a coincidence, we can only wonder, that Jung was the son of a Protestant minister, Reverend Paul Jung? Whether or not Reverend Paul Jung actually practiced the "Cure of Souls" is not known, although it is certain that Jung's father was interested in psychiatry and had worked as the chaplain at the mental hospital Friedmatt in Basel. Be that as it may, Jung related in his autobiography how, when he was a young resident at the University Psychiatric Hospital of the Burghölzli in Zurich, he examined a young woman with a severe depression that had been diagnosed as "dementia praecox" and whose prognosis was considered poor.[34] Jung, however, had doubts about the diagnosis. From his new Word Association Test he received clues from the patient that hinted at a gloomy personal story, and finally the woman revealed her secret. She had been in love with a young man who did not seem to care for her, whereupon she had married another man, only to learn five years later that the first young man had actually been in love with her and had regretted that she had married someone else. This was the beginning of the woman's depression. Then, at a later date, while her little daughter was once in the bathtub, she had let the girl suck a sponge filled with dirty water; the little one caught typhoid fever and died, and then the depression worsened. Jung explained to the woman that her illness was related to her inability to discuss that traumatic secret; the patient was then rapidly relieved, and two weeks later she left the hospital as cured. Since that time he had the opportunity of effecting numerous cures of the same kind. All those who knew Jung or who followed his teaching know the importance he attributed to the pathogenic secret. However, he considered it only a preliminary part of the complete psychotherapeutic treatment. Jung also believed that in order to be effective, the confession of a secret must be met by absolute secrecy on the part of the therapist. Jung felt that he was morally not allowed to tell his patients' secrets to any of his colleagues. It is, as it were, the therapy "of the secret by the secret."

General Considerations on the Pathogenic Secret

This brings us finally to a comparison of the meaning of the pathogenic secret to the priest and to the psychiatrist. A perusal of any treatise of moral

---

[34] Jung, *Erinnerungen, Träume, Gedanken*, 121–24.

theology—say, for instance, the *Practical Instruction to Confessors* by Saint Alphonse of Liguori—shows that in the Catholic church the secret of confession is considered absolute, which means that in no case and under no circumstances is the priest allowed to tell anybody whatever he has heard under the "seal" of confession.[35] In very difficult matters he may consult one of his superiors, but he must tell the matter even to the superior in such a way that the personality of the penitent cannot be identified. The confessor is forbidden to refer to these matters, even in talking with his penitent, and he should be careful to avoid ever giving the impression that he may be referring to something heard in confession. Needless to say, there is no question of a priest taking notes, keeping a record book of his penitents, or writing accounts of his experience as a confessor. That the secret of Catholic confession is absolute also means that it must be kept even at the risk of the priest's life and that divulging the secret would be considered an extremely severe infringement on the part of the priest. On the other hand, the secret of confession extends to the penitent himself, who is not allowed to tell under confession, for instance, the names of his accomplices. It is interesting to note that in a French sociological study about treason published in 1951, André Thérive states that he found no instance in which a former priest revealed anything heard in church confession.[36]

Similarly, the physician's professional secret—which is one of the tenets of the Hippocratic oath—is a traditional article of faith taught by medical deontology. It has, however, never been as absolute as the secret of the priest, firstly because it is not endowed with the dimension of the sacred, and secondly for many practical reasons. The extension of medical insurance and of welfare medicine inescapably entails its gradual limitation. However, there is a category of patients who expect a more rigorous observation of professional secrecy when going to their physician, and these are the clients of psychotherapists. Do these patients always get absolute secrecy?

Unfortunately, in this matter a strange development has taken place in recent decades. When the analyzed patient lies on the couch and tells the analyst whatever comes to his or her mind, he knows that the analyst is writing notes. But what happens to these case notes? Are they not then dictated to a secretary, recorded by her in a case history that is then classified in some filing cabinet? And who has the keys to the file cabinets? What if government or private agencies make inquiries? And will these files be open to the medical historians of the future, as happened, for instance, to the case histories of Nietzsche? Moreover, a psychotherapist nowadays

---

[35] Saint Alphonse de Liguori, "Instruction pratique pour les confesseurs," in *Oeuvres* (Paris, Vivès, 1877), 7:436–59.
[36] André Thérive, *Essai sur les trahisons* (Paris, Calmann-Lévy, 1951), 100–101.

most often belongs to a hospital psychiatric staff or psychoanalytic institute. The psychiatrist may have to report everything to his supervisor, or to a group in which his patient's history will be discussed and analyzed, so that the whole staff will necessarily know about many confidential matters.

New techniques of observation have also provided psychotherapists with a whole armamentarium of one-way vision rooms, microphones, and tape recorders that can be hidden in a suitcase or elsewhere. A psychotherapy patient can never be sure that his utterances will not be recorded and kept in some form or another. There is even a historical instance of a textbook of psychoanalysis that had just been published when a patient, who was browsing in a bookstore, found the textbook, recognized his own case history, literally ran to his lawyer, and had the entire issue of the book seized by order of the court and then destroyed.

It is unlikely that this matter escapes the concern of patients. Many of them may not worry about it, and some of them will no doubt tell the psychotherapist that they don't mind about the one-way vision room, the microphone, or the tape recorder. But we can be sure that these same patients will not convey to the psychotherapist those pathogenic secrets they would confess to the priest with a higher standard of secrecy. Actually, pathogenic secrets are often kept hidden by patients undergoing psychotherapeutic treatments for remarkably long periods of time. I remember once having heard Wilhelm Stekel contend that there are certain things that a patient will *never* tell his analyst even after whole years of analysis. On the other hand, I know of two instances in which a patient who had revealed a dangerous secret to his analyst discovered that that most confidential matter had seeped through, probably through the indiscretion of a medical supervisor. I could also tell the authentic story of a psychologist, working in an institution for juvenile delinquents, who obtained one day a surprising confidence from one of the boys, whose behavior from that day on improved notably. Upon pressure from the director of the institute, the psychologist halfheartedly consented to tell what the confidential matter was at a meeting of the team. Everyone promised to keep the secret, but apparently someone did not, because the story got back to the boy from outside; he became incensed against the "traitor" and immediately fell back into his delinquent behavior.

There is much more to say on this intriguing topic, but I notice that I have left the field of medical history and am encroaching on that of professional ethics. Historical investigation of a problem can at times not only have an interest in its own right, but can also focus attention on a problem of pressing actuality.

APPENDICES

Appendix A

The Discovery of the Unconscious:
Table of Contents

Appendix B

Report on My Study Trip to Europe, Summer of 1963

HENRI F. ELLENBERGER

[*Editor's note*: Beginning in the late 1950s, Ellenberger developed a distinctive style of historical research. This method consisted of intensive reading in a wide range of European libraries and archives during the summer months, preceded by an elaborate preparatory correspondence to librarians and archivists, and followed by a continuation of his research activities at these institutions through the mail. The document below, a summary of Ellenberger's research itinerary for 1963 and the shortest of his summer travelogues, gives an indication of this style of work.]

I left Montreal on the SS *Arcadia* on May 17 and arrived in Le Havre, France, on May 25.

Le Havre (May 25)

I had already established contact by mail with the *archiviste départemental* and the director of the lyceum in Le Havre, whom I had asked to assist me in finding information about Pierre Janet's sojourn there (1882–1889). Thanks to the efforts of these two gentlemen, I came across an unpublished lecture, "On the Teaching of Philosophy," by Janet. A perusal of two Le Havre newspapers from that period showed that Janet's famous hypnotic experiments and the visit of a delegation of the Society for Psychical Research [of Britain] had remained unnoticed by the press. This fact is all the more interesting because there was at that time much talk about hypnosis on account of demonstrations of that phenomenon staged publicly in Le Havre.

Paris (May 26–June 15)

From May 26 to June 15 I stayed in Paris, where I had already arranged by mail for meetings with a number of people who were disposed to assist me in my research.

The Early History of Mesmerism

I first contacted M. Robert Amadou, who is preparing a much-needed edition of the complete works of Franz Anton Mesmer. I received from him a number of hints regarding further explorations.

Essential to my research was a trip to the village of Buzancy, near Soissons, where the Marquis de Puységur in 1784 obtained "Mesmeric sleep" (that is, hypnosis) for the first time on a patient of the name Victor Race. I had the great pleasure of getting acquainted with the Vicomte du Boisdulier, a direct descendant of the Marquis de Puységur. He showed me a number of documents, some of them unpublished and pertaining to the Marquis de Puységur and to his family. I learned from him that the rich library and the family archives of the Puységurs had been destroyed during World War I and the chateau itself during World War II. The famous elm tree that Puységur had magnetized in order to obtain many of his cures survived until 1939, when it was broken during a storm, just a few weeks before a film on Mesmer was to be shot in that region. The inhabitants of the village collected pieces of the bark and still keep them. In one of the homes, I was shown a piece of that tree, which is supposed to have preventive and curative properties.

The mayor of Buzancy, M. Guillemot, under whose guidance I visited the village and the ruins of the chateau, introduced me to the departmental archivist in Soissons, thanks to whom I found the birth and death certificates of Victor Race and the names of his children and learned that he still had descendants living in Soissons. After the death of Victor Race, the Marquis de Puységur erected a monument on his tomb in the Buzancy cemetery to the "doyen des somnambules de France." This monument was destroyed at an unknown date.

Following that visit, I came to the conclusion that the history of the discovery of hypnotic sleep cannot be understood outside of its sociological context. The Marquis de Puységur was a powerful feudal landholder. The Race family (as I was told by the Vicomte du Boisdulier) had been at the service of the Puységurs for many a generation. It is unlikely that Puységur could have magnetized so many inhabitants of Buzancy had it not been for the tremendous social and mental dependency of the population upon their lord.

Charcot and the History of Hysteria

Professor [Paul] Castaigne of the Salpêtrière, Charcot's remote successor [in the Chaire des Maladies du Système Nerveux] introduced me to the Bibliothèque Charcot, that is, to Charcot's personal library, which he had bequeathed to the Salpêtrière. To my regret, I found this library in a most pitiful and dilapidated state, although it contains many rare and valuable works. In regard to Charcot's unpublished manuscripts, which are supposedly being kept in that library, all I could find were manuscripts of already published works of his, some notes about patients, some sketches and drawings, but none of the unpublished literary works about which there was much talk after Charcot's death.

I had hoped to be able to study the files of some of Charcot's patients, especially of those who had served as prototypes of his descriptions of hysteria. The medical files of that period are no longer in the Salpêtrière but in the general Archives de l'Assistance Publique. M. Pierre Jean of the Ministère de la Santé Publique authorized me to research in these archives. However, the organization of the archives is such that it would be extremely difficult to identify particular files, and my time would never have sufficed for this task.

Pierre Janet's Career

My inquiry regarding Janet's background and academic career in Paris was very successful. I had already contacted Janet's two daughters, Madame Pichon-Janet and Mademoiselle Fanny Janet. These two ladies were extremely kind and cooperative. They gave me a wealth of information about their father as well as a number of photographs. I also received valuable information about Janet from the Collège Sainte-Barbe, where he went to school as a boy, from the École Normale Supérieure, and above all from the Collège de France, where Janet taught for forty years and where the archivist was willing to put at my disposal Janet's entire file. I also interviewed two men who had been in prolonged personal contact with Janet: Professor Jean Delay of the Clinique Sainte-Anne and Dr. Ignace Meyerson.

Strasbourg (June 15–19)

The city of Strasbourg played a very important role in the history of animal magnetism: the Marquis de Puységur was appointed commander of the artillery regiment there in 1785 and opened a flourishing school of magnetism. Essential to my research was the fact that all of the cures of the years 1785 to 1789 had been recorded with the names of the magnetizers and of the patients. The reports on those cures are extremely rare (not even the Bibliothèque Nationale possesses a copy). I was able to look through those documents at the Strasbourg Public Library and was confirmed in my assumption that in most cases the magnetizer was a nobleman and the cured patient either a peasant or a servant. The Strasbourg Public Library also possesses a unique collection of early French and German publications about Mesmerism.

I also took advantage of my stay in Strasbourg to make inquiries about Pierre Janet's maternal side of the family. (His mother, Fanny Hummel, had been a native of Strasbourg.)

Basel (June 19–20)

The two days I spent in Basel were most productive. I had a long interview with Dr. Kurt von Sury, president of the Swiss Society of Jungian Psychology and lifelong disciple and personal friend of C. G. Jung, who gave me a great deal of biographical information about Jung. I went to Kleinhüningen, once a farmers' and fishermen's village and now a suburb of Basel, which is the place where Jung spent his childhood and youth. Thanks to the present-day Protestant minister of the town, I was able to have an interview with an old woman there who in spite of her eighty years had an astonishing clarity of mind. She had known Jung as a youth and gave me much information about his childhood as well as about his parents. I also interviewed an old lady in Basel who gave me information about Jung's young female cousin [Helene Preiswerk], the medium on whom he made his first experiments. Finally, I got information from the Basel University Library, where the librarians, whom I had contacted in advance, were most helpful.

Zurich (June 21–24)

In Zurich, I had already contacted several prominent Jungians. Dr. C. A. Meier, director of the Jung Institute, had given me permission—which is rarely granted to a foreigner—to make a perusal of the Institute's collection of Jung's unpublished seminars. The collection of these typewritten seminars covers whole shelves and constitutes a very large collection (the ten volumes of the seminars on Nietzsche's *Thus Spoke Zarathustra* alone make some 2,000 to 3,000 typewritten pages). It was a Tantalus torture to have so little time at my disposal to study that immense and rich material. I was told that excerpts and digests of these unpublished seminars will probably be published in a few years.

I also had very interesting and fruitful interviews with Dr. C. A. Meier himself and with Mrs. Aniela Jaffé, C. G. Jung's former secretary and editor of his autobiography.

Munich (June 24–30)

I left Zurich early on June 24, arrived in Munich in the evening, and spent the whole week at the Munich University Institute for the History of Medicine, where I was very well received by its director, Professor Werner Leibbrand, and his wife [Anne-Marie Wettley]. I was invited to participate in a seminar devoted to Paracelsus. The Institute's library is rich in psychiatric publications of the eighteenth and early nineteenth centuries, and I found many rare publications that yielded much information and that I had been unable to find in North America. Professor Leibbrand and his wife also gave me many useful hints regarding other fields of my research.

Vienna (June 30–July 26)

The four weeks I spent in Vienna were also extremely fruitful, mainly thanks to the generous help of Frau Professor Erna Lesky, head of the Vienna University Institute for the History of Medicine.

The Cultural and Medical Background of Psychoanalysis

My main concern was to investigate the social, medical, and cultural context in which psychoanalysis took its roots. Frau Professor Lesky provided me with a firsthand orientation in that field: in a most generous manner, she put at my disposal the manuscript of a book she is presently writing on the history of medicine in Vienna in the nineteenth century. I found there a general picture of the Viennese medical and psychiatric milieu of the second half of the nineteenth century.

Taking advantage of the great wealth of the Institute's library, I studied a range of authors in order to ascertain the possible extent of their influence upon early psychoanalysis. Frau Professor Lesky pointed out to me that in the 1870s and 1880s, relations between Charcot and the Viennese medical world were much closer than is usually believed. I dare say that the early history of psychoanalysis takes on a somewhat different shape when placed in its proper historical context.

The Story of "Anna O."

The story of Bertha Pappenheim, whose case was described by Breuer under the pseudonym of "Anna O.," is of particular importance because she is considered to be the prototype of a neurosis cured by cathartic therapy and is also considered to be the matrix from whence the whole of psychoanalytic therapy was developed. I started an investigation on the life of Bertha Pappenheim, beginning with the

Archives of the City of Vienna. I was thus able to gather information about her family background, her parents, and relevant dates, and I identified the house in which she lived and where the historical cathartic cure was performed by Breuer. Time did not permit me to go much further, but this investigation will be pursued by correspondence and with the help of one of the archivists who became interested in the matter.

Freud and Adler

Investigations into Freud's and Adler's backgrounds were started while I worked in the Archives of the City of Vienna, where I also secured documentary evidence about Adler's family background. A study of Adler's genealogy will be pursued with the help of an archivist.

Sofia, Bulgaria (July 27–August 3)

Shortly before my departure from Europe, I decided to alter my itinerary and to accept an invitation from Professor N. Schipkowensky of the University Psychiatric Clinic in Sofia. Dr. Schipkowensky, to whom I had turned for information regarding the early development of psychoanalysis in Russia and the Slavic countries, pointed out to me that rich material on that topic could be found at the Sofia University Library. I accepted his invitation to come to Sofia before I left Vienna, and he had arranged with the university libraries to have all the relevant material prepared ahead of time and put at my disposal in a specially reserved room. Furthermore, that material which was not available in Sofia had been listed for me with the help of medical librarians in Russia.

This stay in Sofia proved to be one of the most exciting parts of all of my research. As Dr. Schipkowensky had already pointed out to me by mail, psychoanalysis had developed widely at the time when it was officially prohibited in Russia. I found in Sofia not only the Russian translations of Freud and of the first psychoanalysts, but quite a number of publications by native Russian psychoanalysts. The same was true for Bulgaria, and I had the feeling that Russian psychoanalysts had even anticipated some later advances of psychoanalysis in the Western world. Once more, I was exposed to the Tantalus ordeal of having too great a wealth of material to take in during such a short time. I want to emphasize the help given to me by Dr. Schipkowensky and by the librarians in translating and summarizing for me those publications that were not provided with summaries in western European languages.

During my stay, I also had the opportunity to visit the University Psychiatric Clinic of Sofia and to talk with the psychiatrists to clarify in what ways their outlook on dynamic psychiatry differs from our own.

Vienna (August 3–5)

The Institute for the History of Medicine was closed during the month of August. I spent these days making arrangements with the kind archivist for the continuation of my research by mail. I also had the opportunity to visit Professor Viktor Frankl's University Psychiatric Polyclinik and was very much interested by demonstrations

of his new psychotherapeutic method of "paradoxical intention." Professor Frankl
had previously been a disciple of Adler's and had left him in 1927. I interviewed him
on the specific topic of Adlerian psychotherapy and existential psychotherapy.

Zurich (August 6–8)

Unfortunately, the Jung Institute was also closed at that time. However, the University Library was open, and I took advantage of those days to look through some
rare psychiatric books and articles.

Dornach (August 8–15)

My investigations at the Jung Institute and especially the perusal of Jung's unpublished seminars has shown me striking similarities between several basic concepts of Jung's psychology and of Rudolf Steiner's anthroposophy. It appeared to be
a rewarding problem to tackle, and I decided therefore to spend a few days at the
"Goetheanum," the central anthroposophic institute and headquarters of the anthroposophic movement. The Goetheanum contains not only the Rudolf Steiner
archives, but a large and rich philosophical library. Thanks to the courtesy of the
librarians, I was able to gain access to the typewritten copies of Rudolf Steiner's
unpublished lectures, which are accessible nowhere else. I soon came to the conclusion that neither had Jung influenced Steiner nor Steiner influenced Jung, so that it
should probably be assumed that they both drew on one or more common sources.
These common sources could be nothing but certain Romantic philosophers of the
early nineteenth century, whom I was able to identify thanks to the help of the
Dornach librarians.

Another accidental and unexpected find was the fact that Rudolf Steiner had
been well acquainted with Josef Breuer in Vienna and was very favorably impressed
by him, which is obvious from the way he praises him.

Geneva (August 15–18)

I had contacted several people in Geneva prior to my journey. I worked mostly at
the Geneva University Public Library, where I found some rare publications, and
made inquiries about Flournoy's medium "Helen Smith."

Zurich (August 18–25)

At this point, the Jung Institute was open again for a few hours a day, and I was able
to pursue the investigation I had started earlier, while working at the same time at
the Zurich University Library. On August 23, I went to Küsnacht, where I was the
guest of Mr. and Mrs. Franz Jung (Jung's son who is now living in his father's
house). I already knew the house where I had, years ago, been the guest of C. G.
Jung himself. I now had the opportunity to visit in detail C. G. Jung's remarkable
library and was also shown photographs and other documents about him.

Paris (August 26–September 8)

During this time, I attended the International Congress of Adlerian Psychology, which was being held in Paris. This congress afforded me the chance to talk to a number of people who had come from various countries and who had been personally acquainted with Alfred Adler.

The remainder of this period was spent mainly at the Bibliothèque Nationale, where I found several facts about the period 1885–1886 in medical journals and newspapers which, I believe, throw a new light on Freud's visit to Paris during that period.

Appendix C

Henri F. Ellenberger: Complete Writings in the History of Psychiatry

THE BIBLIOGRAPHY below is limited to the writings of Henri Ellenberger of a historical nature. In addition to these, Ellenberger is the author of over 120 publications on medical topics as well as approximately 190 book reviews, many of which concern historical subjects. Where possible, I have cited editions of articles in the English language, although many of these essays have also appeared in other languages. Copies of Ellenberger's full bibliography may be obtained from the author or the editor.

Books

La psychiatrie suisse (Series of articles published between 1951 and 1953 in *L'évolution psychiatrique*) (Paris, Imprimerie Poirier-Bottreau, [1954]).

Criminologie du passé et du présent (Montreal, Presses de l'Université de Montréal, 1969).

The Discovery of the Unconscious: The History and Evolution of Dynamic Psychiatry (New York, Basic Books, 1970). Editions and translations: *The Discovery of the Unconscious: The History and Evolution of Dynamic Psychiatry* (London, Allen Lane, 1970); *La scoperta dell'inconscio: Storia della psichiatria dinamica*, 2 vols. (Turin, Boringhieri, 1972); *Die Entdeckung des Unbewussten*, 2 vols. (Bern, Hans Huber, 1973), with a reprint in Zurich by Diogenes Verlag in 1985; *El descubrimiento del inconsciente (Historia y evolución de la psiquiatría dinámica)* (Madrid, Editorial Gredos, 1974); *A la découverte de l'inconscient: Histoire de la psychiatrie dynamique* (Villeurbanne, Simep-Éditions, 1974); *Muishiki no Hakken* (Rikido-Seishin-Igaku-Hattatsu Shi, Anri Erenberuga-Cho, Kimura Bin, Nakai Hisao Kenyaku, Kobundo, 1980).

Les mouvements de libération mythique et autres essais sur l'histoire de la psychiatrie, with a Preface by Jacques Dufresne (Montreal, Éditions Quinze, 1978). Translation: *I movimenti di liberazione mitica* (Turin, Liguori, 1986).

Articles

"La psychothérapie de Janet," *L'évolution psychiatrique*, special issue in commemoration of Pierre Janet, 15, no. 3 (July–September 1950), 465–84.

"A propos du '*Malleus Maleficarum*,'" *Schweizerische Zeitschrift für Psychologie*, 10, no. 2 (1951), 136–48.

"The Life and Work of Hermann Rorschach (1884–1922)," *Bulletin of the Menninger Clinic*, 18, no. 5 (September 1954), 172–219.

"A Psychiatrist's Informal Tour of Europe," *Menninger Quarterly*, 8–9 (1954–1955), 10–23.

"Fechner and Freud," *Bulletin of the Menninger Clinic*, 20, no. 4 (July 1956) 201–14.

"The Ancestry of Dynamic Therapy," *Bulletin of the Menninger Clinic*, 20, no. 6 (November 1956), 288–99.

"The Unconscious before Freud," *Bulletin of the Menninger Clinic*, 21, no. 1 (January 1957), 3–15.

"Psychiatric Problems as Reflected in the History of German Literature" (Unpublished lecture presented to the Kansas Modern Language Association, Manhattan, Kansas, April 13, 1957).

"The Scope of Swiss Psychology," in Henry P. David and Helmut von Bracken, eds., *Perspectives in Personality Theory* (New York, Basic Books, 1957), 44–64

"A Psychiatrist's Vacation in Europe," *T.P.R.* (*Temperature, Pulse, Respiration*), 18, no. 7 (November 1957), 5–13.

"A Clinical Introduction to Psychiatric Phenomenology and Existential Analysis," in Rollo May, Ernest Angel, and Henri F. Ellenberger, eds., *Existence: A New Dimension in Psychiatry and Psychology* (New York, Basic Books, 1958), 92–124.

"La psychiatrie et son histoire inconnue," *L'union médicale du Canada*, 90, no. 3 (March 1961), 281–89.

"L'existentialisme et son intérêt pour la psychiatrie," *L'union médicale du Canada*, 90, no. 9 (September 1961), 936–47.

"Histoire de la psychopathologie en Occident," *Critique*, 18, no. 182 (July 1962), 641–55.

"Les mouvements de libération mythique," *Critique*, 19, no. 190 (March 1963), 248–67.

"Les illusions de la classification psychiatrique," *L'évolution psychiatrique*, 28, no. 2 (April–June 1963), 221–42.

"L'autobiographie de C. G. Jung," *Critique*, 20, nos. 207–8 (August–September 1964), 754–79.

"Charcot and the Salpêtrière School," *American Journal of Psychotherapy*, 19, no. 2 (April 1965), 253–67.

"Mesmer and Puységur: From Magnetism to Hypnotism," *Psychoanalytic Review*, 52, no. 2 (Summer 1965), 137–53.

"The Pathogenic Secret and Its Therapeutics," *Journal of the History of the Behavioral Sciences*, 2, no. 1 (January 1966), 29–42.

"The Evolution of Depth Psychology," in Iago Galdston, ed., *Historic Derivations of Modern Psychiatry* (New York, McGraw-Hill, 1967), 159–84.

"La conférence de Freud sur l'hystérie masculine (15 octobre 1886): Étude critique," *L'information psychiatrique*, 44, no. 10 (1968), 921–29.

"The Concept of Creative Illness" [1964], *Psychoanalytic Review*, 55, no. 3 (1968), 442–56.

"La vie et l'oeuvre de Pierre Janet," in *Hôpital Pierre Janet à Hull: Ouverture officielle et journée scientifique* (Hull, 1969).

"Methodology in Writing the History of Dynamic Psychiatry," in George Mora and Jeanne L. Brand, eds., *Psychiatry and Its History: Methodological Problems in Research* (Springfield, Ill., Charles C. Thomas, 1970), 26–40.

"Histoire de l'anxiété: Contribution de la psychiatrie dynamique," in *Proceedings of the Fifth World Congress of Psychiatry* (Mexico City, 1971), 678–82.

"Discours prononcé par le docteur Henri F. Ellenberger à l'occasion de l'inauguration du nouvel Institut Philippe Pinel de Montréal," *Annales internationales de criminologie*, 10, no. 2 (1971), 387–92.

"The Story of 'Anna O.': A Critical Review with New Data," *Journal of the History of the Behavioral Sciences*, 8, no. 3 (July 1972), 267–79.

"Moritz Benedikt (1835–1920)," *Confrontations psychiatriques*, 11 (1973), 183–200.

"La notion de *Kairos* en psychothérapie," *Annales de psychothérapie*, 4, no. 7 (1973), 4–14.

"Pierre Janet, philosophe," *Dialogue: Canadian Philosophical Review/Revue philosophique canadienne*, 12, no. 2 (June 1973), 254–87.

"Psychiatry from Ancient to Modern Times," in Silvano Arieti, ed., *American Handbook of Psychiatry*, 2d ed., 2 vols. (New York, Basic Books, 1974), 1:3–27.

"Développement historique de la notion de processus psychothérapique," *L'union médicale du Canada*, 105, no. 12 (December 1976), 1820–30.

"L'histoire d'"Emmy von N.': Étude critique avec documents nouveaux," *L'évolution psychiatrique*, 42, no. 3 (July–September 1977), 519–40.

"Carl Gustav Jung: His Historical Setting," in Hertha Riese, ed., *Historical Explorations in Medicine and Psychiatry* (New York, Springer, 1978), 142–49.

"Pierre Janet and His American Friends" [1973], in George E. Gifford, Jr., ed., *Psychoanalysis, Psychotherapy and the New England Medical Scene, 1894–1944* (New York, Science History Publication, 1978), 63–72.

"From Justinus Kerner to Hermann Rorschach: The History of the Inkblots" (Unpublished manuscript, available in printed form in Japanese in *Rorschach Japonica*, 23 [September 1981], 1–8).

"Histoire de la psychiatrie," in R. Duguay, H. F. Ellenberger, et al., eds., *Précis pratique de psychiatrie* (Montreal, Chenelière and Stanké, 1981), 1–12.

"Evolution of Ideas about the Nature of the Psychotherapeutic Process in the Western World" [1979], in *History of Psychiatry: Proceedings of the Fourth International Symposium on the Comparative History of Medicine—East and West* (Tokyo, Saikon, 1982), 1–28.

"The Story of Helene Preiswerk: A Critical Study with New Documents," *History of Psychiatry*, 2, no. 5 (March 1991), 41–52.

Bibliographical Essay _____

SCHOLARLY LITERATURE on the history of psychiatry has burgeoned dramatically over the past fifteen years. This scholarship deals with psychiatry in its past theoretical, therapeutic, and institutional aspects and in a broad range of cultural, geographical, and chronological settings. A comprehensive account of the new psychiatric historiography is obviously impossible, and unnecessary, in this context. Rather, the aim of this bibliographical narrative is threefold: to display the lines of influence of Henri Ellenberger's work on subsequent professional commentary about psychiatric history; to indicate the current state of scholarly work on the subjects about which Ellenberger wrote the most; and to furnish interested readers with references for learning more about many of these topics. The texts recorded below have by no means all been inspired by Ellenberger (although a not inconsiderable number do reveal a clear and demonstrable debt to his work). However, all of them deal more or less directly with figures, themes, or ideas that Ellenberger studied during his lifetime. In the main, the bibliography is limited to titles in English, French, and German, with a strong emphasis on the secondary literature of the past twenty years.

Since 1970, nothing even remotely approximating *The Discovery of the Unconscious* has been published in any language. In its cultural and geographical scope, its synthesis of voluminous primary source materials, and its interpretive individuality, the book remains distinctive. However, many general histories of academic psychology have appeared during this period. Generally speaking, these works, which are often designed to serve large American undergraduate audiences, consist of informative and factually straightforward chapters about the major figures, theories, and movements in the history of psychology from, say, Plato and Aristotle to Wundt, James, or Watson. Examples are Thomas Hardy Leahey, *A History of Psychology: Main Currents in Psychological Thought*, 2d ed. (Englewood Cliffs, N.J., Prentice-Hall, 1987); Daniel N. Robinson, *An Intellectual History of Psychology* (Madison, University of Wisconsin Press, 1986); David Hothersall, *History of Psychology* (Philadelphia, Temple University Press, 1984); Clarence J. Karier, *Scientists of the Mind: Intellectual Founders and Modern Psychology* (Urbana, University of Illinois Press, 1986); Raymond E. Fancher, *Pioneers of Psychology*, 2d ed. (New York, Norton, 1990); and Robert I. Watson, Sr., and Rand B. Evans, *The Great Psychologists: A History of Psychological Thought*, 5th ed. (New York, Harper Collins, 1991). Perhaps the most substantial of the works in this mold is D. B. Klein's *A History of Scientific Psychology: Its Origins and Philosophical Backgrounds* (New York, Basic Books), which appeared the same year as Ellenberger's book. A French study along these lines, somewhat more noteworthy for its interpretations than its American counterparts, is Fernand-Lucien Mueller's *Histoire de la psychologie*, 4th ed., rev. and enl., 2 vols. (Paris, Payot, 1976). Far and away the most ambitious of the recent projects of this sort is *Die Psychologie des 20.Jahrhunderts* (Zurich and Munich, Kindler, 1976–1981), which consists of

380   BIBLIOGRAPHICAL ESSAY

sixteen 1,000-page volumes written by many contributors and covering a very wide range of subjects. It is unfortunate that this admirable enterprise is limited in scope to the twentieth century.

If histories of academic psychology have proliferated during the past two decades, the same cannot be claimed for *medical* psychology. Interestingly, despite the rush of publications in recent years about psychiatry's past, no full-scale history of the field, along the lines of the earlier volumes by Zilboorg, Leibbrand and Wettley, or Ellenberger, has been forthcoming. One ongoing, multiauthored work that canvasses some of the same territory as Ellenberger's book is Josef Rattner, ed., *Pioniere der Tiefenpsychologie* (Vienna, Europaverlag, 1979). Rattner's first volume includes chapters on Freud, Jung, and Adler (although not on Janet), along with nine other figures. A second volume in the series is listed under the title *Klassiker der Tiefenpsychologie* (Munich, Psychologie Verlag Union, 1990). Also, the tenth volume of *Die Psychologie des 20.Jahrhunderts*, entitled *Ergebnisse für die Medizin*, deals intelligently with theoretical linkages between clinical psychology and psychiatry.

In addition to these general works, several studies have appeared in recent decades presenting intellectual-historical accounts of psychological medicine in individual countries, such as Henri Baruk, *La psychiatrie française de Pinel à nos jours* (Paris, Presses Universitaires de France, 1967), and German E. Berrios and Hugh Freeman, eds., *British Psychiatry's Strange Past: 150 Years of British Psychiatry, 1841–1991* (London, Gaskell, 1991). Other works proffer broadly conceived studies of psychiatric ideas, attitudes, and practices in their medical, social, and cultural contexts during particular periods. An exemplary study along these lines is Roy Porter's *Mind Forg'd Manacles: A History of Madness in England from the Restoration to the Regency* (London, Athlone, 1987). Perhaps the fullest study of nineteenth-century European psychiatric systems since Ellenberger's book can be found in two complementary volumes by Paul Bercherie entitled *Les fondements de la clinique: Histoire et structure du savoir psychiatrique* (Paris, Navarin, 1980) and *Genèse des concepts freudiens: Les fondements de la clinique II* (Paris, Navarin, 1983). Still other historians have chosen to focus biographically on the lives of individual authors or on the narrative history of a single movement, such as in Reuben Fine's *A History of Psychoanalysis* (New York, Columbia University Press, 1979) and Elisabeth Roudinesco's *La bataille de cent ans: Histoire de la psychanalyse en France*, 2 vols. (Paris, Ramsay, 1982, 1986). A large literature has also appeared over the last twenty years on the history of the asylum, much of it taking the form of institutional case studies.

Overwhelmingly, the new historiography of psychiatry has assumed periodical and monographic forms as scholars strive first to master their subject matters factually before advancing to synthesis. In the English-speaking world, a portion of the best of this writing has been gathered usefully into collections, such as Andrew Scull, ed., *Madhouses, Mad-Doctors, and Madmen: The Social History of Psychiatry in the Victorian Era* (Philadelphia, University of Pennsylvania Press, 1981); W. F. Bynum, Roy Porter, and Michael Shepherd, eds., *The Anatomy of Madness: Essays in the History of Psychiatry*, 3 vols. (London, Tavistock, 1985–1988); and Edwin R. Wallace IV and John Gach, eds., *Handbook for the History of Psychiatry* (New Haven, Yale University Press, forthcoming?). A valuable work of general reference, which offers an array of thematic and chronological chapters, is the *Nouvelle histoire de la psychiatrie* (Toulouse, Privat, 1983), compiled under the direction of Jacques Postel and Claude Quétel.

Of all the subjects in the history of psychiatry and psychology that Ellenberger addressed, none has attracted as much scholarly attention as the life and work of Sigmund Freud. Since the publication of *The Discovery of the Unconscious* and Ellenberger's essays on Fechner, Benedikt, Anna O., and Emmy von N., historians have learned a great deal more about Freud, including about the early formation of his thought and his case histories. As a result, parts of Ellenberger's work on psychoanalytic history are dated today. At the same time, many of his formulations about Freud remain pertinent, and a portion of the historical scholarship on psychoanalysis since 1970 reveals the strong influence of his work.

The *Standard Edition of the Complete Psychological Works of Sigmund Freud*, translated from the German under the general editorship of James Strachey in collaboration with Anna Freud and assisted by Alix Strachey and Alan Tyson, 24 vols. (London, Hogarth Press, 1953–1974), which appeared during the years when Ellenberger was doing his most detailed historical research, remains the basic source for Freud's psychoanalytic corpus. The final volume in the set, of indexes and bibliographies, was published in 1974, and is invaluable. The *Standard Edition* has also now been supplemented by two highly useful works of reference, Samuel A. Guttman, Randall L. Jones, and Stephen M. Parrish, *The Concordance to the Standard Edition of the Complete Psychological Works of Sigmund Freud*, 6 vols. (Boston, G. K. Hall, 1980); and Alexander Grinstein, *Sigmund Freud's Writings: A Comprehensive Bibliography* (New York, International Universities Press, 1977). The standard Freud bibliography in German, compiled by Ingeborg Meyer-Palmedo, which forms the last volume of the *Studienausgabe* published by Fischer, has also now been impeccably reedited and brought up to date by Gerhard Fichtner. The citation is Ingeborg Meyer-Palmedo and Gerhard Fichtner, eds., *Freud—Bibliographie mit Werkkonkordanz* (Frankfurt am Main, S. Fischer, 1989).

Biographically, Freud has been better served than any figure in the history of the mental sciences, although the writing of his life remains, of necessity, highly controversial. Following the early position staked out by Siegfried Bernfeld, Ilse Bry, and Ellenberger, nearly all Freud scholars today acknowledge the manifold shortcomings of Ernest Jones's *The Life and Work of Sigmund Freud*, 3 vols. (New York, Basic Books, 1953, 1955, 1957). They also concede its indispensability, both as a source of firsthand observations about Freud's life and as a means of access to important primary materials that for other scholars remain under prohibition at the Sigmund Freud Archives. In 1972, Max Schur, Freud's private physician during his later years, published a poignant biographical account under the title *Freud: Living and Dying* (New York, International Universities Press). In 1980, Ronald W. Clark, the well-known British biographer, produced a large general account, *Freud: The Man and the Cause* (New York, Random House, 1980). And a major new comprehensive biography has recently appeared, Peter Gay's *Freud: A Life for Our Time* (New York, Norton, 1988). In its conversance with psychoanalytic theory, its integration of historical with biographical information, its interpretive judiciousness, and its fluency and elegance of style, Gay's study is likely to remain the most appealing and

authoritative biography for many years to come. Gay incorporates into his narrative much of the scholarship on Freud's life and work from the last two decades,
which he also reviews in a lively and detailed bibliographical essay (pp. 741–86).

The early history of psychoanalysis has been the subject of close, systematic
study by scholars during the past generation. Piece by piece, the intricate intellectual inheritance of Freudian theory is being reconstructed as "the historical Freud"
comes into focus. A very useful gathering of essays on the subject is Laurence
Spurling, ed., *Sigmund Freud: Critical Assessments*, vol. 1, *Freud and the Origins of
Psychoanalysis* (London and New York: Routledge, 1989). In particular, Ellenberger's belief that many figures and philosophies from Freud's educational years
and early career merit serious, independent study has been widely adopted. A
model study in this regard is Albrecht Hirschmüller's biographical and intellectual-
historical study, *Physiologie und Psychoanalyse in Leben und Werk Josef Breuers*
(Bern and Stuttgart, Hans Huber, 1978), now accessible as *The Life and Work of
Josef Breuer: Physiology and Psychoanalysis* (New York and London, New York
University Press, 1989). Hirschmüller, who teaches at the Institute for the History
of Medicine at Tübingen University, has emerged in the past decade as the leading
historian of early psychoanalysis. He has also written "Die Wiener Psychiatrie der
Meynert-Zeit: Untersuchungen zu Sigmund Freuds nervenärztlicher Ausbildung"
(Doctoral diss., Eberhard-Karls-Universität, Tübingen, 1989), a meticulous investigation based on quantitative archival data of Meynert's clinic for nervous diseases
at the University of Vienna Hospital during the 1880s. Other studies along these
lines include Francis Schiller, *A Möbius Strip: Fin-de-Siècle Neuropsychiatry and
Paul Möbius* (Berkeley, University of California Press, 1982) and Phyllis Gross-
kurth, *Havelock Ellis: A Biography* (New York, Knopf, 1980). For Krafft- Ebing,
one work, rarely cited but very good, is Annemarie Wettley's *Von der "Psychopathia Sexualis" zur Sexualwissenschaft* (Stuttgart, Enke, 1959). The beginnings of
a general intellectual biography of Krafft-Ebing, which examines his work on
neurology and forensic psychiatry as well as sexology, will soon be available in
Renate Hauser, "Sexuality, Neurasthenia and the Law: Richard von Krafft-Ebing
(1840–1902)" (Doctoral diss., University College London, 1993). A biography of
Wilhelm Fliess, Freud's intellectual confidant during the later half of the 1890s, is
also under way by Peter Swales. The recent literature on Charcot is discussed below.

In much the same way that Ellenberger brought to attention the significance of
Fechner and Benedikt, other scholars have of late busied themselves uncovering the
role of other figures in the beginnings of Freud's thought. The intellectual influence
of Freud's undergraduate philosophy and psychology professor has been explored
in James R. Barclay, "Franz Brentano and Sigmund Freud," *Journal of Existentialism*, 5 (1964), 1–36; and Raymond E. Fancher, "Brentano's *Psychology from an
Empirical Standpoint* and Freud's Early Metapsychology," *Journal of the History
of the Behavioral Sciences*, 13 (1977), 207–27. Anne Harrington makes a persua-
sive case for the role of Hughlings Jackson and the English neurological school in
Medicine, Mind, and the Double Brain: A Study of Nineteenth-Century Thought
(Princeton, Princeton University Press, 1987), chap. 8. On the significance of the
German neurologist and sexologist Albert Moll, whose contribution Ellenberger
noted, see the remarkably concise presentation by C. Schröder, "Ein Lebenswerk
im Schatten der Psychoanalyse? Zum 50. Todestag des Sexualwissenschaftlers,

Psychotherapeuten und Medizinethikers Albert Moll (1862–1939)," *Wissenschaftliche Zeitschrift Karl Marx Universität Mathematisch naturwissenschaftliche Reihe*, 38 (1989), 434–44. And Lucille B. Ritvo's *Darwin's Influence on Freud: A Tale of Two Sciences* (New Haven, Yale University Press, 1990), especially chap. 9, brings to light the part played by Carl Claus, Freud's professor of comparative zoology at the University of Vienna and an energetic popularizer of the theories of Haeckel and Darwin. An invaluable source of historical information for studying many of these individuals is the massive study by Ellenberger's good friend Erna Lesky, *The Vienna Medical School of the 19th Century* [1965], translated from the German by L. Williams and I. S. Levij (Baltimore, Johns Hopkins University Press, 1976). Lesky's compendium may now be read in conjunction with Helmut Wyklicky and M. Skopec, *200 Jahre Allgemeines Krankenhaus in Wien* (Vienna, Jugend & Volk, 1984). An excellent shorter piece in this same vein, which acknowledges the obligation of all psychoanalytic scholars to Ellenberger, is George Rosen, "Freud and Medicine in Vienna: Some Scientific and Medical Sources of His Thought," *Psychological Medicine*, 2 (1972), 332–44.

Concerning other intellectual determinants of psychoanalytic theory, the broad influence of the Anglo-French Enlightenment tradition on Freud has been emphasized in many works, most recently and convincingly in Gay's biography. The idea that psychoanalysis was an outgrowth of European Romanticism has met with a mixed reception among scholars over the past two decades. No systematic study has appeared. However, on the influence of the Romantic vitalist tradition, refer to Madeleine Vermorel and Henri Vermorel, "Was Freud a Romantic?" *International Review of Psycho-Analysis*, 13 (1986), 15–37. On a related subject, many critics and historians have come to agree that Freud's intellectual connections to German philosophy, despite his public professions of dislike for metaphysics, were much more complex than previously believed. The widest-ranging study to date is Paul-Laurent Assoun's *Freud, la philosophie et les philosophes* (Paris, Presses Universitaires de France, 1976). Freud's relationship to the Kantian and neo-Kantian metaphysical traditions within the German-language sciences is the subject of John C. Traficante, "The Intellectual Origins of Psychoanalysis: Kant, Kantian Naturalism and the Formation of Psychoanalysis" (Doctoral diss., Columbia University, 1982). The significance of Schopenhauer and Nietzsche for the environment of ideas out of which Freud emerged—a point that Ellenberger insisted on—has been probed from a philosophical viewpoint by Margret Kaiser-El-Safti in *Der Nachdenker: Die Entstehung der Metapsychologie Freuds in ihrer Abhängigkeit von Schopenhauer und Nietzsche*, vol. 13 of *Conscientia: Stüdien zur Bewusstseins-Philosophie* (Bonn, Bouvier, 1987) and from a literary-critical perspective in a second work by Paul-Laurent Assoun entitled *Freud et Nietzsche* (Paris, Presses Universitaires de France, 1980). David S. Luft examines the cultural appeal of Schopenhauer in Freud's time in "Schopenhauer, Austria and the Generation of 1905," *Central European History*, 16 (1983), 53–75. On the influence of the German literary classics, consult Didier Anzieu, "The Place of Germanic Language and Culture in Freud's Discovery of Psychoanalysis between 1895 and 1900," *International Journal of Psychoanalysis*, 67 (1986), 219–26. The historical contextualization of particular areas of Freud's work during the late nineteenth century is also proving illuminating. For a case in point, see Stephen Kern's "The Discovery of

Child Sexuality: Freud and the Emergence of Child Psychology, 1880–1910" (Doctoral diss., Columbia University, 1972). Kern presented the core of his research a year later in "Freud and the Discovery of Child Sexuality," *History of Childhood Quarterly*, 1 (1973), 117–41.

Ellenberger was also at pains in *The Discovery of the Unconscious* to place Freud (and Adler) during the first half of his career in the overlapping social and cultural worlds of *fin-de-siècle* Vienna and Jewish life in central Europe in the postemancipation era. Both subjects have since been explored in much greater depth. Readers may consult William M. Johnston, *The Austrian Mind: An Intellectual and Social History, 1848–1938* (Berkeley, University of California Press, 1972); Marsha L. Rozenblit, *The Jews of Vienna, 1867–1914: Assimilation and Identity* (Albany, State University of New York Press, 1983); Ivar Oxaal, Michael Pollak, and Gerhard Botz, eds., *Jews, Anti-Semitism, and Culture in Vienna* (London, Routledge and Kegan Paul, 1987); and Steven Beller, *Vienna and the Jews, 1867–1938: A Cultural History* (Cambridge, Cambridge University Press, 1989). Among other things, the works of Rozenblit and Beller establish a point made by Ellenberger, namely, the ethnic and sociocultural diversity among professional and intellectual Jews in Vienna in particular and Austria generally during this period. An engaging set of essays on cultural and political life in turn-of-the-century Vienna, which has done much to arouse scholarly interest in the field, is Carl E. Schorske's *Fin-de-Siècle Vienna: Politics and Culture* (New York, Vintage, 1981). See especially chap. 4, Schorske's well-known essay "Politics and Patricide in Freud's *Interpretation of Dreams*." A second cultural and psychological portrait of the young Freud, much influenced by Schorske's essay, is William J. McGrath, *Freud's Discovery of Psychoanalysis: The Politics of Hysteria* (Ithaca, N.Y., Cornell University Press, 1986).

Freud's relationship to the literary culture of his time, another large and complex issue that interested Ellenberger greatly, has been the subject of many specialized studies. Two recent, full, and very informative studies in the Ellenbergian tradition are Jeffrey Berman, *The Talking Cure: Literary Representations of Psychoanalysis* (New York, New York University Press, 1985); and Barry Richards, *Images of Freud: Cultural Responses to Psychoanalysis* (New York, St. Martin's Press, 1989). Alexander Grinstein's *Freud at the Crossroads* (Madison, Conn., International Universities Press, 1990) attempts to survey the subject comprehensively.

On Gustav Theodor Fechner, a substantial volume of writing has appeared since Ellenberger's essay of 1956; the bulk of this commentary, however, concerns Fechner's work in experimental psychology. To my knowledge, the only general book-length intellectual biography is still Johannes E. Kuntze, *Gustav Theodor Fechner: Ein deutsches Gelehrtenleben* (Leipzig, Breitkopf & Härtel, 1892). Kuntze's study includes good coverage of Fechner's "crisis" (chap. 5) as well as a bibliography of Fechner's writings (pp. 363–72). On Fechner's life, early psychoanalytic scholars, while paying little attention to Fechner's theoretical contributions, were less loathe to psychobiographize him, as in Hermann Imre's *Gustav Theodor Fechner: Eine psychoanalytische Studie über individuelle Bedingtheiten wissenschaftlicher Ideen* (Leipzig, Internationaler Psychoanalytischer Verlag, 1926). More recently, see also Marilyn E. Marshall, "Biographical Genre and Biographical Archetype: Five Studies of Gustav Theodor Fechner," *Storia e critica della psicologia*, 1 (1980),

197–210. Two additional articles on the psychodynamic aspects of Fechner's work are William R. Woodward, "Fechner's Panpsychism: A Scientific Solution to the Mind-Body Problem," *Journal of the History of the Behavioral Sciences*, 8 (1972), 367–86; and Lothar Sprung and Helga Sprung, "Gustav Theodor Fechner: Directions and Misdirections in the Establishment of Psychophysics," *Zeitschrift für Psychologie*, 186 (1978), 439–54. To my knowledge, the only study since Ellenberger's of Fechner's intellectual influence on Freud is Franz Buggle's and Paul Wirtgen's detailed analysis, "Gustav Theodor Fechner und die psychoanalystischen Modellvorstellungen Sigmund Freuds: Einflüsse und Parallelen," *Archiv für die gesamte Psychologie*, 121 (1969), 148–201.

In contrast to Fechner and many other figures in early psychoanalytic history, Moritz Benedikt has remained almost entirely unknown. None of Benedikt's writings is currently in print in any language, and there has been no further scholarly research on his life or thought. Surprisingly, Ellenberger's 1973 article about Benedikt in *Confrontations psychiatriques* has yet to enter mainstream psychoanalytic historiography, and Benedikt has not received consideration in subsequent biographies of Freud. An exception is Erna Lesky, who alerted Ellenberger in the first place to Benedikt's importance. See Lesky's pages on Benedikt in *The Vienna Medical School of the 19th Century*, 350–53, 358ff. Among other facts, Lesky brings to light an article of Benedikt's dating from 1880 that deals with Mesmerism and cataleptic states and that provides yet another of Ellenberger's links between the "old" and the "new" dynamic psychiatries. Incidentally, Ernest Jones relates, tantalizingly, in *The Life and Work of Sigmund Freud* (1:100) that the unpublished letters of Freud to his fiancée, Martha Bernays, include a memorable depiction of Benedikt.

A quantity of the recent historical literature on Freud has taken as its subject specific episodes in the intellectual history of psychoanalysis, including several events and texts that Ellenberger addressed. A case in point is the scholarship on Freud's lecture on male hysteria to the Vienna Society of Physicians in 1886. Freud's original presentation to the Gesellschaft der Ärzte, it will be recalled, has been lost. However, since Ellenberger wrote about this subject in 1968, the contemporary stenographical accounts of the lecture meeting have been assembled and reprinted in "Quellentexte," *Luzifer-Amor: Zeitschrift für Geschichte der Psychoanalyse*, 1 (1988), 156–75. As stated in the Introduction, Ellenberger's analysis of these sources has been hotly contested by two distinguished psychoanalysts: Léon Chertok, "Sur l'objectivité dans l'histoire de la psychanalyse: Premiers ferments d'une découverte," *L'évolution psychiatrique*, 35 (1970), 537–61; and K. R. Eissler, *Talent and Genius: The Fictitious Case of Tausk Contra Freud* (New York, Quadrangle Books, 1971), 351–58. The same year that Ellenberger published his article, additional information about the Society of Physicians was provided by K. Sablik in "Sigmund Freud und die Gesellschaft der Ärzte in Wien," *Wiener klinische Wochenschrift*, 80 (February 9, 1968), 107–10. For the general history of the Society, see Karl Hermann Spitzy, ed., *Gesellschaft der Ärzte in Wien 1837–1987* (Vienna and Munich, Wilhelm Maudrich, 1987–1988). And for a study of Freud's role during the 1890s in another, specifically psychiatric, professional organization, the Verein für Psychiatrie und Neurologie in Wien, see Renate Hauser,

"Krafft-Ebing and Freud," *History of Psychiatry* (forthcoming) as well as Edward Shorter, "The Two Medical Worlds of Sigmund Freud," in Gelfand and Kerr, *Freud and the History of Psychoanalysis*, 59–78.

Kenneth Levin situates Freud's thinking on this matter in the context of the German-language medical sciences of the time in "Freud's Paper 'On Male Hysteria' and the Conflict between Anatomical and Physiological Models," *Bulletin of the History of Medicine*, 48 (1974), 377–97. Esther Fischer-Homberger reconstructs the late-nineteenth-century debate between French and German physicians over the nature of post-traumatic neurosis in *Die traumatische Neurose: Vom somatischen zum sozialen Leiden* (Bern, Hans Huber, 1975), especially pp. 105–70. And Ingeborg Hartung of Tübingen University is currently writing a dissertation on the history of pre-Freudian medical research on male hysteria in Germany and Austria. Freud's interest in this subject during the 1880s was largely inspired by the work of Charcot and the French school. On this topic, one could do worse than consult Mark S. Micale, "Charcot and the Idea of Hysteria in the Male: Gender, Mental Science, and Medical Diagnosis in Late Nineteenth-Century France," *Medical History*, 34 (1990), 363–441; and idem, "Hysteria Male/Hysteria Female: Reflections on Comparative Gender Construction in Nineteenth-Century France and Britain," in Marina Benjamin, ed., *Science and Sensibility: Gender and Scientific Enquiry, 1780–1945* (Oxford, Basil Blackwell, 1991), 200–239. Further, Charcot's clinical lectures on this subject have now been anthologized in Jean Martin Charcot, *Leçons sur l'hystérie virile*, with an Introduction by Michèle Ouerd (Paris, S.F.I.E.D., 1984).

Ellenberger was also one of the first historians to place a strong accent on Freud's early neurophysiological work, especially the so-called "Project for a Scientific Psychology" of 1895. The importance of this document for understanding the origins of psychoanalytic theory is now universally acknowledged. The most extensive analysis to date is Karl H. Pribram and Merton M. Gill, *Freud's "Project" Reassessed: Preface to Contemporary Cognitive Theory and Neuropsychology* (New York, Basic Books, 1976). An excellent general exposition of Freud's thought that stresses the significance of this text is Richard Wollheim's *Sigmund Freud* (London, Fontana, 1971), chap. 2, a volume in the Modern Masters series.

No period in Freud's intellectual evolution interested Ellenberger more than the 1890s. Three general studies trace Freud's gradual, dramatic turn during this decade from a neurological to a psychological conceptualization of the mind: Walter A. Stewart, *Psychoanalysis: The First Ten Years, 1888–1898* (London, G. Allen and Unwin, 1969); Kenneth Levin, *Freud's Early Psychology of the Neuroses: A Historical Perspective* (Pittsburgh, University of Pittsburgh Press, 1979); and Jacques Nassif, *Freud. L'inconscient. Sur les commencements de la psychanalyse* (Paris, Galilée, 1977). In detail of coverage and intelligence of analysis, these have now been superseded by Albrecht Hirshmüller's new study, *Freuds Begegnung mit der Psychiatrie: Von der Hirnmythologie zur Neurosenlehre* (Tübingen, Diskord, 1991).

In "The Concept of Creative Malady" (1968) as well as other writings, Ellenberger studied the continual interaction during the later 1890s of Freud's systematic psychological self-analysis, his personal relationship with Fliess, and his intense intellectual creativity. Crucial for Ellenberger in understanding this association was the Freud/Fliess correspondence, which is now available in an annotated and unexpurgated edition, *The Complete Letters of Sigmund Freud to Wilhelm Fliess, 1887–1904*, translated and edited by Jeffrey Moussaieff Masson (Cambridge, Mass., Harvard University Press, 1985). The German edition of the letters, which appeared in 1986 as *Briefe an Wilhelm Fliess 1887–1904*, includes a number of items left out of the English version. This is an extraordinarily interesting set of documents that amply confirms Ellenberger's emphasis on the exceptionally intimate connection between autobiography and the origins of psychoanalytic theory. On many pages, the Freud/Fliess letters may well be read as illustrations of "creative neurosis" in action.

The definitive study of Freud's self-analysis, and one of the most intriguing books in the Freud literature, is Didier Anzieu's *L'auto-analyse: Son rôle dans la découverte de la psychanalyse par Freud, sa fonction en psychanalyse* (Paris, Presses Universitaires de France, 1959). Anzieu's book was later revised and reissued as *L'auto-analyse de Freud et la découverte de la psychanalyse*, new ed., 2 vols. (Paris, Presses Universitaires de France, 1975), and is now accessible as *Freud's Self-Analysis*, translated from the French by Peter Graham (London, Hogarth Press and the Institute of Psychoanalysis, 1986). For a second set of reflections, consider Jules Glenn, ed., *Freud and His Self-Analysis* (New York, Jason Aronson, 1979). Valuable information about this matter may also be found in the fourth chapter of Schur's *Living and Dying*. On the autobiographical content, overt and covert, in *The Interpretation of Dreams* in particular, there is much material in Anzieu as well as in Alexander Grinstein, *Sigmund Freud's Dreams*, 2d ed. (New York, International Universities Press, 1980).

Psychoanalytic *Rezeptionsgeschichte* is yet another subject and methodology that Ellenberger helped to pioneer and that has since developed fruitfully. Exemplary scholarly work in this mold has been done by Hannah Decker. Decker's two studies, "The Medical Reception of Psychoanalysis in Germany, 1894–1907: Three Brief Studies," *Bulletin of the History of Medicine*, 45 (1971), 461–81, and "The *Interpretation of Dreams*: Early Reception by the Educated German Public," *Journal of the History of the Behavioral Sciences*, 11 (1975), 129–41, were later combined with additional historical data into *Freud in Germany: Revolution and Reaction in Science, 1893–1907*, in *Psychological Issues*, vol. 10, monograph 41 (New York, International Universities Press, 1977). Nor is Decker alone in investigating this topic. A project to examine in their entirety contemporary reactions to Freud's writings is currently in progress by Thomas Köhler. The first volume of Köhler's study, *Das Werk Sigmund Freuds—Entstehung, Inhalt, Rezeption*, entitled *Von der hypnotischen Suggestionsbehandlung zur Theorie des Traumes* (Frankfurt am Main, Fachbuchhandlung für Psychologie, 1987), includes information about the reception of Freud's early essays on the psychoneuroses as well as his books. Furthermore, a generous sampling of reviews of Freud's books from all stages of his career, rendered into English, has recently appeared under the title *Freud without Hindsight: Reviews of His Work (1893–1939)*, selected and edited by Norman Kiell, with translations from the German by Vladimir Rus and the French by Denise Boneau (Madison, Conn., International Universities Press, 1988).

These reviews make for fascinating reading. Interestingly, Kiell's systematic reading in this genre causes him to pursue a counter-revisionist argument, namely, that many of Freud's early texts *were* received with hostility. The debate goes on.

This may also be the best place to consider Frank Sulloway's *Freud, Biologist of the Mind: Beyond the Psychoanalytic Legend* (New York, Basic Books, 1979). Sulloway's 600-page study represents the most detailed and intelligent analysis to date of the intellectual origins of Freudian thought from the perspective of the professional historian of science. Significantly, perhaps no piece of scholarship on Freud owes a more extensive intellectual debt (regularly acknowledged) to Ellenberger than Sulloway's book. In the fifth and sixth chapters of his volume, Sulloway demonstrates conclusively that the work of Fliess, particularly on the theme of universal bisexuality and in its general sexual mysticism, was far more consequential for the origins of psychoanalysis than acknowledged by Jones. In a similar vein, Sulloway emphasizes the previously underestimated importance of Albert Moll's writings, such as *Untersuchungen über die Libido sexualis* (1897), for Freud's thinking. And in chapters 8 and 9, following Ellenberger's lead, he reviews the pre-Freudian medical literatures on sexology and dream psychology as backgrounds for understanding Freud's work.

Most noteworthy is Sulloway's historiographical revisionism. Combined with the intellectual-historical parts of *Freud, Biologist of the Mind* is a polemic against what Sulloway perceives as the idealizing self-historiography of the psychoanalytic profession and the actions of its members to propagate a highly favorable image of their founder. The principal target of Sulloway's critique is Jones. In his account of Freud's early career, Sulloway foregrounds many of the same episodes that Ellenberger highlights. Moreover, the very subtitle of his book—"Beyond the Psychoanalytic Legend"—recalls Ellenberger's concern with the formation of legends in the history of science and, before this, of Van Gennep's *La formation des légendes*. In drawing extensively on Ellenberger's precedents, Sulloway, it should be added, schematizes and polemicizes Ellenberger's work. For the clearest illustration of this practice, see *Freud, Biologist of the Mind*, supplement to chap. 13, pp. 489–95, where the author presents a "Catalogue of Major Freud Myths." These "myths" number twenty-six, and in the list of sources of rebuttals to each myth, Ellenberger's writings appear liberally. Sulloway's book represents one working out of Ellenberger's ideas, and his sharp programmatic revisionism, shared today by many nonanalytic historians, may be contrasted instructively with the work of other Freud scholars (such as Decker, Hirschmüller, and Gay). The historiographical processing of Ellenberger's work, in other words, has been diverse.

As is evident from two essays in this collection, Ellenberger was continually concerned to bring to prominence the work of the "French school" in the history of psychology. Since Ellenberger's article "Charcot and the Salpêtrière School," Charcot studies have developed energetically. Ellenberger's modest essay of 1965, with its outstanding offering of primary sources, remains an important, if preliminary, piece of work for Charcot scholars today. Unfortunately, Ellenberger's call for a major intellectual biography of Charcot has not been fulfilled, although a triauthored study by Toby Gelfand, Christopher Goetz, and Michel Bonduelle is under way. The only general books remain Georges Guillain, *J. M. Charcot (1825–1893):*

Sa vie, son oeuvre (Paris, Masson, 1955; English translation, 1959), which stresses the neurological work of the 1860s and 1870s; and A.R.G. Owen, *Hysteria, Hypnosis and Healing: The Work of J. M. Charcot* (London, Dobson, 1971), which separates out Charcot's later writings on psychological and parapsychological topics. Both studies are useful but seriously limited.

In lieu of the large general scholarship that exists for Freud, there are numerous studies of specific facets of Charcot's work and life. An analysis of high quality of Charcot's scientific methodology is Alain Lellouch, "La méthode de J. M. Charcot (1825–1893)," *History and Philosophy of the Life Sciences*, 11 (1989), 43–69. On the relationship of emotional temperament and intellectual style—a link that Ellenberger often made—see A. Lellouch and C. Villard, "La personnalité de J.-M. Charcot (1825–1893) (Étude psycho-grapho-biographique sur manuscrits inédits)," *Histoire des sciences médicales*, 22 (1988), 97–105; and idem, "La personnalité de J.-M. Charcot (1825–1893) (Analyse critique morpho-psychologique et biographique)," in the same journal, 107–13. Christopher Goetz has provided translations with commentaries of a selection of Charcot's *leçons du mardi* from the 1880s, the celebrated bedside clinical lessons, in *Charcot, the Clinician: The Tuesday Lessons* (New York, Raven Press, 1987); and a nineteenth-century British translation of a volume of Charcot's formal medical lectures has recently been reprinted as part of the Tavistock Classics in the History of Psychiatry: Jean-Martin Charcot, *Clinical Lectures on Diseases of the Nervous System*, translated by Thomas Savill [1889], edited and with an Introduction by Ruth Harris (London, Routledge and Kegan Paul, 1991). Freud's full, complex, evolving intellectual relationship with Charcot has yet to be analyzed in full. However, some very good work has already been done in Ola Andersson, *Studies in the Prehistory of Psychoanalysis* (Stockholm, Norstedts, 1962), chaps. 2–4; Jean-Bernard Pontalis, *Entre Freud et Charcot* (Paris, Gallimard, 1977); and " 'Mon Cher Docteur Freud': Charcot's Unpublished Correspondence to Freud, 1888–1893," with annotations, translations, and commentary by Toby Gelfand, *Bulletin of the History of Medicine*, 62 (1988), 563–88.

On other topics, a perceptive study of the Charcotian model of hysteria is provided in Étienne Trillat's *Histoire de l'hystérie* (Paris, Seghers, 1986), chap. 6. On the so-called School of the Salpêtrière, Jean-Louis Signoret discusses the figures in the famous painting of Charcot and his students in "Variété historique: Une leçon clinique de la Salpêtrière (1887) par André Brouillet," *Revue neurologique*, 139 (1983), 687–701. More importantly on this topic, Bernard Brais, in "The Making of a Famous Nineteenth-Century Neurologist: Jean-Martin Charcot (1825–1893)" (Master's thesis, University College London, 1990), unites a mass of historical information drawn from original sources about the origins and evolution of the Charcot school. Brais's thesis reveals the importance of the intense and highly rivalrous world of medical politics under the French patronal system for understanding Charcot and his circle.

Charcot's dramatic visualization of hysteria in medical photographs and past works of art has become a source of interest for professional art historians lately. See, for instance, Georges Didi-Huberman's glossy *Invention de l'hystérie: Charcot et l'iconographie photographique de la Salpêtrière* (Paris, Macula, 1982), a convenient, if sensationalistic, selection of documents. Also now available is an attractive edition of Jean-Martin Charcot and Paul Richer, *Les démoniaques dans l'art*, introduced by Pierre Fédida and with a postface by Didi-Huberman (Paris, Macula, 1984). The *Démoniaques* of Charcot and Richer may be read in conjunction with Jacqueline Carroy-Thirard, "Possession, extase, hystérie au XIXe siècle," *Psychanalyse à l'université*, 5 (1980), 499–515. Highly congruent with Ellenberger's presentation of Charcot's psychological work are two recent studies by Anne Harrington, "Hysteria, Hypnosis, and the Lure of the Invisible: The Rise of Neo-Mesmerism in *fin-de-siècle* French Psychiatry," in Bynum, Porter, and Shepherd, *The Anatomy of Madness*, 3:226–46; and "Metals and Magnets in Medicine: Hysteria, Hypnosis, and Medical Culture in *fin-de-siècle* Paris," *Psychological Medicine*, 18 (1988), 21–38. Harrington examines the scientific research programs of Charcot, Victor Dumontpallier, and Jules Bernard Luys and, as her use of the term *neo-Mesmerism* indicates, locates extensive parallels between the work of these late-nineteenth-century physicians and their predecessors working on animal magnetism.

Ellenberger was also the first scholar to bring to attention the extensive cultural and popular dissemination of Charcot's ideas. Today, the most ambitious cultural contextualization of the work of French psychologists at this time is Debora Leah Silverman's *Art Nouveau in Fin-de-Siècle France: Politics, Psychology, and Style* (Berkeley, University of California Press, 1989). See especially pp. 83–91. For literary representations of Charcot and his work, a highly suggestive essay is Carroy-Thirard's "Hystérie, théâtre, littérature au dix-neuvième siècle," *Psychanalyse à l'université*, 7 (1982), 299–317, while Toby Gelfand takes a look at the imaging of the Salpêtrière in one popular French novel of the period in "Medical Nemesis, Paris, 1894: Léon Daudet's *Les morticoles*," *Bulletin of the History of Medicine*, 60 (1986), 155–76. Incidentally, the recent spate of publications about this subject includes a fictionalized historical novel about Charcot, directly reminiscent of the tales of Claretie and Daudet. See Philippe Meyer, *Sommeils indiscrets* (Paris, Olivier Orban, 1990). For the history of hysteria as a cultural trope in nineteenth-century France generally, refer to Mark S. Micale, *Hysteria's Histories: A Study of Disease and Its Interpretive Traditions* (Princeton, Princeton University Press, forthcoming), sec. 2. On Charcot and his late essay on faith healing, see J. Postel and M. Postel, "J.-M. Charcot et 'la foi qui guérit,'" *Histoire des sciences médicales*, 20 (1986), 153–56. Finally, interesting work is currently being done on the precipitous posthumous decline of Charcot. Refer to Christopher G. Goetz, "The Salpêtrière in the Wake of Charcot's Death," *Archives of Neurology*, 45 (1988), 444–47; Brais, "Making of a Famous Nineteenth-Century Neurologist," chap. 6; and Mark S. Micale, "On the 'Disappearance' of Hysteria: A Study in the Clinical Deconstruction of a Diagnosis," *Isis* (forthcoming).

Next, there is Pierre Janet. Ellenberger's call for a revival of Janet studies, which seemed most improbable two decades ago, has in recent years become a striking reality. The situation is described clearly by the Australian psychiatrist Paul Brown. "In 1960," writes Brown, "following the centennial year of his birth, Janet's work was quietly celebrated by his French followers. At that stage, he was virtually forgotten and unknown. Only thirty years later, in the centennial year of the publication of his first major work, *L'automatisme psychologique*, there are now four centers of Janet scholarship: in France, Holland, the United States, and Australia. In the year surveyed [1989], important aspects of Janet's *oeuvre* were the subject of editorial and leading articles in the *American Journal of Psychiatry*, the journal *Dissociation*, a special section of the *Journal of Traumatic Stress*, and . . . of a twenty-article monograph of the Société Pierre Janet and the Société Médico-Psychologique. The turning point in Janet scholarship came in fact in 1970 with Ellenberger's seminal publication, *The Discovery of the Unconscious*. Ellenberger's magisterial chapter, entitled 'Pierre Janet and Psychological Analysis,' rekindled scholarly interest." (Brown, "Pierre Janet: Alienist Reintegrated," *Current Opinions on Psychiatry*, 4 [1991], 389–95, quotation on p. 389).

As Brown indicates, something like a renaissance of scholarly interest in Janet's psychological work is now in progress. In 1970, the Société Pierre Janet was founded in Paris, partly under the impulse of Ellenberger's work. Over the last twenty years, the Society, working primarily with the publishing house of Masson, has edited and republished seven of Janet's books. The citations are: *L'automatisme psychologique* [1889] (Paris, Masson, 1973; reedition, 1989); *De l'angoisse à l'extase* [1926–1928], 2 vols. in 1 (Paris, Masson, 1988); *La médecine psychologique* [1923] (Paris, Masson, 1980; reedition, 1988); *L'état mental des hystériques* [1893–1894] (Marseille, Jeanne Laffitte Reprints, 1983); *L'évolution psychologique de la personnalité* [1929] (Paris, Masson, 1984; reedition, 1988); *Les médications psychologiques* [1919], 3 vols. in 1 (Paris, Masson, 1986; reedition, 1988); and *Névroses et idées fixes* [1898] (Paris, Masson, 1990). Several works were also reprinted in the United States during the mid-1970s: *Psychological Healing: A Historical and Clinical Study* [1925], 2 vols. (New York, Arno Press, 1976); *Les obsessions et la psychasthénie* [1903], 2 vols. (New York, Hafner, 1976); *Principles of Psychotherapy* [1919] (New York, Arno Press, 1976); and *The Mental State of Hystericals* [1901] (Washington, D.C., University Publications of America, 1977). For a discussion of the circumstances surrounding this burst of publications in France, see the statement by the current president of the Société Pierre Janet, Henri Faure, "La réédition des oeuvres de Pierre Janet," *Bulletin de psychologie*, 41 (1988), 477–81.

As Brown also suggests, the revival of Janet studies has been led by physicians, whose concern proceeds from the lively medical interest today in consciousness and dissociation, psychological automatisms, and post-traumatic stress disorders. The new Janet literature examines the clinical, theoretical, conceptual, and experimental aspects of Janet's work in these three areas. In the spring of 1989, a symposium was held in Paris entitled "Centenaire de '*L'automatisme psychologique*' 1889–1989." The papers delivered at this event, which were outstanding and which extended far beyond a consideration of this one Janet title, were published simultaneously in 1989 as a special issue of the *Annales médico-psychologiques* (vol. 147, pp. 935–1016), the leading French psychiatric journal, and as *L'automatisme psychologique de Pierre Janet: 100 ans après* (Paris, Masson, 1989). In the *Annales médico-psychologiques* issue, see in particular H. Maurel, "Approche historique de la notion d'automatisme en psychiatrie," 946–50, which traces the history of this idea in French psychiatry from the mid–nineteenth century to Lacan. For an American appreciation of this text, consult J. C. Nemiah, "Janet Redivivus: The Centenary of *L'automatisme psychologique*," *American Journal of Psychiatry*, 146 (1989), 1527–29.

On Janet and dissociation, the literature is expanding rapidly. Perhaps most important is Onno van der Hart and Barbara Friedman, "A Reader's Guide to Pierre Janet on Dissociation: A Neglected Intellectual Heritage," *Dissociation*, 2 (1989), 3–16. Van der Hart and Friedman offer a detailed rendition of the evolution of the dissociation concept through seven major works of Janet, emphasizing Janet's use of illustrative clinical cases. See also Onno van der Hart and Rutger Horst, "The Dissociation Theory of Pierre Janet," *Journal of Traumatic Stress*, 2 (1989), 397–412. Among other useful overviews, there is Campbell Perry and Jean-Roch Laurence, "Mental Processing Outside of Awareness: The Contributions of Freud and Janet," in Kenneth S. Bowers and Donald Meichenbaum, eds., *The Unconscious Reconsidered* (New York, Wiley, 1984), 9–48; and F. W. Putnam, "Pierre Janet and Modern Views of Dissociation," *Journal of Traumatic Stress*, 2 (1989), 413–29.

Concerning the study of Janet's ideas on post-traumatic psychopathology, the leading figure today is again Onno van der Hart of the Institute for Psychotrauma in Utrecht, the Netherlands. See in particular Onno van der Hart, Paul Brown, and Bessel A. van der Kolk, "Pierre Janet's Treatment of Post-traumatic Stress," *Journal of Traumatic Stress*, 2 (1989), 379–95, which provides a major presentation of Janet's model of trauma processing. Another important piece of work may be found in L. Crocq and J. de Verbizier, "Le traumatisme psychologique dans l'oeuvre de Pierre Janet," *Bulletin de psychologie*, 41 (1988), 483–85. Crocq and Verbizier make a statistical and clinical review of some six hundred of Janet's cases during the 1890s, half of which, they argue, involved traumatic psychogenesis. On the continuing relevance of Janet's dynamic psychotherapeutic ideas (the subject of an early essay by Ellenberger), refer to P. Marchais, "Pierre Janet, précurseur," *Annales médico-psychologiques*, 147 (1989), 969–72. And for current interest among clinicians in Janet's work on other specialized topics, see Roger K. Pitman, "Pierre Janet on Obsessive Compulsive Disorders," *Archives of General Psychiatry*, 44 (1987), 226–32; and Harrison G. Pope, Jr., James I. Hudson, and Jean-Paul Mialet, "Bulimia in the Late Nineteenth Century: The Observations of Pierre Janet," *Psychological Medicine*, 15 (1985), 739–43. Henri Baruk's "Signification de l'oeuvre de Pierre Janet," *Annales médico-psychologiques*, 147 (1989), 940–41; and Henri Ey's "Pierre Janet: The Man and His Work," in Benjamin B. Wolman, ed., *Historical Roots of Contemporary Psychology* (New York, Harper and Row, 1988), chap. 9, are general statements by leading French psychiatrists about Janet's significance today.

As with Charcot, there exists no "life and times" of Janet. Therefore, for biographical information readers must still rely heavily on Ellenberger's chapter in *The Discovery of the Unconscious*. For an overall exposition of Janet's *oeuvre, Die Neurosen und die dynamische Psychologie von Pierre Janet* (Basel, Benno Schwabe, 1951) by Leonhard Schwartz, the Basel neurologist who first awakened Ellenberger's interest in Janet, remains perhaps the best source. Schwartz's book, which appeared in French translation in 1955, has subsequently been supplemented by Claude Prévost, *La psycho-philosophie de Pierre Janet* (Paris, Payot, 1973), a work that is far more indebted to Ellenberger than its occasional footnotes suggest. For Janet's clinical methodology and epistemology, a sophisticated study is J. Fursay-Fusswerk, "Le croire et la croyance chez Pierre Janet, fil conducteur vers une psychiatrie d'avenir," *Annales médico-psychologiques*, 147 (1989), 952–55. It is likely that in the near future other aspects of Janet's work will also emerge from oblivion.

The question of the personal and intellectual relations between Janet and Freud continues to rankle scholars on both sides of the controversy. There are currently two book-length studies, and they are *Freud et Janet: Étude comparée* (Toulouse, Privat, 1971) by Henri-Jean Barraud, and *Janet, Freud et la psychologie clinique* (Paris, Payot, 1973) by Claude M. Prévost. An attempt to defuse the debate on this issue has been made by M. Laxenaire in "Les relations Janet-Freud: Pourquoi la guerre?" *Annales médico-psychologiques*, 147 (1989), 1004–7. Laxenaire finds important theoretical complements between the ideas of the two men. Reaching conclusions similar to those of Ellenberger, M. B. Macmillan has examined the issue of intellectual priority in "Delboeuf and Janet as Influences in Freud's Treatment of Emmy von N.," *Journal of the History of the Behavioral Sciences*, 15 (1979), 299–309. Macmillan has also published a second, substantial comparative study, "Freud and Janet on Organic and Hysterical Paralyses: A Mystery Solved?" in O. Zentner, ed., *Papers of the Freudian School of Melbourne: Australian Psychoanalytic Writings* (Melbourne, The Freudian School of Melbourne, 1988), 11–31. Macmillan argues in this context that Freud's notion of hysterical conversion originated in Janet's cases of Lucie, Marie, and Marcelle rather than Breuer's Anna O. or Freud's Emmy von N. See also Léon Chertok, "La découverte de la méthode cathartique," *Bulletin de psychologie*, 14 (November 5, 1960), 33–36. Finally, Ellenberger strove to prove that a current of Janetian psychology runs through the thinking not only of Freud but of many twentieth-century depth psychologists. This insight has been beautifully borne out in two recent studies by the American Jungian analyst John R. Haule. The references are "Archetype and Integration: Exploring the Janetian Roots of Analytical Psychology," *Journal of Analytical Psychology*, 28 (1983), 253–67; and "From Somnambulism to the Archetypes: The French Roots of Jung's Split with Freud," *Psychoanalytic Review*, 71 (1984), 635–59. In virtually all of the new Janet studies, Ellenberger is cited as the key pioneering scholar.

According to Ellenberger, the only overview of the history of psychiatry in Switzerland before the appearance of his *La psychiatrie suisse* was A. Zolliker's "Zehn Jahre schweizer Psychiatrie (1937–1947)," *Folia psychiatrica, neurologica et neurochirurgica neerlandica*, 53 (1949), 122–36. Since Ellenberger's articles of the early 1950s, no general account of the subject has appeared. A short and concise article, similar to Ellenberger's essay in this collection, may be found in Oskar Diethelm, "Switzerland," in John G. Howells, ed., *World History of Psychiatry* (New York, Brunner/Mazel, 1975), 238–55. Also relevant is Manfred Bleuler, "Some Aspects of the History of Swiss Psychiatry," *American Journal of Psychiatry*, 130 (1973), 991–94. Ellenberger's proposition that there exists an independent national tradition of psychiatry in the country is the topic of intelligent analysis in Jakob Wyrsch, "Schweizerische Psychiatrie?" *Schweizer Archiv für Neurologie, Neurochirurgie und Psychiatrie*, 112 (1973), 487–520. Wyrsch sides with Ellenberger on this question, extending the Swiss tradition back to Paracelsus in the first half of the sixteenth century.

Beyond this, a steady stream of monographs and articles, generally very competent in scholarship and devoted to the historical role of individual Swiss writers, institutions, and cities, has appeared over the past two decades. The development of psychiatric theory and practice at the most celebrated Swiss psychiatric facility is the subject of a set of essays assembled by Eugen Bleuler's son. See Manfred Bleuler, ed., *Kantonale psychiatrische Universitätsklinik Burghölzli 1870–1970* (Zurich, 1970). Erwin H. Ackerknecht, a venerable presence for many years in the teaching of medical history in the Zurich community, examined one episode in the history of the Burghölzli in "Gudden, Huguenin, Hitzig: Hirnpsychiatrie im Burghölzli 1869–1879," *Gesnerus*, 35 (1978), 66–78. The personal letters of the founding figure of the Zurich school have also been printed as Auguste Forel, *Briefe, Correspondence, 1864–1927*, edited by H. H. Walser (Bern, Hans Huber, 1968).

For a recent study of a major Swiss center with a very different psychological tradition, consult Thomas Haenel, *Zur Geschichte der Psychiatrie: Gedanken zur allgemeinen und Basler Psychiatriegeschichte* (Basel, Birkhäuser Verlag, 1982). Three institutional case studies of governmental asylums are John E. Staehelin, *Geschichte der kantonalen Heil- und Pflegeanstalt Friedmatt* (Zurich, Eckhardt & Pesch, 1933); Jakob Wyrsch, *Hundert Jahre Waldau* (Bern, Hans Huber, 1955); and, more recently, Hans Walser, *Hundert Jahre Klinik Rheinau 1867–1967* (Aarau, Schweizerische Gesellschaft für Geschichte der Medizin und der Naturwissenschaften, 1970). One very relevant institutional study that Ellenberger surprisingly overlooked is Ludwig Binswanger's privately printed *Zur Geschichte der Heilanstalt Bellevue in Kreuzlingen, 1857–1932* (Zurich, [1932?]). In the last half-decade, Hans Walser, professor of medical history at the University of Zurich, has emerged as the leading historian of Swiss psychiatry. In addition to the monograph cited above on Rheinau, he has also published "Schweizer Psychiatrie im 19.Jahrhundert," *Gesnerus*, 29 (1972), 183–95; and "Die 'deutsche Periode' (etwa 1850–1880) in der Geschichte der schweizer Psychiatrie und die moderne Sozialpsychiatrie," *Gesnerus*, 28 (1971), 47–55.

Despite the intrinsic interest of the subject, a full history of the Swiss psychoanalytic movement remains unwritten. Walser's "Psychoanalyse in der Schweiz," in *Die Psychologie des 20.Jahrhunderts*, 2:1192–1218, provides a factually dense review of the main figures and organizations during the pre– and post–World War I years. Similarly, interest in Freud's ideas in Zurich, Bern, and Basel has been canvassed by Fritz Meerwein in "Reflexionen zur Geschichte der Schweizerischen Gesellschaft für Psychoanalyse in der deutschen Schweiz," *Schweizerische Gesellschaft für Psychoanalyse Bulletin*, 9 (1979), 25–39. Mireille Cifali of the University of Geneva is currently researching a book on the history of psychoanalysis in the Genevan community. In a local publication, Cifali has already published three highly interesting pieces: "Le fameux couteau de Lichtenberg," *Le Bloc-notes de la psychanalyse*, 4 (1984), 171–88, which deals with Jung, Freud, and controversies over psychology and religion in Switzerland; "Théodore Flournoy, la découverte de l'inconscient," *Le Bloc-notes de la psychanalyse*, 3 (1983), 111–36, which examines the relationship of the ideas of the Genevan psychologist Flournoy with Freud; and "Entre Genève et Paris: Vienne," *Le Bloc-notes de la psychanalyse*, 2 (1982), 91–130, which looks at representations of psychoanalytic themes in the cultural arts of *la Suisse Romande* during the 1920s. This last essay documents in detail Ellenberger's assertion that literary intellectuals led the way in the importation of

Freud's work into France. Cifali has also coedited a new edition of Flournoy's book, *Des Indes à la planète Mars*, introduced and annotated by Marina Yaguello and Mireille Cifali (Paris, Seuil, 1983). Also, a reedition of the early English translation of this fascinating work, accompanied by an extensive introductory essay by Sonu Shamdasani, is currently in progress at Princeton University Press. Another leading figure in the French-Swiss school, Édouard Claparède, is currently being studied by the Italian scholar Carlo Trombetta. Most substantially, see Trombetta, *Édouard Claparède: Psicologo* (Rome, Armando, 1989).

On Oskar Pfister, a major figure in the history of psychoanalysis in Switzerland and (briefly) Ellenberger's own analyst, no full biography exists. In its place, refer to Hans Zulliger, "Oskar Pfister 1873–1956," in Franz Alexander, Samuel Eisenstein, and Martin Grotjahn, eds., *Psychoanalytic Pioneers* (New York, Basic Books, 1966), 169–79; and to the autobiographical statement "Oskar Pfister," in Erich Hahn, ed., *Die Pädagogik der Gegenwart in Selbstdarstellungen*, 2 vols. (Leipzig, Felix Meiner, 1926–1927), 2:161–207. An important compilation of documents on this subject is Heinrich Meng and Ernst L. Freud, eds., *Psychoanalysis and Faith: The Letters of Sigmund Freud and Oskar Pfister*, translated from the German by Eric Mosbacher (New York, Basic Books, 1963). Unfortunately, this is only a limited and expurgated selection of the complete unpublished Freud/Pfister letters. According to Gay (*Freud: Life for Our Time*, 756), a quantity of Pfister's unpublished correspondence is housed at the Zentralbibliothek in Zurich.

Two book-length studies of the personal and intellectual relationship between Pfister and Freud have recently been completed in Europe. See Jacques Besson, "Freud et le pasteur Pfister" (Doctoral diss., University of Lausanne, 1986); and E. Nase, *Oskar Pfister und die Anfänge der Psychoanalyse: Fallstudien eines Theologen* (Frankfurt am Main, Hain, 1989). An interesting discussion of the disagreement between these two long-standing friends over religious matters during the late 1920s is also available in H. Newton Malony and Gerald North, "The Future of an Illusion—The Illusion of a Future: An Historic Dialogue on the Value of Religion between Oskar Pfister and Sigmund Freud," *Journal of the History of the Behavioral Sciences*, 15 (1979), 177–86. And a recent examination of the Swiss tradition of lay psychoanalysis has been made by Pier Cesare Bori in "Oskar Pfister, 'pasteur à Zurich' et analyste laïque," *Revue internationale de l'histoire de la psychanalyse*, 3 (1990), 129–43. On a related topic, John S. Cornell, "When Science Entered the Soul: German Psychology and Religion 1890–1914" (Doctoral diss., Yale University, 1990) is a fine monographic study of "psychologies of religion" in Germany, Austria, and Switzerland during the period before the First World War.

A second figure of importance for the Swiss psychoanalytic movement is Ludwig Binswanger. Binswanger's memoirs, including letters to Freud, appeared in 1956 as *Erinnerungen an Sigmund Freud*. The English translation is *Sigmund Freud: Reminiscences of a Friendship* (New York, Grune and Stratton, 1957). For a detailed comparative study of the two men, try Christian Laugwitz, "Ludwig Binswanger und Sigmund Freud: Persönliche Beziehung und sachliche Divergenz" (Doctoral diss., Faculty of Medicine, University of Würzburg, 1986).

Binswanger's greatest significance for psychiatric history, of course, lies not in his relation to Freud but in his role as the founding figure of existential analysis, the primary source of Ellenberger's interest in him, too. Binswanger was a beloved

figure in the Swiss psychiatric community, and his death in 1966 aroused considerable interest in his writings within both medical and philosophical circles. The best
introduction to the man and his work seems to be Josef Rattner, "Ludwig Binswanger," in Rattner, ed., *Pioniere der Tiefenpsychologie*, 221–46. Roland Kuhn's
"Die aktuelle Bedeutung des Werkes von Ludwig Binswanger," *Zeitschrift für
klinische Psychologie und Psychotherapie*, 20 (1972), 311–21, is an informative,
appreciative study by a former colleague. Monographs include Hans Kimmich,
"Anthropologie und Menschlichkeit: Der Beitrag Ludwig Binswangers zur Hu-
manisierung der Psychiatrie" (Doctoral diss., Faculty of Medicine, University of
Göttingen, 1978); and Bradley Seidman, *Absent at the Creation: The Existential
Psychiatry of Ludwig Binswanger* (New York, Libra Publications, 1983). A useful
collection of Binswanger's writings in one volume is *Being-in-the-World: Selected
Papers of Ludwig Binswanger*, translated from the German and with an Introduc-
tion by Jacob Needleman (London, Souvenir Press, 1975), while Binswanger's
major work of existential analysis has recently been republished by an American
firm—Ludwig Binswanger, *Über Ideenflucht* [1922] (New York, Garland, 1980).
For a full listing of his writings, consult Germaine Sneessens, "Bibliographie de
Ludwig Binswanger," *Revue philosophique de Louvain*, 64 (1966), 594–602.

Concerning general expositions of existential analysis and phenomenological
psychiatry, the volume edited by May, Angel, and Ellenberger remains as good as
any. The introductory essays by May and Ellenberger, which amount to a quarter of
the volume, are perceptive and quite interpretive. Another succinct presentation
can be located in Wolfgang Blankenburg's entry, "Die Daseinanalyse," in *Die
Psychologie des 20.Jahrhunderts*, 3:941–64. The standard history of the movement in English is Herbert Spiegelberg's *Phenomenology in Psychology and Psychiatry: A Historical Introduction* (Evanston, Ill., Northwestern University Press,
1972), which includes detailed discussions of major and minor European and
American figures as well as an extensive bibliography. Ludger Riem's *Das daseins-
analytische Verständnis in der Medizin: Von seinem Beginn bei Ludwig Binswanger bis zur Gründung des 'Daseinsanalytischen Institutes für Psychotherapie
und Psychosomatik' in Zürich* (Herzogenrath, Murken-Altrogge, 1987) is another
general narrative study. Incidentally, these two psychiatric movements remain very
much alive today and, among other activities, publish major journals, *The Review
of Existential Psychology and Psychiatry* and *The Journal of Phenomenological
Psychology*.

Interest in the work of Hermann Rorschach took off dramatically in the late
1930s, peaked during the 1950s, and continues at a high level at present, not least
of all in the United States. Today, there are entire textbooks and work manuals of
Rorschachian psychology. Yearly international congresses take place, the proceedings of which are published intermittently as *Rorschachiana*. A large literature
exists on Rorschach's projective techniques in particular, almost all of which, sorry
to say, is devoid of any historical dimension. Two exceptions appear to be Giancarlo
Quarneti, "Il metodo di H. Rorschach e i fondamenti teorici di esso nella storia
della psicologia sperimentale," *Rivista di storia della medicina*, 16 (1972), 207–26
(for readers with the language); and Diane E. Jonte-Pace, "From Prophets to Perception: The Origins of Rorschach's Psychology," *Annals of Psychoanalysis*, 14
(1986), 179–203. Rorschach's *Meisterstück* (according to Ellenberger) can be read

in a reliable translation from the German by Paul Lemkau and Bernard Kronenberg under the title *Psychodiagnostics: A Diagnostic Test Based on Perception*, 6th ed. (New York, Grune and Stratton, 1964). A handsome re-reprint of this edition of the work appeared in 1990 as part of the Classics in the History of Psychiatry and Behavioral Sciences series from Gryphon Press. A comparative look at two figures dealt with by Ellenberger is taken by Robert S. McCulley in *Jung and Rorschach: A Study in the Archetype of Perception*, 2d ed. (Dallas, Spring Publications, 1987), while a revisiting of a subject that Ellenberger addressed may be found in Marcel Weber, "Kerners 'Kleksographien' und Rorschachs 'Psychodiagnostik,'" *Gesnerus*, 41 (1984), 101–9. Interesting in light of Ellenberger's comments about the interaction of the artistic and scientific forms of creativity is B. H. Friedman, "Hermann Rorschach as Artist," *Arts Magazine*, 53 (1979), 128–34.

Few themes dealt with in Ellenberger's work have developed more promisingly in recent years than the medicohistorical study of the patient. Ellenberger's statement on this subject, "The Unknown History of Psychiatry," dates from 1961. In 1985, a major programmatic call within the profession was sounded for a new and more "patient-centered" medical historiography. See Roy Porter, "The Patient's View: Doing Medical History from Below," *Theory and Society*, 14 (1985), 175–98. At the First European Congress on the History of Psychiatry and Mental Health, Porter enlarged upon this statement in "Listening to Insanity" (Lecture delivered at 's Hertogenbosch, the Netherlands, October 26, 1990). He has also edited *Patients and Practitioners: Lay Perceptions of Medicine in Pre-industrial Society* (Cambridge, Cambridge University Press, 1985), with a valuable methodological introduction. A thorough and intelligent analysis of the methodological possibilities, and problems, inherent in this approach may be found in Guenter B. Risse and John Harley Warner, "Reconstructing Clinical Activities: Patient Records in Medical History," *Social History of Medicine* (forthcoming). A general tour through this subject may be found in Edward Shorter's entertaining *Doctors and Their Patients: A Social History* (New Brunswick, N.J., Transaction Books, 1991).

Implicit in "The Unknown History of Psychiatry" is the project of a historical psychology of doctor-patient relations, an idea that by and large remains undeveloped today. However, we have by now acquired a literature on the historical sociology of the doctor-patient encounter. Foremost in this regard are Michael Balint, *The Doctor, His Patient, and the Illness* (New York, International Universities Press, 1957); Pedro Lain Entralgo, *Doctor and Patient*, translated from the Spanish by Frances Partridge (London, Weidenfeld and Nicolson, 1969); and Martin S. Straum and Donald E. Larsen, eds., *Doctors, Patients, and Society: Power and Authority in Medical Care* (Waterloo, Ontario, Wilfred Laurier University Press, 1982). For some thoughts on how to conceptualize the history of doctor-patient relations specifically in the history of psychiatry, see Mark S. Micale, "Hysteria and Its Historiography: The Future Perspective," *History of Psychiatry*, 1 (1990), 70–80, which builds explicitly on Ellenberger's 1961 article.

The study of individual patients in the history of psychiatry has also recently become a pastime of certain historians. The history of psychoanalysis has again attracted the most attention. Mark Kanzer and Jules Glenn, eds., *Freud and His Patients* (New York, Jason Aronson, 1980) provides a collection of essays combining theoretical and historical information about Freud's major published case histories. Gerhard Fichtner's *Freuds Patienten* (Tübingen, Institute für Geschichte der Medizin, 1979) is a work in progress, currently in typescript form, that promises to be important. From the analysands' perspective, see Paul Roazen, "Freud's Patients: First Person Accounts," in Toby Gelfand and John Kerr, eds., *Freud and the History of Psychoanalysis* (Hillsdale, N.J., Analytic Press, 1992).

At this point, Anna O. is probably the most researched case in psychiatric history. General studies of her life include Dora Edinger, *Bertha Pappenheim: Freud's Anna O.* (Highland Park, Ill., Congregation Solel, 1968); Lucy Freeman, *The Story of Anna O.* (New York, Walker, 1972); and Ellen M. Jensen, *Streifzüge durch das Leben von Anna O./Bertha Pappenheim: Ein Fall für die Psychiatrie— Ein Leben für Philanthropie* (Frankfurt am Main, ZTV, 1984). The most authoritative pronouncement on the subject is Hirschmüller's previously cited *Life and Work of Josef Breuer*, which places the case of Anna O. in the context of Breuer's medical career. Hirschmüller's book is deeply researched and judiciously argued and is equipped with an exhaustive bibliography. His analysis of Pappenheim's case appears on pp. 95–132. Taking as his starting point Ellenberger's study of Anna O. in 1972—"without doubt we have Ellenberger to thank for giving a decisive impetus in this direction," the author writes (p. 97)—Hirschmüller returned to the Bellevue Sanatorium in Kreuzlingen and located over a dozen additional documents pertaining to the case. Along with Breuer's medical report that Ellenberger had disinterred earlier, Hirschmüller reproduces these documents in translation on pp. 276–303. In addition, Hirschmüller has located the archival evidence that eluded Ellenberger—entries in the admissions registry indicating that Pappenheim, after her months of residence at Kreuzlingen, was hospitalized three additional times later in the 1880s at the Inzersdorf Sanatorium near Vienna (pp. 115–16).

A medical literature concerned to rediagnose Pappenheim's case has also appeared in recent years. A representative sampling of this work may be found in Max Rosenbaum and Melvin Muroff, eds., *Anna O.: Fourteen Contemporary Reinterpretations* (New York, Free Press, 1984). A sophisticated study of this sort, which again draws specifically on medical information accumulated by Ellenberger, is Alison Orr-Andrawes's "The Case of Anna O.: A Neuropsychiatric Perspective," *Journal of the American Psychoanalytic Association*, 35 (1987), 387–419.

Ellenberger's discovery that Pappenheim did not recover after her long, intense, private psychotherapy, as Breuer and Freud contended, but rather suffered serious and prolonged relapses has by now been integrated into the historical literature of psychoanalysis. Scholars have imputed a range of motives to Breuer and Freud, and at this point the subject makes for an interesting historiographical study in its own right. Gay, for example, observes that Breuer in his published account of the case "compressed with little warrant a difficult, often disrupted time of improvement into a complete cure" (*Freud: A Life for Our Time*, 66). Hirschmüller assesses the matter with equanimity and ends up terming the idea of Pappenheim's cathartic cure "a myth" (*Life and Work of Josef Breuer*, 131; see also pp. 107–8, 116). The harshest judgments contend that these new facts undermine the credibility of Breuer and Freud as well as the scientific status of psychoanalysis. For this view, refer to E. M. Thornton, *Freud and Cocaine: The Freudian Fallacy* (London, Blond and Briggs, 1983), chap. 8; J. N. Isbister, *Freud, An Introduction to His Life and Work* (Oxford, Polity Press, 1985), 54–67; and Fritz Schweighofer, *Das Privattheater der Anna O.: Ein psychoanalytisches Lehrstück, ein Emanzipationsdrama* (Munich, E. Reinhardt, 1987).

Ellenberger's pioneering, detective-like researches on the cases of Anna O. and Emmy von N. have also served as a model for research on Freud's other early patients. By now, the identities of all the patients in the *Studies on Hysteria*, with one exception—the English governess "Miss Lucy R."—have been established. Much fascinating material about the personal and medical biographies of these psychoanalytic patients is being uncovered. Ola Andersson, who initially identified the patient Emmy von N. and communicated this information to Ellenberger, later published the results of his research in "A Supplement to Freud's Case History of 'Frau Emmy von. N.' in Studies on Hysteria 1895," *Scandinavian Psychoanalytic Review*, 2 (1979), 5–16. Further analyses of the case include Clemens de Boor and Emma Moersch, "Emmy von N.—Eine Hysterie?" *Psyche*, 34 (1980), 265–79; W. W. Meissner, "Studies on Hysteria—Frau Emmy von N.," *Bulletin of the Menninger Clinic*, 45 (1981), 1–19; Oskar Wanner, "Die Moser vom 'Charlottenfels,' " *Schweizer Archiv für Neurologie, Neurochirurgie und Psychiatrie*, 131 (1982), 55–68; and idem, "Sigmund Freud und der Fall Emmy von N.," *Schaffhauser Nachrichten*, 105 (May 6, 1977), 17–19.

On the lives of other patients in the *Studies on Hysteria*, see Gerhard Fichtner and Albrecht Hirschmüller, "Freuds 'Katharina'—Hintergrund, Entstehungsgeschichte und Bedeutung einer frühen psychoanalytischen Krankengeschichte," *Psyche*, 39 (1985), 220–40; Peter J. Swales, "Freud, His Teacher, and the Birth of Psychoanalysis," in Paul Stepansky, ed., *Freud: Appraisals and Reappraisals*, 3 vols. (Hillsdale, N.J., Analytic Press, 1986), 1:3–82; and idem, "Freud, Katharina, and the First 'Wild Analysis,' " in Stepansky, *Freud: Appraisals and Reappraisals*, 3:80–164. In his book on Breuer, Hirschmüller includes documents pertaining to two additional patients of Breuer's, "Emma L." and "Clara B." (pp. 309–12). He has also dug up the case of a severe hysteric—"Nina R."—seen by Freud and Breuer at the Bellevue Sanatorium but not included in the *Studien*. See "Eine bisher unbekannte Krankengeschichte Sigmund Freuds und Josef Breuers aus der Entstehungszeit der 'Studien über Hysteria,' " *Jahrbuch der Psychoanalyse*, 10 (Bern, Hans Huber, 1978), 136–68. A similar case is discussed in L. Z. Vogel's "The Case of Elise Gomperz," *American Journal of Psychoanalysis*, 46 (1986), 230–38.

An entire subliterature on Freud's later major published cases exists. Much of this writing is clinical and theoretical in orientation or, increasingly, feminist and literary-critical. For specifically biographical and medicohistorical studies, there is Hannah S. Decker, *Freud, Dora, and Vienna 1900* (New York, Free Press, 1990); Patrick J. Mahony, *Freud and the Rat Man* (New Haven, Yale University Press, 1986); William G. Niederland, *The Schreber Case: Psychoanalytic Profile of a Paranoid Personality* (New York, Quadrangle Books/New York Times Book Co., 1974); and Hans Israëls, *Schreber: Father and Son* [1980], translated from the Dutch by the author (Madison, Conn., International Universities Press, 1989).

Frank J. Sulloway's "Reassessing Freud's Case Histories: The Social Construction of Psychoanalysis," *Isis*, 82 (1991), 245–75, is a hard-hitting critique informed by the contemporary sociology of science.

The paradigmatic patients of other major dynamic theorists are also being investigated today. Jung's dissertation, inspired largely by Helene Preiswerk and entitled *Zur Psychologie und Pathologie sogenannter occulter Phänomene: Eine psychiatrische Studie* (Leipzig, Mutze, 1902), has been translated by R.F.C. Hull and printed in the *Collected Works of C. G. Jung*, 2d ed. (Princeton, Princeton University Press, 1970), vol. 1, *Psychiatric Works*, 3–88. A full biographical study of this patient has also been made by Stefanie Zumstein-Preiswerk, *C. G. Jungs Medium: Die Geschichte der Helly Preiswerk*, with a Foreword by Heinrich Balmer (Munich, Kindler, 1975). (Zumstein-Preiswerk, Helene Preiswerk's niece, initially approached Ellenberger to coauthor this book with her.) For a detailed review of Zumstein-Preiswerk's book, and a discussion of issues surrounding Jung's dissertation, consult James Hillman, "Some Early Background to Jung's Ideas: Notes on C. G. Jungs Medium by Stephanie Zumstein-Preiswerk," *Spring: An Annual of Archetypal Psychology and Jungian Thought* (1976), 123–36. William B. Goodheart provides a further provocative analysis of this case in "C. G. Jung's First 'Patient': On the Seminal Emergence of Jung's Thought," *Journal of Analytical Psychology*, 29 (1984), 1–34. Goodheart gives a full account of the theoretical yield of Jung's experiments with Preiswerk and then goes on to argue that she was to Jung as Emma Eckstein was to Freud. See also M. Ebon, "Jung's First Medium," *Psyche*, 7 (1976), 3–15. Jung's most brilliant patient has been studied by Aldo Carotenuto, *A Secret Symmetry: Sabina Spielrein between Jung and Freud*, translated from the Italian by Arno Pomerans, John Shepley, and Krisha Winston (New York, Pantheon, 1982). Spielrein is also the subject of a second major study, John Kerr's *A Most Dangerous Method: Sabina Spielrein, Jung, and Freud* (New York, Knopf, 1993). Kerr's book ranges more widely than its title suggests and includes, among other things, much material on the rise of the Zurich school of psychology during the early twentieth century. For additional references on Jung, see below.

Scholarly interest in Janet's early patients is beginning to develop, too. John R. Haule investigates Janet's case of "Madeleine," a "psychotic mystic," in " 'Soulmaking' in a Schizophrenic Saint," *Journal of Religion and Health*, 23 (1984), 70–80. Similarly, the life of "Léonie," one of Janet's most important cases in *Psychological Automatisms*, is currently under investigation by Martin Stanton at the University of Kent. Catherine Muller (a.k.a. "Helen Smith"), the gifted medium who served as the subject of Flournoy's *From India to the Planet Mars* (1900), is being studied by Mireille Cifali. And Sonu Shamdasani, an independent researcher in London, is working on Miss Frank Miller, the cultured and beautiful American patient who contributed decisively to Jung's thinking about mythology and symbolism. See Shamdasani, "A Woman Called Frank," *Spring: An Annual of Archetypal Psychology and Jungian Thought* 50 (1990), 26–56, as well as "Miss Frank Miller, Jung, and Her Psychiatrists: Jung's Paradigm Case of Schizophrenia as Seen through American Confinement" (Essay presented to the New York Hospital–Cornell Medical Center, April 3, 1991). Finally, on a patient from the early history of dynamic psychiatry, there is Frank Pattie, "A Mesmer-Paradis Myth Dispelled,"

American Journal of Clinical Hypnosis, 22 (1979), 29–31, which attempts to revise Ellenberger's account of Mesmer's patient Maria Theresia Paradis.

This may also be the best place to observe the recent flood of feminist scholarship on the history of medicine, including on nervous disorders among many of the patients described by Ellenberger. The feminist scholarship on psychiatric history has a historiographical evolution of its own, and Ellenberger is not really a part of it. However, quite a few pieces of work in this camp have focused, like Ellenberger's article about Fanny Moser and her daughters, on the familial situations of female patients in past patriarchal societies. For social and cultural background, two sensitive and informative studies are Elaine Showalter, *The Female Malady: Women, Madness, and English Culture, 1830–1980* (New York, Pantheon, 1985), and Esther Fischer-Homberger, *Krankheit Frau: Zur Geschichte der Einbildungen* (Darmstadt, Luchterhand, 1984). Feminist literature on psychoanalysis has been of uneven quality and is continuing to grow rapidly. Representative works include Jane Gallop's *The Daughter's Seduction: Feminism and Psychoanalysis* (London, Macmillan, 1982) and Charles Bernheimer and Claire Kahane, eds., *In Dora's Case: Freud—Hysteria—Feminism* (New York, Columbia University Press, 1985). A widely cited study emphasizing social and familial circumstances in the American setting (with observations that correspond readily with Ellenberger's picture of the Mosers) is Carroll Smith-Rosenberg's "The Hysterical Woman: Sex Roles and Role Conflict in 19th-Century America," *Social Research*, 39 (1972), 652–78. See also Marc H. Hollender, "Conversion Hysteria: A Post-Freudian Reinterpretation of 19th-Century Psychosocial Data," *Archives of General Psychiatry*, 26 (1972), 311–14.

On Pappenheim in particular, the feminist commentary is extensive. A sampling should include Dianne Hunter, "Hysteria, Psychoanalysis, and Feminism: The Case of Anna O.," *Feminist Studies*, 9 (1983), 464–88; Showalter, *The Female Malady*, chap. 6; and Schweighofer, *Das Privattheater der Anna O.* Some relevant historical information is also contained in Marion A. Kaplan's *The Jewish Feminist Movement in Germany: The Campaigns of the Jüdischer Frauenbund, 1904–1938* (Westport, Conn., Greenwood Press, 1979). A review of the feminist historiography on the functional nervous disorders may be found in Mark S. Micale, "Hysteria and Its Historiography: A Review of Past and Present Writings," 2 pts., *History of Science*, 27 (1989), 319–31. Janet Oppenheim's *"Shattered Nerves": Doctors, Patients, and Depression in Victorian England* (New York, Oxford University Press, 1991), a richly detailed and highly informative study, represents the first synthetic study of the "nervous culture" of the Victorians.

On a related subject, the experiences of Preiswerk, Miss Frank Miller, and Helen Smith were part of the larger phenomenon of female mediumship in the second half of the nineteenth century. Two recent studies have explored this subject from a feminist standpoint. See Ann Braude, *Radical Spirits: Spiritualism and Women's Rights in Nineteenth-Century America* (Boston, Beacon Press, 1989); and Alex Owen's superb study, *The Darkened Room: Women, Power and Spiritualism in Late Victorian England* (Philadelphia, University of Pennsylvania Press, 1990). Owen's sixth chapter, on relations between academic medicine and the world of mediumship during the closing decades of the century, is of particular interest.

The work of Alfred Adler has failed to generate over the past two decades a scholarly literature comparable in quantity to that about Freud or Jung. Nor can Adler studies be said to be undergoing a revival, as with Janet. Nevertheless, a number of publications of high quality have appeared. Many of Adler's writings remain in print today in both German and English editions. The standard biography, which is quite defensive in tone, still seems to be Phyllis Bottome's *Alfred Adler: Apostle of Freedom* [1939], 3d rev. ed. (London, Faber and Faber, 1957). Two recent surveys of Adler's work are Joseph Rattner, *Alfred Adler*, translated from the German by Harry Zohn (New York, Frederick Ungar, 1983); and Ronald Wiegand, *Alfred Adler und danach: Individualpsychologie zwischen Weltanschauung und Wissenschaft* (Munich, E. Reinhardt, 1990). In 1983, Paul E. Stepansky provided a full and intelligent intellectual-historical study under the title *In Freud's Shadow: Adler in Context* (Hillsdale, N.J., Analytic Press, 1983). In the introduction of his book, Stepansky discusses Ellenberger's chapter on Adler in *The Discovery of the Unconscious*. Following Ellenberger's lead, he then begins his analysis with a consideration of Adler's premedical writings. More recently, Stepansky has contributed the entry on Adler in *Handbook for the History of Psychiatry* (forthcoming). For a second major study of Adler's thought, we now have Bernhard Handlbauer's *Die Entstehungsgeschichte der Individualpsychologie Alfred Adlers* (Vienna, Geyer, 1984), which appeared as the twelfth volume in the series Veröffentlichungen des Ludwig-Boltzmann-Institutes für Geschichte der Gesellschaftswissenschaften. The first section of Handlbauer's book has also been printed with revisions as *Die Adler-Freud-Kontroverse* (Frankfurt, Fischer Taschenbuch, 1990).

There also exist numerous studies of specialized aspects of Adler's thought. The masked religious component in his writings is the subject of Jochen Ellerbrock, *Adamskomplex: Alfred Adlers Psychologie als Interpretation christlicher Überlieferung* (Frankfurt am Main, Peter Lang, 1985). The influence of Nietzsche on Adler, a point that Ellenberger underscored, had previously been pursued by F. G. Crookshank, *Individual Psychology and Nietzsche* (London, C. W. Daniel Co., 1933). And the significance of Adler's early years in Vienna during the late Hapsburg Empire is examined in Almuth Bruder-Bezzel, *Alfred Adler: Die Entstehungsgeschichte einer Theorie im historischen Milieu Wiens* (Göttingen, Vandenhoeck & Ruprecht, 1983). Also, on this point, see again the books by Rozenblit, Keller, and Oxaal et al. cited previously on the cultural and professional world of Viennese Jews during the *fin de siècle*. Unlike the literature on psychoanalysis, Adler studies by and large have remained the preserve of Adlerian therapists. A summation of theoretical interests among Adlerians up until the early 1970s is contained in Harold H. Mosak, ed., *Alfred Adler: His Influence on Psychology Today* (Park Ridge, N.J., Noyes Press, 1973), while a compilation of Adlerian literature may be found in Harold H. Mosak and Birdie Mosak, eds., *A Bibliography for Adlerian Psychology* (Washington D.C., Hemisphere, 1975). The primary periodical organ for the movement is *Individual Psychology: The Journal of Adlerian Theory, Research, and Practice*.

Like psychoanalysis, Jungian analysis today forms an international movement with its own training centers, textbooks, and publications and with well over a thousand practitioners. Jung's collected writings are available as *C. G. Jung: Gesammelte Werke*, 20 vols. (Zurich and Stuttgart, Rascher, 1958–1987). Thanks to the generosity of Mary and Paul Mellon, who were personally acquainted with Jung, the Bollingen Foundation, named for the small village in Switzerland where Jung had a private rural retreat, was established in the early 1940s. The Foundation has provided for the publication of *The Collected Works of C. G. Jung*, 20 vols. (1953–1983), edited by Herbert Read, Michael Fordham, and Gerhard Adler. (The volumes in this collection that appeared during the years 1943 to 1960 were published by Pantheon Books, during 1960 to 1969 by the Bollingen Foundation and Random House, and from 1969 to the present by Princeton University Press.) The most complete listings of Jung's writings are *C. G. Jung: Bibliographie*, edited by Lilly Jung-Merker and Elisabeth Rüf (Olten, Switzerland, Walter-Verlag, 1983), included as vol. 19 of *C. G. Jung: Gesammelte Werke*; and *General Bibliography of C. G. Jung's Writings*, compiled by Lisa Ress with collaborators (Princeton, Princeton University Press, 1979), the nineteenth volume of the *Collected Works*. A revised edition of this bibliography, published in 1991, is exceptionally thorough and records through 1990 all of Jung's publications in German and English, including articles, paperback editions, and translations. The final, twentieth volume of the complete works, *General Index to the Collected Works*, compiled by Barbara Forryan and Janet M. Glover (1979), indexes all volumes in the series by paragraph.

As with Janet and Adler, there is no biography of Jung comparable in importance or quality to the volumes of Jones and Gay for Freud. For a compact, reliable, and psychiatrically informed synopsis of Jung's life and thought, try Anthony Storr, *C. G. Jung*, Modern Masters series (London, Fontana, 1973). More detailed biographically are Vincent Brome's *Jung* (New York, Atheneum, 1978); Paul J. Stern's *C. G. Jung—The Haunted Prophet* (New York, G. Braziller, 1976); and Barbara Hannah's highly sympathetic *Jung: His Life and Work, A Biographical Memoir* (New York, G. P. Putnam, 1976). Peter Homans's sensitive study *Jung in Context: Modernity and the Making of a Psychology* (Chicago, University of Chicago Press, 1979) focuses on the psychological and sociological factors in the formation of Jung's thought. The most recent general life is Gerhard Wehr, *Jung: A Biography*, translated from the German by David M. Weeks (Boston, Shambhala, 1987). A general intellectual biography is in progress by Sonu Shamdasani. Ellenberger's chapter on Jung in *The Discovery of the Unconscious* retains its importance for Jung scholars today.

A number of Jungian texts that Ellenberger stressed have also now become accessible. As previously mentioned, Jung's dissertation forms the first volume of the *Collected Works*. On Jung's other early medical writings, see J. Hillman, "Three Early Papers of C. G. Jung," *Spring: An Annual of Archetypal Psychology and Jungian Thought* (1973), 171–79; and Aubrey Lewis, "Jung's Early Work," *Journal of Analytical Psychology*, 2 (1957), 119–36. Ellenberger also paid close attention to the lectures on theology, psychology, spiritism, and philosophy that Jung delivered during his undergraduate years at Basel University to his student fraternity, the Zofingia. These have now been gathered and translated as *The Zofingia Lectures*, translated by Jan Van Heurck, *Collected Works* (1985), supp. vol. A. A source that Ellenberger was the first to consult in manuscript form and that he believes was key to the formation of Jung's philosophical and psychological thought has now been translated and published. See C. G. Jung, *Nietzsche's Zarathustra: Notes of the Seminar Given in 1934–1939*, edited by James L. Jarrett

(Princeton, Princeton University Press, 1988). A similar set of Jung's lectures on dreams and dream analysis was printed a few years earlier under the editorship of William McGuire. For the influence of two figures on Jung that Ellenberger insisted on, refer to "C. G. Jung—Bachofen, Burckhardt, and Basel," *Spring: An Annual of Archetypal Psychology and Jungian Thought* (1976), 137–47.

Many readings dealing with specialized aspects of the Jungian psychological system also exist. Jung's work on religious psychologies is treated by Murray Stein, *Jung's Treatment of Christianity: The Psychotherapy of a Religious Tradition* (Wilmette, Ill., Chiron Publications, 1985); and Herbert Unterste, *Theologische Aspekte der Tiefenpsychologie von C. G. Jung* (Dusseldorf, Patmos Verlag, 1977). Another important statement is Eugene Taylor's "Jung in His Intellectual Setting: The Swedenborgian Connection," *Studia Swedenborgiana*, 7 (1991), 47–69. Taylor, who derives his title from Ellenberger's essay "Carl Gustav Jung: His Historical Setting" (1978), maintains that many aspects of Jungian psychology may more profitably be interpreted as continuations of the mediumistic psychologies of Flournoy, Frederick Myers, and William James than as divergences from psychoanalytic theory. Two other studies by Taylor in the Ellenbergerian tradition are "C. G. Jung and the Boston Psychopathologists, 1902–1912," *Voices*, 21 (1985), 131–44; and "William James and C. G. Jung," *Spring: An Annual of Archetypal Psychology and Jungian Thought* (1980), 157–69. For Jung and another relevant topic, see the interesting comparative study of Nandor Fodor, *Freud, Jung, and Occultism* (New Hyde Park, New York University, 1971).

On the troubling issue of Jung and the German Third Reich, valuable background information may be found in two excellent and responsible studies, Geoffrey Cocks's *Psychotherapy in the Third Reich: The Göring Institute* (New York, Oxford University Press, 1985); and Regine Lockot's *Erinnern und Durcharbeiten: Zur Geschichte der Psychoanalyse und Psychotherapie im Nationalsozialismus* (Frankfurt, Fischer Taschenbuch, 1985). The story of German psychiatrists, psychotherapists, and psychoanalysts during the Nazi years has become a subject of enormous interest (and sensitivity) among young German historians of medicine today, and it is likely that more information regarding Jung will be forthcoming. Already available is Aryeh Maidenbaum and Stephen A. Martin, eds., *Lingering Shadows: Jungians, Freudians, and Anti-Semitism* (Boston, Shambhala, 1991), an outstanding collection of essays that emerged out of two conferences on the subject held in Paris and New York in 1989.

The historic relationship between Jung and Freud continues to generate commentary, much of it heated and polemical, from the Jungian and Freudian camps alike. In the last decade, three book-length studies have appeared: George B. Hogenson, *Jung's Struggle with Freud* (Notre Dame, Ind., University of Notre Dame Press, 1983); Linda Lewis Donn, *Freud and Jung: Years of Friendship, Years of Loss* (New York, Scribners, 1988); and Duane Schultz, *Intimate Friends, Dangerous Rivals: The Turbulent Relationship between Freud and Jung* (Los Angeles, Jeremy P. Tarcher, 1990). Since Ellenberger published his essays and book chapter on Jung, a set of documents basic to this subject has been published, namely, *The Freud/Jung Letters: The Correspondence between Sigmund Freud and C. G. Jung*, translated from the German by Ralph Manheim and R.F.C. Hull (Princeton, Princeton University Press, 1974). Ably edited by William McGuire, this collection includes over

350 letters spanning a period of seven years. A thoughtful study comparing the ideas of the two men is Liliane Frey-Rohn, *From Freud to Jung: A Comparative Study of the Psychology of the Unconscious* [1969], translated from the German by Fred E. Engreen and Evelyn K. Engreen (New York, G. P. Putnam, 1974). See also Patrick Vandermeersch, *Unresolved Questions in the Freud/Jung Debate on Psychosis, Sexual Identity and Religion* (Louvain, Belgium, Louvain University Press, 1991). A recent reflection on three of the main figures presented in *The Discovery of the Unconscious* can be found in Walter Kaufmann, *Discovering the Mind*, 3 vols. (New York, McGraw-Hill, 1980), vol. 3, *Freud versus Adler and Jung*.

The evolution of Analytical Psychology since Jung has also spawned a large literature of its own. For a readable account of the spread of Jung's ideas in the years following his death, see Andrew Samuels, *Jung and the Post-Jungians* (London, Routledge and Kegan Paul, 1985). An important reference work for the literature of Jungian psychology is Joseph F. Vincie and Margreta Rathbauer-Vincie, eds., *C. G. Jung and Analytical Psychology: A Comprehensive Bibliography* (New York, Garland, 1977).

A number of historical movements antedating the work of Janet, Freud, Adler, and Jung that Ellenberger emphasized in his writings have also been studied at much greater length and with great profit in the past generation. The most striking example concerns Mesmerism. There still exists no edition of Mesmer's collected writings in any language. However, two good selections of Mesmeriana are available in *Franz-Anton Mesmer: Le magnétisme animal*, works published by Robert Amadou, with commentary and notes by Frank A. Pattie and Jean Vinchon (Paris, Payot, 1971); and *Mesmer et son secret: Textes choisis et présentés par R. de Saussure* (Toulouse, Privat, 1971). To my knowledge, the only English-language collection is *Mesmerism: A Translation of the Original Scientific and Medical Writings of F. A. Mesmer*, compiled and translated by George Bloch (Los Altos, Calif., W. Kaufman, 1980). Similarly, there is no authoritative biography of Mesmer (although the unpublished manuscript for such a biography, by Frank Pattie of the University of Kentucky, is said to exist). In contrast, popular, sensationalistic accounts of Mesmer's life abound. The least unreliable of these appears to be Vincent Buranelli's *The Wizard from Vienna: Franz Anton Mesmer* (New York, Coward, McCann and Geoghegan, 1975). A succinct and accurate conspectus of Mesmer's life may be found in Robert Darnton's "Mesmer, Franz Anton," in Charles Coulston Gillispie, ed., *Dictionary of Scientific Biography*, 16 vols. (New York, Scribners, 1974), 9:325–28. Bernhard Milt's *Franz Anton Mesmer und seine Beziehungen zur Schweiz: Magie und Heilkunde zu Lavaters Zeit* (Zurich, Leeman, 1953) is an earlier, mildly psychoanalytic biographical account that deals with Mesmer's years in Switzerland.

The great significance of Mesmer's work in the history of dynamic psychiatry is now widely acknowledged. Max Bihan's "Quelques arguments pour la réhabilitation d'Anton Mesmer," *Histoire des sciences médicales*, 8 (1974), 627–32, is a programmatic statement that appeared soon after *The Discovery of the Unconscious*. The particular line of evolution in the nineteenth-century history of dynamic psychiatry that Ellenberger traced out—from Mesmer and Puységur to the beginnings of psychoanalysis—has subsequently been rehearsed, with differing emphases on the figures and movements involved, in several writings. Soon after the French publication of Ellenberger's book in 1974, two studies appeared in France, Léon Chertok's and Raymond Saussure's *Naissance du psychanalyste de Mesmer à Freud* (Paris, Payot, 1973; English translation, 1979); and Franklin Rausky's *Mesmer ou la révolution thérapeutique* (Paris, Payot, 1977). For shorter statements, consult Josef Vliegen, "Vom Mesmer bis Breuer," in *Die Psychologie des 20.Jahrhunderts*, 2:687–700; and Heinz Schott, "Mesmer, Braid und Bernheim: Zur Entstehungsgeschichte des Hypnotismus," *Gesnerus*, 41 (1984), 1110–13. Perhaps most importantly, the first comprehensive intellectual-historical study of Mesmerism and its many offshoots is now ready for publication. See Adam Crabtree, *Magnetic Sleep: The Mesmeric Roots of Psychological Healing* (New Haven, Yale University Press, 1993). Crabtree begins his study with Mesmer's medical dissertation of 1766 and continues very thoroughly up to the early writings of Janet, Myers, and Freud. He also explicitly considers Ellenberger the leading figure in this area of study.

The primary source literature on the history of Mesmerism and animal magnetism is vast, and Ellenberger, working during the 1950s and 1960s, had to pick his way through it as best he could. Today, two indispensable bibliographical references exist. First, Eric John Dingwall, ed., *Abnormal Hypnotic Phenomena, A Survey of Nineteenth-Century Cases* (London, Churchill, 1967) is a remarkable (but strangely underused) resource that in four volumes surveys, country by country, the past medical literatures on paranormal phenomena. Dingwall's volumes include extensive coverage of Britain, France, Germany, Russia, Portugal, the United States, and Latin America. Second, Crabtree has also published *Animal Magnetism, Early Hypnotism, and Psychical Research, 1766–1925: An Annotated Bibliography* (White Plains, N.Y., Kraus International Publications, 1988). A labor of scholarly love, this source, which supersedes in completeness numerous earlier bibliographies, runs to over five hundred pages and catalogues approximately two thousand titles in four languages. Crabtree's introductory essay reviews the historiography of Mesmerism and animal magnetism.

Earlier Mesmer scholars tended to limit their discussions to Mesmer's medical theories and practices while Ellenberger stressed Mesmerism as a cultural and popular-medical phenomenon. Another dimension of the subject, the sociopolitical, was explored the same year that Ellenberger finished writing *The Discovery of the Unconscious*. See Robert Darnton's short but fascinating and influential study, *Mesmerism and the End of the Enlightenment in France* (Cambridge, Mass., Harvard University Press, 1968). Probably the finest example of the new Mesmer studies is *Franz Anton Mesmer und die Geschichte des Mesmerismus* (Stuttgart, Franz Steiner, 1985), edited by Heinz Schott of the Medical-Historical Institute in Bonn. This is a collection of twenty essays of high scholarly quality that were delivered at an international symposium commemorating the 250th anniversary of Mesmer's birth. In addition to articles on Mesmer's influence in different countries, the book includes entries on Mesmerism and the occult sciences, Mesmerism and Romanticism, and Mesmerism and homeopathic medicine. Schott's own essay at the end of the volume concludes with a bibliography of the twentieth-century scholarship on Mesmer. The book is dedicated to Ellenberger.

Ellenberger was also the first person to bring to attention the extensive diffusion of Mesmeric ideas and practices outside of Vienna and Paris during the late eighteenth and nineteenth centuries. A subsequent general study of this subject is Ernst Benz's *Franz Anton Mesmer und seine Ausstrahlung in Europa und Amerika* (Munich, Wilhelm Fink, 1976). No thorough examination of the French Mesmerist movement has been written yet. However, an unpublished dissertation from the University of Strasbourg elaborates on Ellenberger's discovery that Alsace-Lorraine was a center of Mesmeric activity during the lifetimes of Mesmer and Puységur. See Jacqueline Levy, "Magnétisme animal et médecine à Strasbourg à la fin du XVIIIe siècle" (Doctoral diss., Faculty of Medicine, University of Strasbourg, 1974).

First-rate historical research concerning Mesmerism and the German-speaking regions has also been done. An excellent overview is Martin Blankenburg's "Der 'thierische Magnetismus' in Deutschland," which is appended to the German translation of Darnton's book entitled *Der Mesmerismus und das Ende der Aufklärung in Frankreich* (Munich, Carl Hanser, 1983), 191–231. For more detail, there is Walter Artelt, *Mesmerismus in Berlin* (Wiesbaden, Akademie der Wissenschaften und der Literatur, 1965); and Paul Hoff, "Der Einfluss des Mesmerismus auf die Entwicklung der Suggestionstheorie in Deutschland" (Doctoral diss., School of Medicine, University of Mainz, 1980). Also, Joost Vijselaar of the Netherlands Institute of Mental Health is completing a dissertation on Mesmeric movements in German-speaking cultures during the first half of the nineteenth century. Vijselaar has also published "Het dierlijk magnetisme in Nederland 1774–1830: Het verhaal van een kortstondige fascinatie [Animal Magnetism in the Netherlands, 1774–1830: The Story of a Short-Lived Fascination]," *Maanblad Geestelijke Volksgezondheid (Dutch Journal of Mental Health)*, 43 (1988), 782–95.

For interest in (and initial suspicion of) Mesmer's ideas across the English Channel, consult Fred Kaplan, " 'The Mesmeric Mania': The Early Victorians and Animal Magnetism," *Journal of the History of Ideas*, 35 (1974), 691–702; Jon Palfreman, "Mesmerism and the English Medical Profession: A Study of a Conflict," *Ethics in Science and Medicine*, 4 (1977), 51–66; and Roy Porter, " 'Under the Influence': Mesmerism in England," *History Today*, 80 (1985), 385–96. Robert C. Fuller, *Mesmerism and the American Cure of Souls* (Philadelphia, University of Pennsylvania Press, 1982) deals with the American scene.

Still other aspects of Mesmerism have also been explored lately. The theoretical origins of Mesmer's ideas are the subject of Ernst Benz, *Franz Anton Mesmer und die philosophischen Grundlagen des 'animalischen Magnetismus'* (Mainz, Akademie der Wissenschaften, 1977). The political and philosophical motivations of scientific academicians in rejecting Mesmeric theory for so long have been explored very suggestively by F. Azouvi in "Sens et fonction épistémologique de la critique du magnétisme animal par les Académies," *Revue d'histoire des sciences et leur application*, 19 (1978), 123–42. And the popular appeal of itinerant magnetizers is considered in Terry M. Parssinen, "Mesmeric Performers," *Victorian Studies*, 21 (1977), 87–104. The cultural history of Mesmerism—again, a subject intriguing to Ellenberger—has been investigated in various of its aspects by Maria M. Tatar, *Spellbound: Studies on Mesmerism and Literature* (Princeton, Princeton University Press, 1978); Fred Kaplan, *Dickens and Mesmerism* (Princeton, Princeton University Press, 1975); and Klaus H. Kiefer, "Goethe und der Magnetismus,"

Philosophia Naturalis, 20 (1983), 264–311, as well as by a number of essayists in Schott, *Mesmer und die Geschichte des Mesmerismus*.

German "Romantic" psychiatry is yet another topic that much engaged Ellenberger and is now receiving renewed attention from historians of medicine. At the same time that Ellenberger was conducting research in this area, Otto M. Marx appreciated the work of the German *Psychiker* in "A Re-evaluation of the Mentalists in Early 19th-Century German Psychiatry," *American Journal of Psychiatry*, 121 (1965), 752–60. Marx has now returned to this subject and published two substantial essays, "German Romantic Psychiatry," 2 pts., *History of Psychiatry*, 1 (1990), 351–81; and 2 (1991), 1–25. Also during the mid-1960s, Ernest Harms argued at length for the importance of J.C.A. Heinroth's work in *Origins of Modern Psychiatry* (Springfield, Ill., Charles C. Thomas, 1967), chaps. 13–16. Heinroth's most important text has now been published in a modern English version. See Johann Christian Heinroth, *Textbook of Disturbances of Mental Life, or Disturbances of the Soul and Their Treatment* [1818], translated from the German by J. Schmorak, 2 vols. (Baltimore, Johns Hopkins University Press, 1975), which includes a splendid and highly informative seventy-page introduction by George Mora. On Justinus Kerner, there now exists a biography in the form of Otto-Joachim Grüsser's *Justinus Kerner 1786–1862: Arzt, Poet, Geisterseher* (Berlin, Springer, 1987). Refer also to the critical appreciation by Uwe Henrik Peters, "Justinus Kerner as a Psychiatric Practitioner. E. T. A. Hoffman as a Psychiatric Theorist," in *Studies in German Romantic Psychiatry* (London, Institute of Germanic Studies, University of London, 1990). For a modern edition of Kerner's most important publication, see *Die Seherin von Prevorst: Eröffnungen über das innere Leben des Menschen und über das Hereinragen einer Geisterwelt in die unsere*, 4th ed. (Stuttgart, Steinkopf, 1980).

Another important expression of the new revisionist interest in German Romantic psychiatry may be found in Edwin Clarke's and L. S. Jacyna's *Nineteenth-Century Origins of Neuroscientific Concepts* (Berkeley, University of California Press, 1987). In their introduction, Clarke and Jacyna, who are concerned equally with the histories of physiology and psychiatry, propose that the literature of German *Naturphilosophie* contains many previously overlooked insights into mind-body relations and accord to this writing a greater scientific merit than earlier historians of science. Two relevant studies of individual figures may be found in Guenter B. Risse, "Kant, Schelling and the Early Search for a Philosophical 'Science' of Medicine in Germany," *Journal of the History of Medicine and the Allied Sciences*, 27 (1972), 145–58; and Kenneth Dewhurst and Nigel Reeves, *Friedrich Schiller, Medicine, Psychology, and Literature* (Oxford, Sandford, 1978). The study of Romantic culture and German-language medicine and science in general is at present developing rapidly. For an exciting and wide-ranging collection of the current work, refer to Andrew Cunningham and Nicholas Jardine, eds., *Romanticism and the Sciences* (New York, Cambridge University Press, 1990).

Ellenberger's interest in the history of individual diagnostic categories has developed impressively, too. Most notable has been the historical commentary on multiple personality. An important work of reference on this subject—Carole Goettman, George B. Greaves, and Philip M. Coons, eds., *Multiple Personality and Dissociation, 1791–1990: A Complete Bibliography* (Atlanta, George B.

Greaves)—appeared in 1991. Before his untimely death, Eric T. Carlson was working toward a general history of this subject from the late eighteenth to the late nineteenth centuries. Carlson had already published "The History of Multiple Personality in the United States: 1. The Beginnings," *American Journal of Psychiatry*, 138 (1981), 666–68; "The History of Multiple Personality in the United States: Mary Reynolds and Her Subsequent Reputation," *Bulletin of the History of Medicine*, 58 (1984), 72–82; and "Multiple Personality and Hypnosis: The First One Hundred Years," *Journal of the History of the Behavioral Sciences*, 25 (1989), 315–22. An excellent sampling of essays on the subject has also been assembled by Jacques M. Quen under the title *Split Minds/Split Brains: Historical and Current Perspectives* (New York, New York University Press, 1986). One of the best-known cases of multiple personality in American medical history is treated at length in Michael G. Kenny, *The Passion of Ansel Bourne: Multiple Personality in American Culture* (Washington, D.C., Smithsonian Institution Press, 1986). See also George B. Greaves, "Multiple Personality: 165 Years after Mary Reynolds," *Journal of Nervous and Mental Disease*, 168 (1980), 577–96; and Carlos S. Alvarado, "Historical Perspectives on Dissociation: A Review of Recent Publications," *Journal of the Society for Psychical Research*, 56 (1990), 159–66. A medical figure of secondary importance that Ellenberger discusses has been studied further by Catherine G. Fine in "The Work of Antoine Despine: The First Scientific Report on the Diagnosis and Treatment of a Child with Multiple Personality Disorder," *American Journal of Clinical Hypnosis*, 31 (1988), 33–39; and the intellectual association of French and American medical authors working on this subject in the late nineteenth century is now being investigated by Paul Dambowic in "Memory Lost and Found: Multiple Personality in Western Culture" (Doctoral diss., Yale University, work in progress).

Furthermore, Adam Crabtree, weaving many case histories into the narrative of his book, examines continuities between the demonological and medicopsychological paradigms of dissociation in *Multiple Man: Explorations in Possession and Multiple Personality* (New York, Praeger, 1985). An interesting survey, very Ellenberger-like, of the cultural applications of psychiatric writing on this subject has been made by Jeremy Hawthorn in *Multiple Personality and the Disintegration of Literary Character: From Oliver Goldsmith to Sylvia Plath* (New York, St. Martin's Press, 1983). And Michael S. Roth has studied a related psychological phenomenon in cultural context in "Remembering Forgetting: *Maladies de la Mémoire* in Nineteenth-Century France," *Representations*, 26 (1989), 49–68. A glance at the documentation of these writings indicates that the authors all learned extensively from Ellenberger's pages in *The Discovery of the Unconscious*.

On the history of hypnosis, two thorough studies of developments in individual countries appeared just as Ellenberger was completing *The Discovery of the Unconscious*. These are Dominique Barrucand's *Histoire de l'hypnose en France* (Paris, Presses Universitaires de France, 1967), which includes an abundant bibliography of French medical titles; and Norbert Purr's "Zur Geschichte des Hypnotismus in Wien im 19. Jahrhundert (1844–1860)" (Doctoral diss., Faculty of Medicine, University of Frankfurt, 1968). The latter study establishes conclusively that a widespread medical interest in hypnotherapeutics existed in Vienna long before the experiments of Krafft-Ebing, Breuer, and Freud. A major new study is also now available in Alan Gauld, *The History of Hypnotism* (Cambridge: Cambridge University Press, 1993). Valuable historical information is also included in Jean-Roch Laurence and Campbell Perry, *Hypnosis, Will, and Memory: A Psycho-Legal History* (New York, Guilford, 1988).

On Puységur, who clearly deserves a study of his own, consult J. Postel and J. Corraze, eds., *Armand Marie-Jacques de Chastenet Marquis de Puységur: Mémoires pour servir à l'histoire et à l'établissement du magnétisme animal* (Paris, Privat, 1986). Lengthy excerpts from the writings of Esdaile and Braid, the mid-nineteenth-century British hypnotists, are reproduced in Maurice M. Tinterow, *Foundations of Modern Hypnosis from Mesmer to Freud* (Springfield, Ill., Charles C. Thomas, 1970). For similar gatherings of primary texts, refer to James Esdaile, *Natural and Mesmeric Clairvoyance*, reprint of the 1852 edition (New York, Arno Press, 1975); and Fred Kaplan, ed., *John Elliotson on Mesmerism* (New York, Da Capo Press, 1982). An interesting secondary study is Nathan Mark Kravis, "James Braid's Psychophysiology: A Turning Point in the History of Dynamic Psychiatry," *American Journal of Psychiatry*, 145 (1988), 1191–1206. Jacqueline Carroy's *Hypnose, suggestion, et psychologie: L'invention de sujets* (Paris, Presses Universitaires de France, 1991) is a characteristically perceptive study of the French scene during the late nineteenth century. On the British parapsychological tradition, a subject about which Ellenberger has had surprisingly little to say, there has again been outstanding work. Important studies include John J. Cerullo, *The Secularization of the Soul: Psychical Research in Modern Britain* (Philadelphia, Institute for the Study of Human Issues, 1982); and Janet Oppenheim, *The Other World: Spiritualism and Psychical Research in England, 1850–1914* (Cambridge, Cambridge University Press, 1985).

The history of European sexology is also arousing much interest today among critics and historians; in the main, this is due to the impetus from Michel Foucault's work rather than Ellenberger's. In contrast, see Yannick Ripa, *Histoire du rêve: Regards sur l'imaginaire des Français au XIXe siècle* (Paris, Olivier Orban, 1988), as well as Rosemarie Sand, "Pre-Freudian Discovery of Dream Meaning: The Achievement of Charcot, Janet, and Krafft-Ebing," in Gelfand and Kerr, *Freud and the History of Psychoanalysis*. Sand is also completing a general study of nineteenth-century theories of the dream. Another highly pertinent piece of scholarship is Ian Dowbiggin's "Alfred Maury and the Politics of the Unconscious in Nineteenth-Century France," *History of Psychiatry*, 1 (1990), 255–87, which elaborates on one of the major dream psychologists first brought to light by Ellenberger.

On theories of the unconscious mind in the immediate pre-Freudian period, material may be found in many secondary works. Directly relevant are Dennis N. Kenedy Darnoi, *The Unconscious and Eduard von Hartmann: A Historico-Critical Monograph* (The Hague, Martinus Nijhoff, 1967); and D. B. Klein, *The Unconscious: Invention or Discovery? A Historico-Critical Inquiry* (Santa Monica, Calif., Goodyear, 1977), chaps. 1–3. The complex intellectual adaptation of Freudian theories of the mind following their transplantation to the New World is the subject of John Seeley's *The Americanization of the Unconscious* (New York, International Universities Press, 1967). For a review of contemporary approaches to the unconscious, see the later chapters of Klein's book as well as Kenneth S. Bowers and Donald Meichenbaum, eds., *The Unconscious Reconsidered* (New York, Wiley, 1984).

The cultural history of psychiatry extends in so many different directions that it is impossible to chart its bibliography with any accuracy. Many books and articles appearing over the last generation have pursued topics touched on by Ellenberger. From the titles listed above, see especially those by McGrath, Grinstein, Beller, Silverman, Cifali, Tatar, Hawthorn, and Carroy-Thirard. Two general sources of value are Enid Rhodes Peschel, ed., *Medicine and Literature* (New York, Neale Watson Academic Publications, 1980); and Lillian Feder, *Madness in Literature* (Princeton, Princeton University Press, 1980). Other studies exploring specific themes set out by Ellenberger include Jacques Borel, *Médecine et psychiatrie balzaciennes; la science dans le roman* (Paris, J. Corti, 1971); Judith Ryan, *The Vanishing Subject: Early Psychology and Literary Modernism* (Chicago, University of Chicago Press, 1991); and two studies in progress, Janet L. Beizer, *Emma's Daughters: The Narrative Uses of Hysteria in France (1850–1900)*; and Elaine Showalter, *Hystories: Studies in Literature, Gender, and Psychology*. For a broad attempt to explore the "cultures of hysteria" of the nineteenth century (primarily in France), see my *Hysteria's Histories*, sec. 2. In particular, I attempt here to continue Ellenberger's investigation of the types of past cultural interactions between psychiatry and imaginative literature and to develop a circular model of influence between the two fields. An intelligent statement about the methodological difficulties inherent in this interdisciplinary project has been provided by G. S. Rousseau in "Literature and Medicine: The State of the Field," *Isis*, 72 (1981), 406–24.

It may also be appropriate at this point to note an important parallel. Ellenberger's work on the cultural history of psychiatry, especially his distinctive blend of cultural history and the history of psychiatric ideas, bears close resemblance to the writings of another masterful critic and historian in the field, also of Swiss background. I am referring to Jean Starobinski. From a wonderfully rich offering, see in particular Starobinski, "La nostalgie: Théories médicales et expression littéraire," in *Studies on Voltaire and the Eighteenth Century*, 27 (1963), 1505–18; idem, "Sur les fonctions de la parole dans la théorie médicale de l'époque romantique," *Médecine de France*, 205 (1969), 9–12; idem, "The Word Reaction: From Physics to Psychiatry," *Diogenes*, 93 (1976), 1–27; idem, "Sur la chlorose," *Romantisme: Revue du dix-neuvième siècle*, 31 (1981), 113–30; idem, "Brève histoire de la conscience du corps," in Robert Ellrodt, ed., *Genèse de la conscience moderne* (Paris, Presses Universitaires de France, 1983), 215–29; and idem, *Le remède dans le mal: Critique et légitimation de l'artifice à l'âge des Lumières* (Paris, Gallimard, 1989). A number of Starobinski's works, like Ellenberger's, are currently being brought today to English-speaking audiences for the first time.

Subsequent historical research has also been conducted on several miscellaneous themes running through Ellenberger's essays. Currently, there exists no systematic exploration of the autobiographical component in the history of psychiatry. The ongoing series *A History of Psychology in Autobiography*, 7 vols. (Worcester, Mass., Clark University Press, 1930–1980), the earlier volumes of which were edited by Carl Murchison, contains much valuable information. See also *Psychiatrie in Selbstdarstellungen*, with a Foreword by Ludwig J. Pongratz (Bern, Hans Huber, 1977), which offers a compendium of short autobiographies by major twentieth-century Swiss, Austrian, and German psychiatrists, many of whom reflect on the subjective element in their work. Similarly, Ellenberger's concept of *les maladies créatrices* has been developed further (without reference to his work) by George Pickering in *Creative Malady: Illness in the Lives and Minds of Charles Darwin, Florence Nightingale, Mary Baker Eddy, Sigmund Freud, Marcel Proust, Elizabeth Barrett Browning* (New York, Oxford University Press, 1974). Many studies explore the idea in the lives of individuals in the history of the arts. A good, psychiatrically oriented example is H. Bower, "Beethoven's Creative Illness," *Australian and New Zealand Journal of Psychiatry*, 23 (1989), 111–16. L. D. Hankoff's "The Hero as Madman," *Journal of the History of the Behavioral Sciences*, 11 (1975), 315–33, develops the same notion in regard to five figures from ancient history and mythology. A stimulating general study of the possible connections between artists and their mental and physical diseases is Philip Sandblom, *Creativity and Disease: How Illness Affects Literature, Art, and Music*, 2d rev. ed. (Philadelphia, G. F. Stickley, 1983). At the same time, Sandblom's study reveals the dangers in positing a direct causal relation between these things. Interestingly, Ellenberger himself, long after writing his article on the concept of creative malady in 1964, found an earlier description of the illness. See Paul Valéry, "Une vue de Descartes," in *Les pages immortelles de Descartes*, selected and with commentary by Paul Valéry (Paris, Corrêa, 1941), 7–66.

Lastly, there are Ellenberger's ideas about studying the formation and function of legends in the historiography of science and the history of psychiatric history-writing. Once again, no general works on these topics have been forthcoming. Moreover, Ellenberger's observations about these matters have at times been appropriated for partisan purposes. The closest things to general studies of the function of historical mythmaking that I know of are Joseph Campbell's *The Hero with a Thousand Faces* [1949], 2d ed. (Princeton, Princeton University Press, 1968); Raphael Samuel, ed., *The Myths We Live By* (London, Routledge, 1990); and P. Smith, *La nature des mythes*, vol. 3 of *L'unité de l'homme*, edited by E. Morin (Paris, Seuil, 1974). A suggestive work on the role of historians in the making and unmaking of social and political myths is Eric Hobsbawm and Terence Ranger, eds., *The Invention of Tradition* (Cambridge, Cambridge University Press, 1983). In the past ten years, historians of science have become attuned to this issue and have produced a handful of provocative studies of individual figures from different branches of science and medicine. See L. S. Jacyna, "Images of John Hunter in the Nineteenth Century," *History of Science*, 21 (1983), 85–108; George Weisz, "The Posthumous Laennec: Creating a Modern Medical Hero, 1826–1870," *Bulletin of the History of Medicine*, 61 (1987), 541–62; and Bernadette Bensaude-Vincent, "A Founder Myth in the History of Sciences? The Lavoisier Case," in Loren Graham, Wolf Lepenies, and Peter Weingart, eds., *Functions and Uses of Disciplinary Histories* (Dordrecht, D. Reidel, 1983), 53–78.

On the history of the interpretation of psychiatry's past, much work remains to be done. However, refer to Thomas J. Schoeneman, "The Role of Mental Illness in the European Witch Hunts of the Sixteenth and Seventeenth Centuries: An Assessment," *Journal of the History of the Behavioral Sciences*, 13 (1977), 337–51; and Gladys Swain, *Le sujet de la folie: Naissance de la psychiatrie* (Toulouse, Privat, 1977), 41–47, 119–71, which deals very suggestively with the historical image of Pinel as psychiatric liberator. As previously noted, image-making in the historiography of psychoanalysis is the subject of Sulloway's *Freud, Biologist of the*

Mind. See especially his introduction, chap. 13, and epilogue. Sulloway may profitably be read along with Paul Roazen, "The Legend of Freud," *Virginia Quarterly Review*, 47 (1971), 33–45; and George Weisz, "Scientists and Sectarians: The Case of Psychoanalysis," *Journal of the History of the Behavioral Sciences*, 11 (1975), 350–64. A collection of articles on this general subject—the complex and manifold ways in which psychiatrists past and present have constructed the historical image of their profession—will shortly be available in the form of Mark S. Micale and Roy Porter, eds., *Discovering the History of Psychiatry* (New York, Oxford University Press, 1993). Of particular relevance in this volume will be Elisabeth Young-Bruehl, "The History of Freud Biography"; Patrick Vandermeersch, "*Les mythes d'origines* in the History of Psychiatry"; and Dora Weiner, "Pinel and the Unchaining of the Insane: History of a Psychiatric Myth." This aspect of Ellenberger's teachings, too, is moving forward.

Index